THE
SCIENCE
OF BLACK HAIR

THE
SCIENCE
OF BLACK HAIR

A COMPREHENSIVE GUIDE TO
TEXTURED HAIR CARE

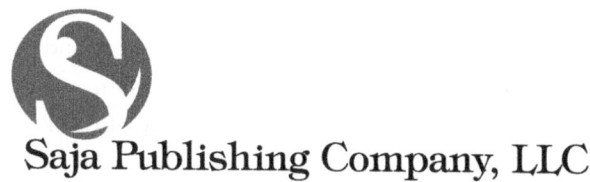

Saja Publishing Company, LLC

AUDREY DAVIS-SIVASOTHY

Published in 2011 by
Saja Publishing Company, LLC.
P. O. Box 2383
Stafford, Texas 77497
www.sajapublishing.com

Printed in the United States of America.
Page and book design by Velin Saramov
Cover design by Quantum Connect Services Pvt. Ltd.
Cover Images courtesy of
© iStockphoto.com (Alejandro Rivera and Noriko Cooper.)

Ordering Information: Special discounts are available on quantity purchases by bookstores, wholesalers, corporations, associations, and others. For details, contact the publisher at the address above or visit us on the web at www.blackhairscience.com.

Publisher's Cataloging-in-Publication Data

Davis-Sivasothy, Audrey, 2011—
The science of black hair:
a comprehensive guide to textured hair care/ Audrey Sivasothy.
p. cm.
Includes bibliographical references and index.
ISBN-978-0-9845184-0-1 (hardcover)
ISBN-978-0-9845184-1-8 (paperback)
ISBN-978-0-9845184-3-2 (hardcover)
ISBN-978-0-9845184-2-5 (paperback)

1. Hair—Care and hygiene. 2. African-American women—Health and hygiene. 3. Hairdressing of Blacks.
    I. Title.
2011903643
First Edition

And the LORD answered me, and said, Write the vision, and make it plain upon tables, that he may run that readeth it.
— Habakkuk 2:2 (KJV)

Read it, and Run!

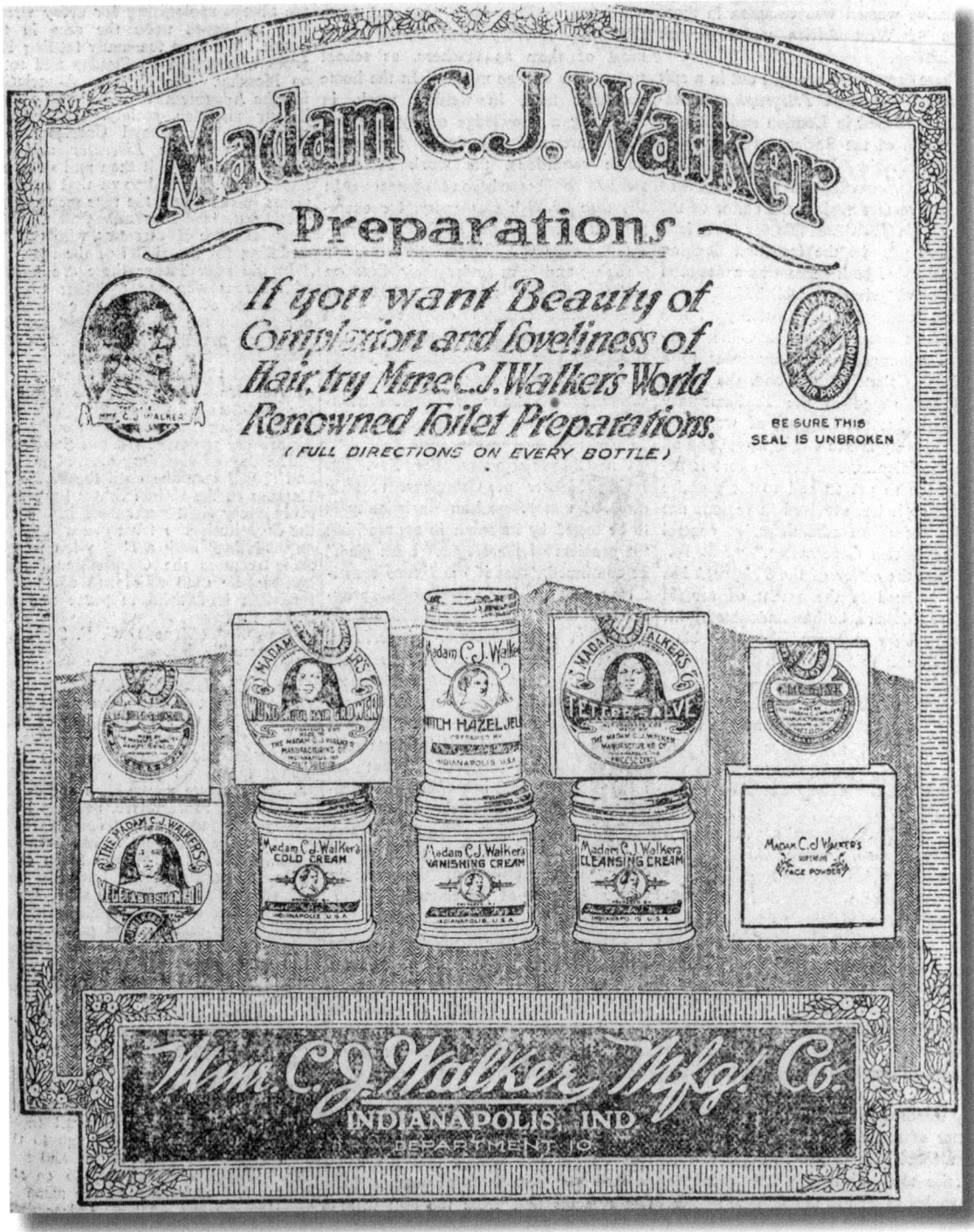

Advertisement (1867-1919) for beauty products sold by Madam C. J. Walker, one of the first African-American millionairesses. Walker, born Sarah Breedlove, rose from cotton-picking on a plantation to working in a laundrette, to founding a hair and cosmetics company.
This advert is from the January 17th, 1920 issue of The New York Age.
©LIBRARY OF CONGRESS/PHOTO RESEARCHERS, INC.

Contents

Foreword

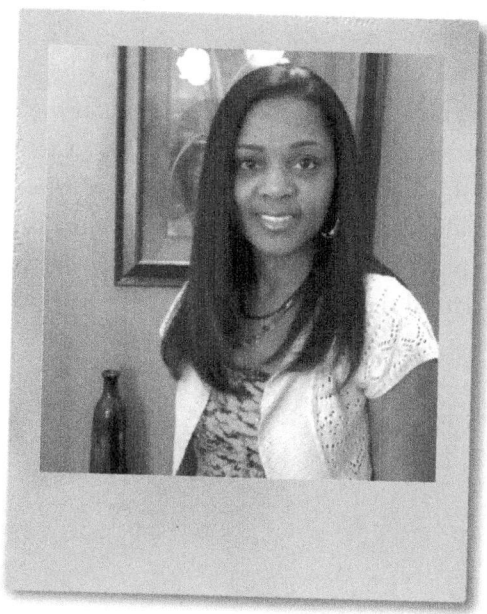

Virginia A. Clayton,
Owner, Master Stylist
Salon N'Richments Alexandria, LA

As a healthy hair cosmetologist for over a decade, I have seen it all. Healthy hair, damaged hair, if you can imagine it—it has walked through my salon doors. *Oh... if those sink bowls and chairs could TALK!* The beauty of my craft is that I get to solve major hair issues and transform them into non-issues for my clients. Clients leave my shop with a new attitude, looking better, feeling better, and ready to face whatever is next in their world! That is my greatest reward.

Although I love "saving the day" for my clients, what I enjoy most, however is working with informed clients. They make my job easier. They bring IN more clients. They ride home from the salon with my voice ringing in their heads, and they go to work! They are reading labels, moisturizing, deep conditioning, and maintaining healthy hair practices in between their visits to me. They are using the type of products I recommend and making educated and informed choices when I am not available. I know that I have done my job when a client can take the knowledge and expertise that I provide and make it work on non-salon days. That's power—and that is why I love Audrey's book, **The Science of Black Hair.**

The Science of Black Hair is in many ways an extension of my *chair talk*. The healthy hair principles and strategies that Audrey shares in this book are put into practice every day in my thriving salon. I am so delighted to see it in print with full commentary and new information to consider. I wholeheartedly recommend this book to my colleagues and clients just the same. We never stop learning, even as stylists—and in the best salons, open feedback between clients and the styling team is encouraged. We learn from each other, and **The Science of Black Hair** has certainly been an educational breath of fresh air for all of us.

The proliferation of weaved styles on the market has been both a blessing and curse to cosmetology. These services are lucrative in this craft, and they also provide clients considerable flexibility with their menu of styling options. However, the rampant abuse of this styling modality cannot be ignored. Sadly, many clients believe that weaves are their only means of having long hair and their REAL hair suffers underneath the style. A healthy hair care intervention like **The Science of Black Hair** is needed now more than ever.

The Science of Black Hair is a beautiful, timeless book with outstanding information and breathtaking images of hair up close and personal. It is like an encyclopedia: a reference guide in every sense of the word. We've needed a book like this—one with a fresh approach to our unique hair care. It is written with a scientific thrust, but is so easy to understand. Unlike many books today, it addresses BOTH prominent black hair textures: relaxed hair and natural hair. Even better, it does not encourage or play into the cultural "hair divide" that often exists between the two textures. It is not preachy, and it doesn't push an agenda. For the price of a salon shampoo and conditioner set or a trip to the salon, it has more than earned a place on my shelf and a prominent place in my salon. What more can I say?

The Science of Black Hair is certainly a treasure, not only for my customers but for me as an African American woman in general who is interested in caring for my own hair. I refer to it, and encourage my clients who wish to know more about this "much fussed-over appendage" to read it as well. Fellow hair masters and stylists at salons worldwide, give YOUR clients a healthy hair advantage by including this book in your salon. Audrey, many thanks for bringing this valuable information together in such a timeless volume at such a critical time for black hair care. Thank you for helping us all to understand, *The Science of Black Hair.*

Virginia A. Clayton
Owner, Master Stylist
Salon N'Richments
1611 Melrose
Alexandria, LA 71303
For appointments: 318.619-9320

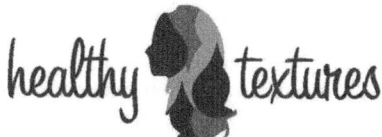

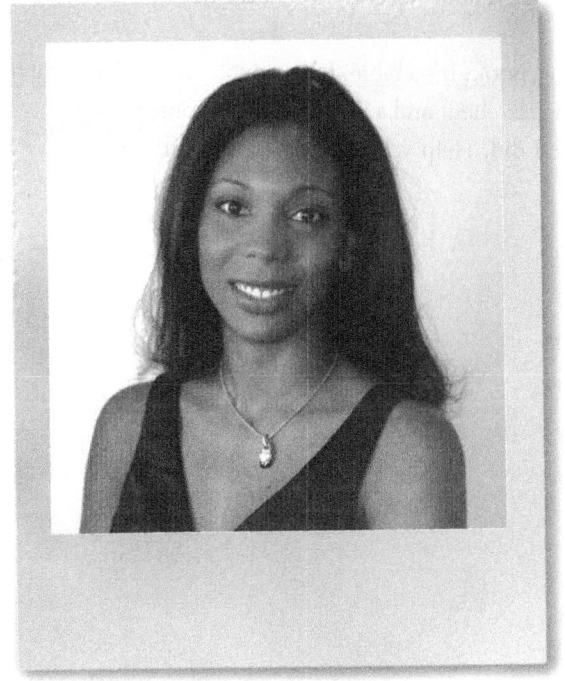

Gennifer Miller, CEO/Founder of Healthy Textures, LLC

Not too long ago, I remember standing in the bathroom, staring at dozens of strands of dry, broken hair all over the floor.

For nearly 15 years, I thought I was doing the right thing. I went to the salon every single week for a blow out, relaxed and trimmed every six weeks and curled my hair every single morning before school or work. Sure, my hair never grew past my shoulders and broke all of the time but... that was normal, *right?*

In my head, yes, it was normal! I'd never really seen black women with long hair (relaxed or natural). And, sure, it was dry and brittle but black women just had hair that felt "like that", *right?* And, yes, I had to take out the broom and dustpan every time I curled my hair to sweep up the stray strands but that's what everyone did, *right?*

In my heart, however, I knew something was wrong. When something breaks, a piece of string, an eggshell, a piece of glass, etc., it is usually due to extreme pressure and/or force. So, what did it mean that *MY* hair was breaking? And was it *really* normal for my hair to feel dry and brittle? Why did women of other races seem to have such soft and shiny hair?

I just didn't understand.

And, THAT was it. I just fundamentally did not understand my hair. I had gone to a stylist faithfully for nearly 15 years. There were long stretches of time, in which I did not even touch my own wet hair. When I did try to do my hair at home, I took my cues from shampoo commercials and glamour magazines. Shampoo, pile the hair on top of your head, rinse and repeat. Condition in the shower and then blow dry and curl. And yet, each week, I still stood upon a graveyard of broken hair strands.

And that day in the bathroom, it finally hit me. Something was wrong, this was not normal and I was going to find out what it was. I decided that I was going to learn how to take better care of my hair and set off on a mission to help women of color avoid the same mistakes I've made.

And yet, with all of the reading and writing I have done on the topic of black hair over the years, I have not come across a more well-researched, exhaustive and comprehensive book as **The Science of Black Hair**.

The Science of Black Hair has consolidated and organized the best information on healthy hair care and has made it both easy to find and easy to understand. This book helps women of color understand WHY their hair is different, why it acts the way it does and how to address its needs. And when we give our hair what it truly needs, it grows, it shines and it thrives.

Understanding the science of our hair helps us truly understand our hair. When you know what frizz really is, you know how to prevent it. When you understand what protein does for the hair, you understand how to use it and when. When you understand what a blow dryer does to the hair, you have a reason to use it sparingly.

The Science of Black Hair is MORE than a book. It's a bible. It's my bible. It will help you become a more educated consumer, a more responsible client and a more cautious home stylist.

Don't set low expectations for your hair like I did. Help your hair realize its full potential. And remember, knowledge.... is power!

Gennifer Miller *aka Macherieamour*
CEO/Founder of Healthy Textures LLC
A Do-It-Yourself Approach to Healthier Hair
www.healthytextures.com

Acknowledgments

The Science of Black Hair is a work that has truly been the creation of many. The list of individuals to whom I owe the utmost gratitude is lengthy. Without their support, this work would simply not have been possible. I first give honor to God, who has provided this Vision and purpose in my life and endowed me with the resources and faculties to fulfill it. You've put the most amazing people in my life. Thank you for this Vision; I am honored to be your vessel. To my earthly father, thanks Dad for EVERYTHING. Without you, this book would have remained a dream deferred.

To Sathyan, my loving, wonderful husband/mentor/financial manager/coach/best friend—my everything. Thank you for being my soft place to fall and my shoulder to cry on. Your name should be on the cover of this book, my love. This project has taught us so much about one another. I look forward to seeing what God will do in our lives as we grow stronger in our faith and service to Him. Thank you for all the time you've spent alone, the meals you've cooked, the clothes you've folded and put away, and the kid shuffling you've done while I wrote this book. I love you, and I never could have done this without your help. To my children, Justin and Anjali, I hope that you will find this book useful and a great source of pride as you grow. Thank you for your patience with Mommy.

To my family and friends (the Louisiana, California and Texas folk who are too numerous to name): Thank you all for always believing in me. Your prayers for me have all been heard! To my aunts, uncles and cousins great and small: I love each and every one of you. Mom, I love you. Thank you for your advice and suggestions throughout this entire process and in life in general. Whenever I've needed you, you have always been there. Thank you for everything, Mom. To Mr. Mike, one of the first real Texans I'd ever met: You're one of the greatest, most down-to-earth people I know.

To Chris: I love you. Keep singing—never, ever stop singing. Hang in there, be encouraged, and never forget the early experiences that shaped us. Brianna, Brian and Brandon: Always follow your dreams.

Special thanks to the editor of *The Science of Black Hair:* Lisa Lawley Nesbitt. Your expert direction and guidance turned a manuscript with potential into a groundbreaking new book. Thank you many times over.

Many thanks to my pastor, William D. Gilliam and Global Impact Ministries (Humble, Texas), for speaking a Word and igniting the fire in this writer that would later become *The Science of Black Hair.*

From the Author

The black hair stories that usually get told are those of the little girl with thick, long hair who lost it all when she became a teenager by experimenting with some combination of coloring, relaxing, weaving or heat styling her hair. But my story is different. Unfortunately, no thick-haired, hair-down-the-back little black girl story exists for me. Growing up, my hair was always an issue. By kindergarten, I'd had my first chemical relaxer, and my hair was simply left to fend for itself. And fend it did. My hair was never thick, and it certainly was never long. It was stringy, choppy and greasy for much of my childhood—and I have pictures to prove it.

Rewind to 1993. Four eight-year-old Caucasian girls stood huddled together in fear, shivering beside a pool. They were quickly joined by an equally panicked mom who had abandoned whatever she had going on in the oven at the time to come bursting through the sliding glass door in response to their screams.

"Snake! Snaaaaaake!" one of my friends yelled out.

"Audrey, GET OUT NOW! another warned. "There's a snaaaake in the pooool!"

I was underwater and could scarcely make out their distorted images on the surface pointing at something terrible in the water. Not wanting to become a victim of whatever monstrosity was following me in the pool that day, I quickly swam to the side of the pool and climbed out. At this point, my friends were crying. I braced myself before turning to face the pool monster.

A snake? I looked around to see what kind of snake possibly could have made its way into this suburban pool. Then, my fear quickly turned to embarrassment. Their "snake" had been my braid. My braid extension had somehow slipped loose from my hair and was floating on the surface of the water behind me as I swam. I was traumatized.

But the trauma would not end at the pool. Once the water had loosened the braids, there would be more *Toyokalan* braid casualties. And rather than gripping my friends with fear, finding and picking up Audrey's braids became a game at that slumber party from hell. My friends giggled as they handed me one fallen braid after another. By this point, my love-hate relationship with my hair was in full swing. This hair that had the power to evacuate an entire group of third graders from a pool would time and again continue to be the source of much distress in my life years later.

Summers I had always welcomed my beloved braid extensions. For me, this was the only chance I thought I had to have long, beautiful hair. With my braids, I finally felt equal to my long-haired friends. Sure, I could not comb this hair, and of course there were the many "snake" scares, but it was all I had. It was my reprieve. With my braids, I could now understand why hair needed to be swept out of the face and tucked behind an ear. I now understood why ponytails were so convenient for those moments where your hair would just "get in the way." I could finally say that I knew the tickle of long hair on my back, even if it happened to be scratchy, synthetic horse hair! Unfortunately, the joy that I always felt with braids was always quickly interrupted when it came time to remove them. Braid by braid, my long hair was stripped away from me, and I was now faced with my own short, damaged hair until the next summer's set of braids. Hair was everything to me then, and because it seemed to fail me at every opportunity— my hair made me feel like I had absolutely nothing. I remember thinking to myself, Why can't my hair be as long as other little girls' hair? What is wrong with mine? Why did my hair have to be like... *this*?

There were very few little black girls going to school with me back then, and so naturally my first inclination was to have hair like all of my friends: the white girls. As a little girl, I remember just staring at their hair in amazement. They all had hair that actually moved. Their ponytails would still be swinging long after their heads had stopped moving, and sadly, I had nothing of my own to swing. I still vividly remember the little tinge of envy I felt when my schoolmates would cut their hair over the summer, and by the time school started again, much of their hair had already grown right back! I wouldn't dare cut mine.

Lord knows, it would be forever trying to grow it back! In retrospect, my impossible desire to have long, flowing hair like my classmates all but consumed me. My dream had me restyling my hair in the elementary and junior high school bathrooms and experimenting with flatirons, gel and curling irons at an early age.

Looking back, I realize that many of the images I had of myself and my hair as a child were simply unhealthy. I secretly despised my hair and the fact that much of my self worth was tied up in it. It wasn't what I wanted, and it embarrassed me. The self-affirming, black-is-beautiful moments in my early life were few and far between. My mother took care of my hair the best way she knew how, and she did her best to affirm me in every way, but her affirmations about me in general back then (as motherly affirmations tend to be with any developing preteen personality) were completely overruled and drowned out by the stronger, more pressing social and media influences I felt around me as a child. I was socialized by the prevailing culture as well as by many well-meaning people into believing that my hair, unless super long or relaxed to the brink of straightness, made me inferior.

I thought that having a relaxer was the key to having hair like my friends' hair—hair that moved—and that other than having to relax it, my hair was exactly the same as theirs. I had no idea that this process was damaging and weakening my hair, even though I clearly remember being burned on many occasions. It was simply "the cost of doing business," and I never made the connection that my styling choices had consequences. I did not know that having a relaxer meant that I'd need to take special steps to maintain my hair's health. Perhaps even more disheartening to me today is the fact that I did not understand that life could go on without relaxers, period. I would be well into my college years before I ever came into contact with my first natural-haired friend.

In high school, the cycle of hair breakage and damage continued. I was relaxing my hair on schedule every eight to ten weeks but had no growth to show for it. Where was all the impossible new growth that was driving me to relax in the first place going? It was breaking, and what wasn't breaking was being clipped off by scissor-happy stylists. It seemed like it was always one step forward, two steps back with my hair. After years and years passed with one disappointment after another, I finally gave up. I simply reached the conclusion that some people were meant to have long hair and some just were not. I, apparently, was one who was not meant to have long hair at all. My hair had never grown more than an inch beyond my shoulders, no matter what I tried... in my entire life. I decided to accept and just live with my permanently thin, breaking shoulder-length hair. After all, it was a blessing to have made it that far, right? From there, I simply moved on with my life, and college was a welcome distraction.

A few years into my undergraduate work, my hair issues would be forced to the forefront once again. I was pregnant with my daughter, and I knew that I could not possibly hope to take care of my own little girl's hair when I had been so grossly unsuccessful caring for my own. I knew that I would need to educate myself quickly to spare her from the hair battles I faced growing up.

I stumbled across my first online hair community in the summer of 2004, and by this point, my frustration with my hair was at an all-time high. The hair-care sites were just what I needed for motivation and support. They were full of information on healthy black hair care, and whole communities of black women were supporting each other day in and day out, challenging one another to grow their hair out natural and relaxed to greater lengths. It was beautiful and encouraging, and without those many ladies I would not be here today. Those sisters inspired me to put my thoughts on hair care together into a book with the hope that this knowledge will continue to be shared in our community.

My own misunderstanding of textured hair cost me dearly over the years. I am fortunate that I have been able to reexamine many of my earlier beliefs about my own head of hair and come to terms with them. My view of textured hair as a rough, indestructible force led me to snatch combs and brushes through it at every turn. I thought my hair was tough and had to be manhandled into place. I thought it could take anything. I was abusing my hair and expecting it to just continue to thrive. But no more!

The book you are holding in your hands is the culmination of years and years of heartbreak and sorrow surrounding my own hair. I am, very much like the majority of you, neither a stylist nor a traditional lab scientist. My background is in Health Science and Policy, a field that concerns itself with developing interventions and programs to improve health outcomes in at-risk populations. As a Health Scientist, many of the health-care interventions I am qualified to address involve larger physical, mental and social health issues such as obesity prevention, drug/smoking cessation and hypertension awareness in at-risk populations. The hair care problems rampant in our community, however, can easily be viewed as a social health issue for which a well-planned and customized intervention would certainly be appropriate. While improper hair care may not carry the threat of increased mortality, it can result in a reduced quality of life and poorer self-image, all of which are primary concerns of Health Scientists. As a primary marker of our personhood and major contributor to our overall appearance, our hair is intimately connected with our well being as people. As superficial as it may appear, no one can deny that hair is very important and its appearance is quite frequently the barometer by which we are judged and even valued in this society.

Sisters, the beauty of our hair lies in its absolute diversity, and this uniqueness should be celebrated and embraced. My hope is that this book will be received, not as a relaxed hair care or natural hair care book, but as a black hair care book that combines the wealth of our experiences so that they can be understood as one. Whether your definition of healthy, vibrant hair is lengthy, cascading locks or hair that simply grows up and out to touch the sky, each of us can achieve the kind of hair that makes heads turn and time stand still. Healthy black hair comes in a variety of styles and forms, and it remains a beautiful expression of each wearer's personality, life and even politics. I hope that by sharing my own knowledge of hair care, you will be able to break the complex cycle of poor hair health that presently runs unchecked in our community. For the black woman, growing longer, healthier hair rarely happens automatically, but with the proper knowledge, it is not an impossibility.

Be blessed.

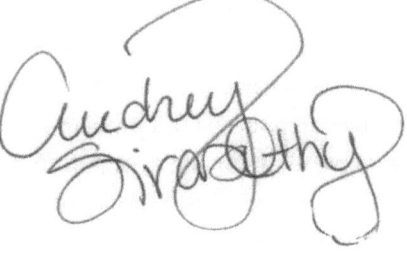

Audrey Davis-Sivasothy

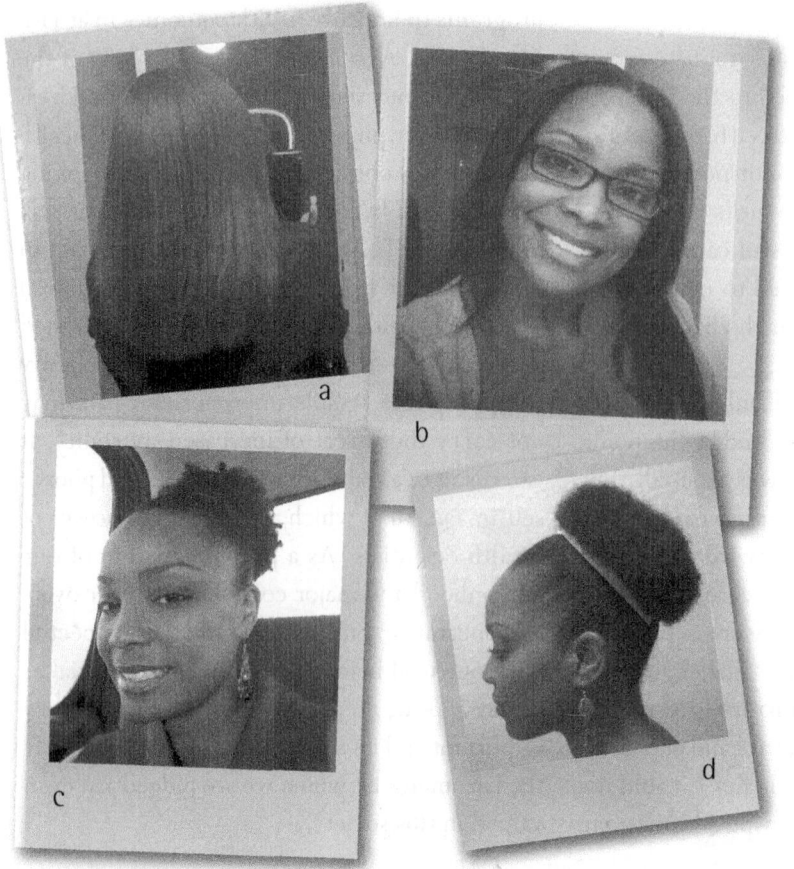

Our hair is so versatile— whether it is worn long and straight, or in its natural state. Photos a & b show my straight hair in January 2010. Photos c & d show my natural hair January 2011 after an eleven month transition to natural hair.

Introduction

Black hair today is in a state of crisis.

If you are like many black women, your hair has been roughly the same length and condition for years regardless of what you have done to it. Shoulder length is occasionally achieved in our community but it is rarely exceeded. To add to the insult, little to no cutting is required to maintain the mediocre lengths that we do achieve. Hair growth, for a majority of black women, simply appears to remain static over time. Rampant, chronic breakage prevents most black hair from ever growing to any point beyond the shoulders. The few black women who have learned to overcome their hair hurdles to achieve lengths beyond the shoulders are often seen as exceptions to the "black hair rule"—endowed with a superior genetic code or precious hair secrets they aren't likely to share. Long hair is such a rare and valued commodity in the black hair community that we are more inclined to seek the packaged hair of others than to develop an understanding of our own hair so that we can unlock its hidden potential. Black hair is in serious trouble.

Successfully achieving and maintaining healthier, longer hair appears to come without a second thought for women of other races and cultures. These women often cut their hair with the understanding that it will grow back quickly—and it often does. This freedom to part with hair on a whim and then recover it quickly is one that many black women simply do not enjoy. Unlike our sisters of other races, black women often find that the return on our "hair investment" from trimming and cutting takes many months—even years—to recover. This poor return on investment instigates a vicious cycle of paranoia and resentment that keeps many black women out of stylists' chairs and away from shears. We hoard our precious hair as we would a rare commodity, and we defend every inch of it, despite its troubled condition. The weariest of us have turned entirely to weaves, putting our real hair out of commission indefinitely—out of sight, out of mind.

Why haven't we been able to achieve healthier hair that grows and retains length successfully? Why must many of us depend on wigs and weaves as crutches to hide our real hair and its damaged state rather than use these hair additions as styling tools consciously chosen on occasion to change up a style?

Hair breakage is the number one enemy of healthy, vibrant black hair. Until we understand the causes of breakage and take steps to control it, we will be unable to add visible length to our hair over time. This book presents a proven method for improving black hair health. It reveals a strategy for identifying and correcting common hair breakage issues, mostly using products you already have at home.

Calming the Misinformation Beast

Years of misinformation have crippled our efforts to grow and maintain healthy heads of hair. Some of us have had hair that has been the same length for years without us ever having cut it. Some of us have never had hair that could be pulled into a ponytail, let alone felt the tickle of hair brushing the middle of our backs. Our lack of information has left many of us in a state of cyclical hair helplessness. Proactive hair care must begin with better education.

Unfortunately, hair-care misinformation runs rampant in the black hair community. Countless individuals capitalize on our lack of basic knowledge about healthy hair. Hair companies have unleashed many products over the years to satisfy this overwhelming demand for healthier, longer, stronger black hair. Some of these hair products are true gems—worth their weight in gold. However, the vast majority of products geared toward our community are utterly useless. Chief among this category of useless products are the mega/super/ultra hair-growth products (often sold with misspelled names like Qwik-GRO) that are formulated to magically grow the hair from the scalp quickly with regular use. People often flock to the web or to local beauty-supply stores to purchase these new hair-growth products, only to find that they have fallen for yet another gimmick. Perhaps you are one of those who hoped, prayed and shelled out countless dollars for products to finally grow your hair to the length of your dreams. I surely was.

If there were a product out there that could deliver what we've all been looking for, there wouldn't be a sister out there with short, broken off, damaged hair. We'd all have long (or big, for my natural ladies) healthy hair! The company behind the miracle product would be rich and would find itself unable to keep the product on the shelves. There would be no need for books like this one. But here it is, a new millennium for hair care, and we have seen no such product that has been able to stand the test of time. In black hair care, *healthy techniques always trump hair products.*

The Science of Black Hair

Welcome to *The Science of Black Hair*, your complete guide to understanding, growing and maintaining healthier black hair. *The Science of Black Hair* is a comprehensive volume, written in textbook style to provide in-depth information about processes specific to black hair care and maintenance. This book is unique because it frames the topic of textured hair care in a way that combines science with testimony. Science is paired with personal experience and observation in a way that allows the reader to connect with the text on a personal level. *The Science of Black Hair* is designed to teach you optimal healthy hair-care strategies based on sound, logical scientific information.

The approach is a sensible one—no speedy hair-growth promises or magical products. We have enough of that today. This book, thoroughly researched and carefully crafted, is truly the first of its kind in the area of black hair science and overall care. Future editions will expand upon our forever growing and changing understanding of hair care. Although the book discusses proper hair maintenance and care, it is not a step-by-step styling book. Detailed styling instructions are therefore beyond the scope of this text.

How Is Our Hair Different?

At the outset of our journey to healthy, vibrant (and long!) hair, we must first understand that our hair is different. Although all hair is chemically composed of the same principal elements, black hair differs from that of other races in the basic shape of the hair fiber and in its composition—that is, is the percentage and distribution of basic compounds. [1] [2] [3] Kinky hair often appears thick, tough and coarse, but because of its inherent physical composition, it is not nearly as strong as it appears. [1] Every twist, bend and curl represents a point of weakness and vulnerability along the hair fiber. Black hair requires extra care, especially if it has been compromised by chemical relaxing or coloring. Black hair's natural tendency toward dryness is another obstacle that must be overcome to achieve longer, healthier hair. Many of us simply do not have the luxury of expecting our hair to gain length as a matter of course. We must take conscious steps to help it along if we want to grow it. Fortunately, with the right information and a proper understanding of textured hair growth and maintenance, we can overcome breakage cycles and achieve healthier hair.

Healthy Hair Begins at Home

You are your greatest hair asset. Unless you have a hairstylist in your pocket, you should never completely write off your own responsibility for basic hair care in favor of complete dependence on someone else. You possess an intimate connection with your hair, and no one can possibly care about the health and quality of your hair like you do! You are in the best position to recognize and address simple hair problems because no person alive knows your hair better than you. You know where it has been, and you know where you would like it to go. You can support this process by ensuring that your fundamental understanding of hair care is solid. *The Science of Black Hair* will help you get to this place.

While a great stylist is certainly an asset to any healthy hair care regimen, the key to achieving an optimal level of hair health ultimately rests in your own hands. You will always need to maintain some degree of control and responsibility for your own healthy hair care because things change. A new job may take you halfway across the country, college may have you in a remote part of the world or your styling goals may simply change over time. What happens if your stylist moves, or can't book you into her schedule for the next few weeks? You must develop some baseline of healthy hair care at home to see you through from visit to visit.

Healthy Hair Is Made Between Stylist Visits

Your stylist's role should be to assist you with hair care by teaching you proper care and maintenance, professionally styling your hair, and expertly identifying and correcting mistakes in your overall hair regimen. They are the providers of expert assistance. Assistance is the key word here. Making or breaking your hair (literally) happens during the many weeks and days that you are not in the chair. The best stylists understand this and usually are genuinely concerned with the state of their clients' hair between visits. Such stylists are gems and will support and encourage your understanding of healthy hair-care practices both in and out of the chair. Stylists are generally very busy people—especially the really good ones! They see your hair only a couple of times a month if you are an extremely faithful client. In the meantime, your hair is being affected by the day-to-day ravages of life: heat, smog, humidity, products and physical manipulation. It is imperative that your hair be appropriately looked after during these in-between times. So yes, healthy hair is made between stylist visits. Your healthy hair makes a stylist's job a lot more enjoyable and will certainly attract more clients to his/her salon.

Hair Care Is an Art... and a Science

Your success with this book will be greatly determined by your dedication to the regimen-building process and your adoption of a long-haul mindset. Growing black hair takes time, dedication, and patience above all else. This book is about learning to know your hair and what it needs to thrive over your lifetime, not about more quick-fix miracle products, miracle stylists or miracle cures. We must begin to take a proactive approach to our hair care. We must strive to curb our dependence on hair weaves and hairpieces as crutches to hide our damaged hair or cover-ups to help us avoid dealing with it. We must resolve to keep hair weaves and hairpieces in their proper places—as fun, quick hair-styling enhancements, tools to protect already healthy, thriving hair, and hair replacements for those of us facing situations that have taken our real hair. No one should feel that they have to wear a weave to have presentable hair; a weave should be a conscious styling choice, not a crutch.

unit 1

The Science of Black Hair

Chapter 1: Scalp and Hair Structure, Function and Characteristics

A hair book is simply not complete without a quick lesson about hair and scalp structure and anatomy. Having a working knowledge of the scientific aspects of hair growth and care is very important. When I started reading books and articles about hair care years ago, I always skimmed anxiously past the diagrams and scientific stuff to get to the "good parts." I wanted to know which products to use. That was it. My philosophy was, Just tell me the secrets and the products, and I'll be on my way! I did not care to know what a cuticle or cortex were until I got tired of hitting walls and failing to find answers about why my hair was breaking and shedding.

When I became interested in learning what separated good hair care from bad hair care, my focus shifted from "Give me the products" to a desire to understand what hair is so that I could bend it to my will. Later on, I found my focus shifting again from wanting to control and force my hair into submission to learning how to work with it and accept it for what it is. I found that knowing the basics of hair anatomy really supported my understanding of how and why some products and methods worked and why others did not. Having a general knowledge of the hard scientific facts will allow you to sift through and weed out false hair information and bogus claims.

Hair is perhaps the most fussed-over appendage on the human body. Each year, companies pour billions of dollars into hair research including product development. Consumers shell out additional billions for the normal care and maintenance required to successfully produce a quality head of hair. The average American woman is said to spend upward of $50,000 on her hair during her lifetime. (4) The black hair care market alone has evolved into a $9-billion industry and continues to grow. (5)

In many societies, hair has considerable social importance, especially for women. The various ways it is styled and worn can reveal much about its wearer. Information about a woman's historical time, the part of the world she calls home, her religion, her age, her politics and her financial status—all can be found wrapped up in how she chooses to present her hair to the world. (6) Within the black community (and for black women in particular), hair has been the source of much socio-political contention. This consciousness—or unconsciousness—continues to shape the way many black women approach their hair.

Yet beyond its immense cosmetic and social importance, hair naturally serves a protective function against environmental stressors including wind, sun, cold, and rain. Endowed with a resistant and strong keratin protein structure, hair is specially equipped to take on a variety of challenges and assaults.

Exploring the Scalp

Understanding the scalp is important to any hair-growing endeavor. The scalp is the birthplace of hair, and if kept in proper condition, it will provide an optimal environment for the follicles to produce quality hair. In order to grow hair that thrives, your scalp skin should remain clean, toned, pliable and positively stimulated. A toned, pliable scalp is flexible and has a healthy network of connective tissues and nourishing blood vessels throughout. This network of

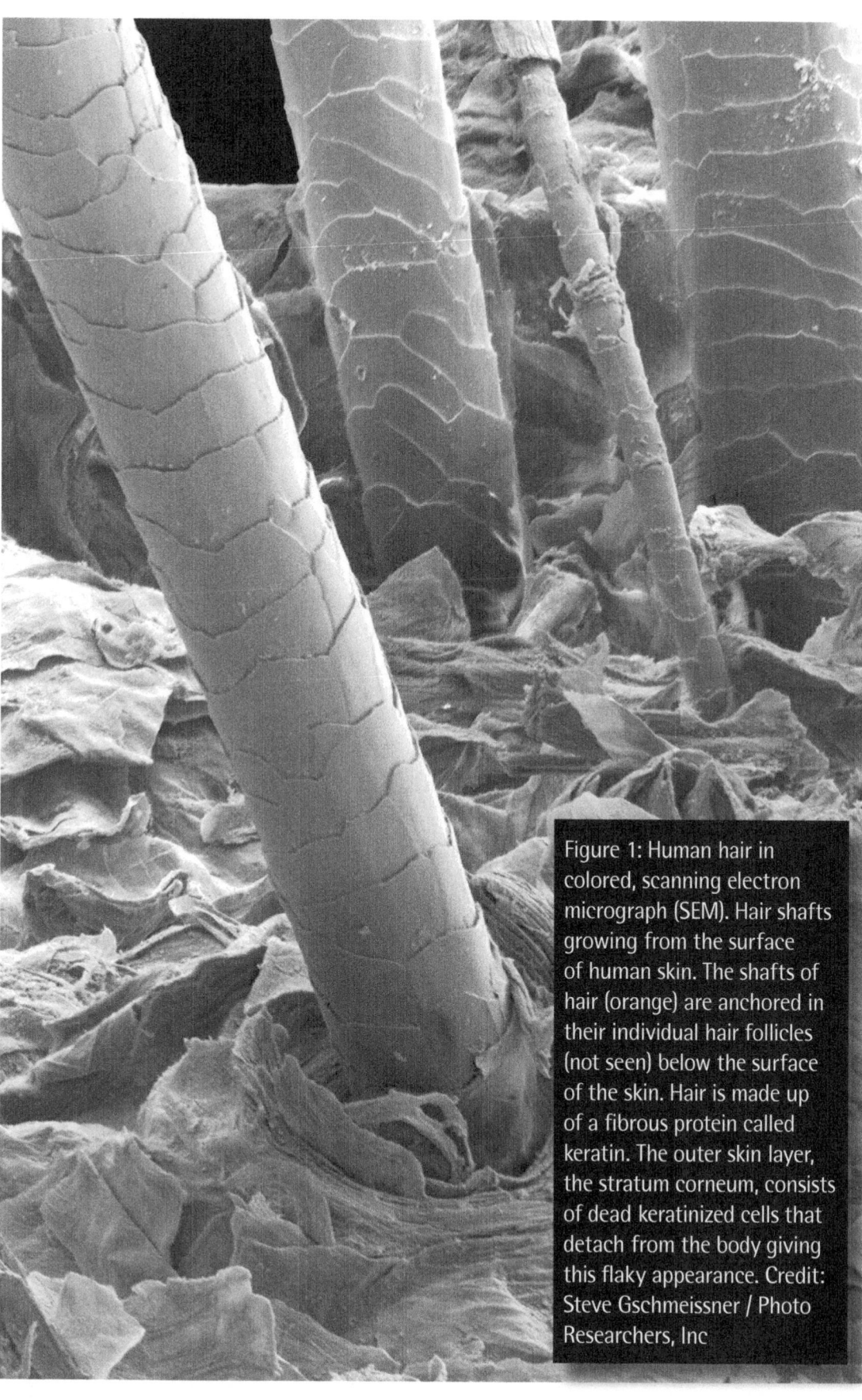

Figure 1: Human hair in colored, scanning electron micrograph (SEM). Hair shafts growing from the surface of human skin. The shafts of hair (orange) are anchored in their individual hair follicles (not seen) below the surface of the skin. Hair is made up of a fibrous protein called keratin. The outer skin layer, the stratum corneum, consists of dead keratinized cells that detach from the body giving this flaky appearance. Credit: Steve Gschmeissner / Photo Researchers, Inc

blood-rich vessels provides critical circulation to the hair follicles. (6) You can increase the pliability of and circulation to your scalp by gently massaging and manipulating it daily.

Like the rest of your skin, the scalp is divided into three layers: the epidermis (uppermost), dermis (middle) and subcutaneous (bottom) layer. (7) The subcutaneous layer houses the scalp's dense supply of blood vessels and fatty tissue. The dermis, or middle layer, contains a network of collagen protein that lends strength and support to skin. The uppermost layer, or epidermis, is roughly fifty cells thick and is the layer we encounter and work with on a daily basis.

Functions of the Scalp Skin

The scalp is heavily vascularized, which means that it has an intricate network of blood vessels moving and carrying nutrients throughout. Because the scalp skin so closely resembles skin on the rest of the body, most general skin features and functions also apply to the scalp. (6) The scalp differs from skin on other parts of the body in that it has larger oil glands and produces more sebum, the body's natural oil. (1)

The epidermis, or top layer of scalp skin, can be further subdivided. Its uppermost layer, known as the stratum corneum, is made up of dead, keratinized (hardened) cells. Like skin cells all over the body, the cells on the surface of the scalp naturally shed as new cells form. Every day, these scalp skin cells shed as minute particles invisible to the naked eye. (1) (8)

The stratum corneum is extremely important. Water housed in the deeper skin layers slowly migrates upward to provide moisture and hydration to the stratum corneum. (9) The next step for moisture in the skin is evaporation into the surrounding environment, which ultimately leaves the skin feeling dry. This is why it is important to hydrate the body from within to fight scalp dryness. If you are dehydrated, your body will supply little moisture

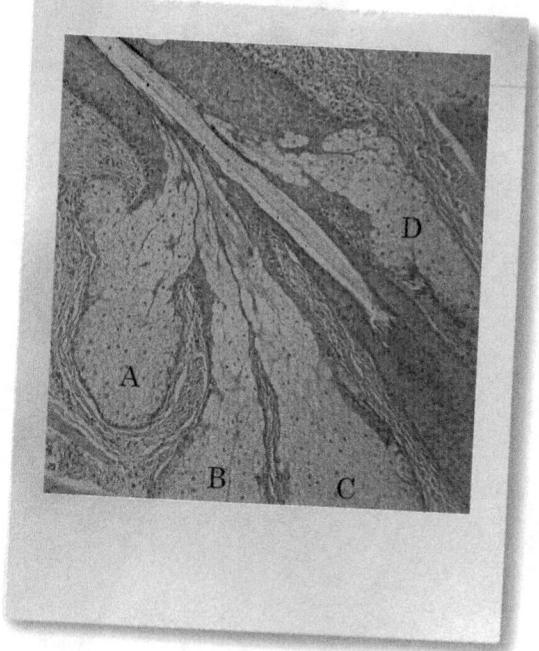

Figure 2: Sebaceous (oil) glands are clearly visible in this photo and denoted by letters A-D. Note the dense network of blood vessels surrounding the hair follicle.

to the upper layers of your skin. You will then have to rely on external moisturizing products to hydrate your scalp.

Although this uppermost skin layer appears smooth to the eye, scanning electron microscopy provides a glimpse of its true glory. Flakes of keratinized cells can be seen forming on the scalp surface (see Figure 1), but we rarely notice the natural flaking process until it is thrown out of sync and we experience dandruff. When the scalp's natural flaking process is disrupted and the moisture content of the scalp skin drops below roughly 10 percent, dandruff and other scaly scalp-irritation issues arise. Dandruff is simply the result of accelerated skin cell turnover at the upper scalp level. (10)

Structures of the Scalp Skin
The Follicle

The follicle (or root) is the birthplace of every new hair. On average, the scalp contains as

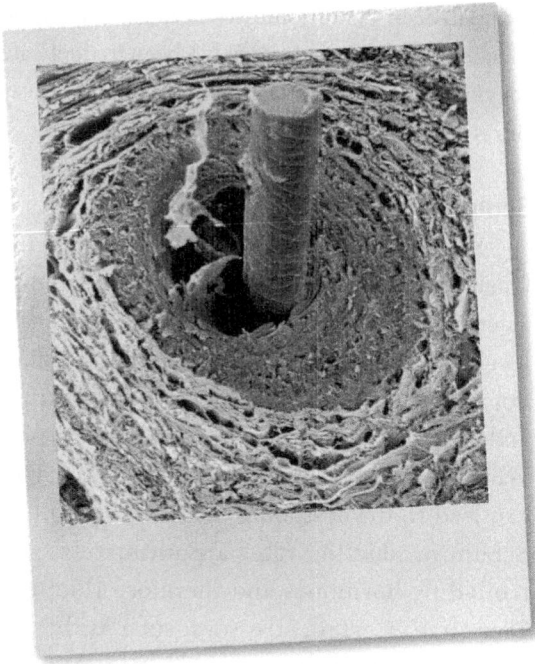

Figure 3: Colored scanning electron micrograph of hair emerging from hair follicle. The hair shaft is covered with a cuticle that contains a hard form of keratin (the protein that is found in hair). At upper center is a shaft of hair surrounded by the epidermis (red), the upper layer of skin.

many as 100,000 individual follicles and hairs. (7) (11) Follicles are located deep within the subcutaneous fatty tissues of the scalp and are nourished by a complex network of blood vessels. The follicles serve as growth bases for the hair, and although they may change over a lifetime, we are born with as many follicles as we will ever have. (11) (12) The number of follicles each of us has is genetically predetermined and is often a function of our natural hair color. Each follicle grows approximately .35 millimeters per day to accommodate the growing hair strand. (1) (8) (11) (13)

The dermal papilla, situated just underneath the hair follicle, contains tiny blood vessels that supply the necessary oxygen, glucose and nutrients required to support hair building and growth at the base of the follicle. The dermal papilla supports the production of key amino acids: the building blocks of protein that are required to support the hair strand. Hormone receptors are present throughout the dermal papilla and have a direct influence on hair growth and shedding during the life of a hair strand. (7)

The base of the hair follicle is also known as the hair bulb. The cells in the hair bulb, fed by an intricate network of capillaries, divide every one to three days—a rate of cell division that surpasses any other in the human body. (11) (14) The hair bulb is also the source of hair color; it contains melanin, the pigment responsible for giving both hair and skin its color.

The replication of cells at the base of the follicle is the continuous process by which our hair grows. As the hair follicle produces new cells, older cells are keratinized (hardened) and forced upward and through the scalp. Once a hair leaves the protection of the hair follicle, it is no longer living tissue.

Each hair follicle is surrounded by inner and outer sheaths that protect and mold it. The erector pili muscle attaches to the outside of the outer root sheath and extends upward to attach to the subcutaneous skin layers (see Figure 5 pg. 30). When the erector pili contracts, hair lifts and stands on end. (1) (11)

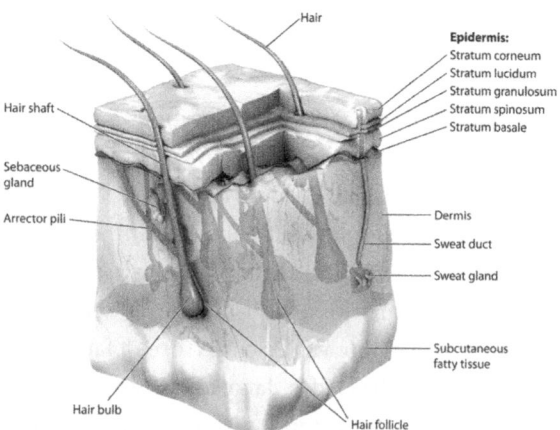

Figure 4: Cross section of skin layers

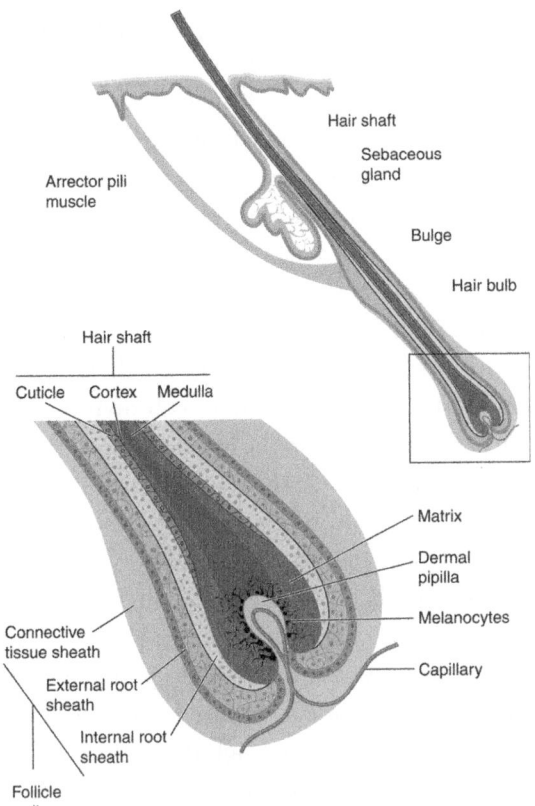

Figure 5: Follicle anatomy and cross section

Sebaceous Glands

The sebaceous (oil) glands are part of the hair follicle (see figure 2). These glands produce sebum, our hair and skin's natural oil, and can be found on every part of the body except the palms of the hands and the soles of the feet. (15) (16)

Sebum

The healthy scalp produces about an ounce of sebum every one hundred days. Sebum comes from the natural breakdown of small cells within the sebaceous glands. Sebum's main job is to condition the skin and act as a barrier to prevent internal moisture loss. Skin-protecting sebum is made up of a highly variable mixture of fatty lipids including glycerides, fatty acids, wax esters, squalene and cholesterol. (You may recognize many of these ingredients as those commonly

found in deep-conditioning treatments. The trend in hair-product development has been to duplicate the composition of natural sebum as the best way of returning hair to its proper condition.)

Scalp dryness

Scalp dryness is a common complaint in the black community, and much of it is related to a genetic lack of sebum production at the scalp level. (8) (Then too, while some of us produce normal amounts of sebum, the natural kinks and bends along our individual hair shafts prevent its easy spread throughout the hair. This can lead to dryness along the hair shaft.) (11) Sebum production rates are ultimately controlled by hormones and therefore fluctuate over time. Certain stressors, such as dietary deficiencies, prescription medications and puberty may increase or reduce normal sebum production levels. (16)

Some individuals may have naturally low sebum production rates, which can be a strong contributor to chronic scalp dryness. For many others, however, scalp dryness may be self-induced. When products are placed directly on the scalp, and are allowed to build up, scalp conditions become unfavorable and problems with scalp dryness and hair growth can arise. The scalp, like any other skin, needs to be able to "breathe." Heavy, oily concoctions inhibit optimal functioning of the scalp by clogging the pores and creating an unhealthy environment for hair growth.

The scalp is essentially an extension of the face. Just as pores on the face can become clogged, hair follicles too can experience obstruction if products are placed directly on them. Heavy oils, pomades and greases are the common culprits, but even the buildup of sebum may cause an issue. When sebum is present on the scalp, it is initially very flexible and moist. However, as the days wear on, this natural oil begins to harden like a wax. Unfortunately, hardened sebum can combine with naturally flaking scalp cells and heavier oils and greases from certain kinds of hair products to create firm obstructions around the entrance of the hair follicle. (17) (18) When something similar happens on the face, a pimple results. On the scalp, hair is simply forced to push through the blockage. In some cases, this blockage can lead to scalp dryness and itchiness, inflammation and miniaturization (shrinking) of the hair follicles, and a decrease in the quality of hair that emerges from the clogged follicles. (16) (19)

Mother Knows Best?

Many of us have fond memories of sitting between Mama or Grandmama's legs as she carefully greased and oiled our scalp. Many of us remember our hair as flourishing in those days. It's easy to connect the thick, healthy hair of our youth with Mama's expert oiling strategy; after all, freshly oiled scalps do look shiny, supple and healthy—temporarily, anyway. More likely, many other factors were at play and contributed more significantly to the healthy hair you recall from childhood.

First and foremost, children tend to have extremely low-manipulation hair regimens. They tend not to use harsh products and treatments such as hairsprays, colors, heat and relaxers that become our mainstays in adulthood. Hair ALWAYS thrives best in low- manipulation environments regardless of products used.

The greasy shine Mama laid on your scalp may have felt good and looked great from her vantage point, but your scalp likely was struggling to maintain its equilibrium and continue its normal daily business of flaking on schedule. The natural flaking process of the scalp simply cannot occur as efficiently with heavy oils obstructing the surface. The flakes then accumulate and become trapped, causing dryness, dandruff and itchy flare-ups.

The proper way to hydrate the scalp and stimulate natural sebum production is simply through frequent cleansing and conditioning of the scalp. Frequent cleansing keeps the scalp skin clear of any obstructing clutter, and hydration (conditioning) keeps it moisturized and supple.

For those who must supplement their scalp oils due to low natural sebum production, or simple aesthetics, a moderate application of a sebum-mimicking oil such as jojoba (pronounced ho-ho-bah) or a light plant-based oil such as coconut to the scalp should do the trick.

Understanding Hair Structure and Form

The shaft—the part of the hair fiber that we see on a daily basis—is composed primarily of keratin protein, lipids, water and different binding materials for these molecules. The hair's protein structure controls its various physical characteristics including its general appearance, its ability to absorb water and chemicals, and its overall strength and quality.

The keratins found in hair are extremely sulfur-rich and are joined together by many, many cystine cross-linkages. Cystine is therefore the most plentiful amino acid in hair and contributes to between 14 and 18 percent of the hair's total composition. Cystine and cysteine are identical amino acids, except that cysteine is free-ranging and has not been cross-linked within the fiber. Hair and fingernails are made from the same keratin components, but nails have a substantially larger amount of cystine cross-linkage. That's why nails tend to be a lot harder and more robust than hair.

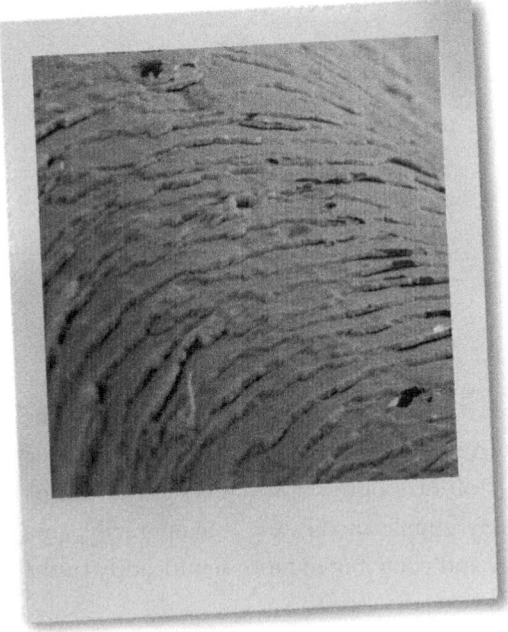

Figure 6: Microscopic image of our hair's surface. Credit: Eye of Science/Photo Researchers, Inc

The keratin found in hair is a resilient protein containing the following amino acids:

Table 1: 18 amino acids found in healthy hair (7) (20)

Alanine	Glycine	Phenylalanine
Arginine	Histidine	Proline
Aspartic Acid	Isoleucine	Serine
Cysteine	Leucine	Threonine
Cystine	Lysine	Tyrosine
Glutamic Acid	Methionine	Valine

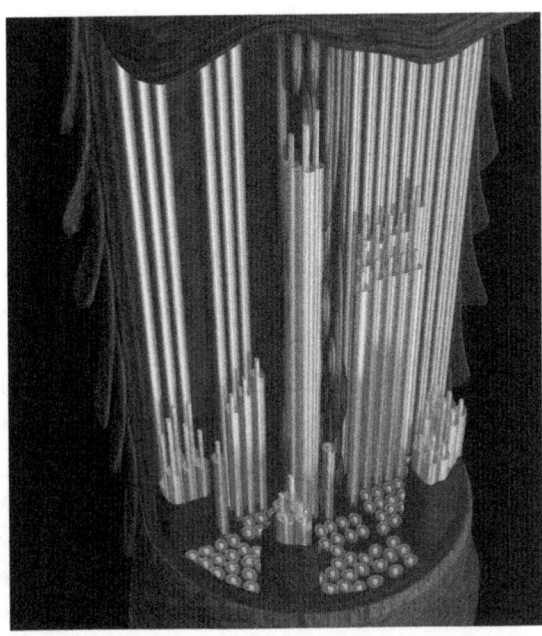

Figure 7: Hair shaft cross-section. Artwork of the internal anatomy of a shaft of human hair. The outer layer, the cuticle, has been partially removed here to reveal the two inner areas, the cortex and the innermost area, the medulla (core) of the hair shaft. The medulla is the brown strand partially seen at the center of the shaft. Most of the image consists of the cortical bundles, which consist of various sizes of fibrils and filaments (yellow and green). Credit: STUDIO MACBETH/PHOTO RESEARCHERS, INC.

Structures of the Hair Fiber

The hair shaft is made up of three layers: medulla, cortex and cuticle.

Internal Structure
Medulla

The medulla—also known as the pith or marrow—is the innermost layer of the hair shaft and is typically only found in thick, coarse hair. (8) (21) Natural blondes and those with thin, fine hair strands typically do not have this inner space in their hair shafts. For now, the medulla has not been shown to be of any particular significance in hair care; it simply makes the hair shafts that contain this space at their heart naturally thicker than those without.

Cortex

If the medulla is absent, the cortex is the innermost portion of the hair shaft and makes up the greatest percentage of the hair fiber, accounting for 80 to 90 percent of its total weight. (7) The cortex is where the hair's strength and elasticity originate. The cortex is comprised of several long, fibrous, highly organized chains of proteins that twist and coil around each other to form the hair fiber's basic structure.

External Structure
Cuticle

The cortex is shielded from the elements by a protective cuticle layer. (1) (8) This outermost layer of the hair shaft is composed of various fatty acids and proteins. Although the cuticle appears to have color, it is colorless. The hair color we see is actually the pigmentation found within the cortex.

The cuticle is made up of five to eleven overlapping sheaths of cells arranged like shingles on a roof; the number of layers reduces significantly from root to tip due to natural weathering and damage. (21) Rather than simply being stacked one upon the other, each layer of cuticle

is attached or anchored to the cortex at its base. Thicker-stranded hair tends to have more overlapping layers with lengthier scales.

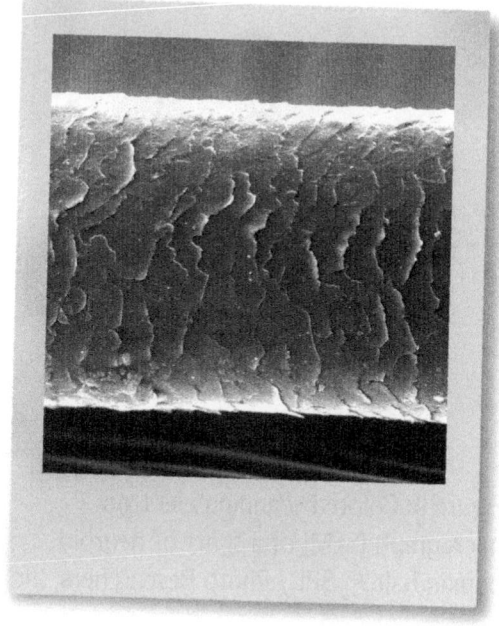

Figure 8: The cuticle is the hair fiber's outer protective barrier. Credit: David Phillips / Photo Researchers, Inc

The healthy appearance of hair depends almost entirely upon the condition of the cuticle. Tattered, worn cuticles reflect light poorly, and increased friction between raised cuticle layers prevents hair from moving well. The farther down the hair shaft we progress, the more vulnerable to damage the hair generally becomes due to lifting and destruction of the cuticle. It is not uncommon for cuticle degradation at the very tip of the hair shaft to be so complete that the cortex is exposed.

Relaxers, hair-coloring products and stripping shampoos all play a great part in wearing away the hair's protective cuticle layers. Aggressive combing and brushing also can damage the outer cuticle layers.

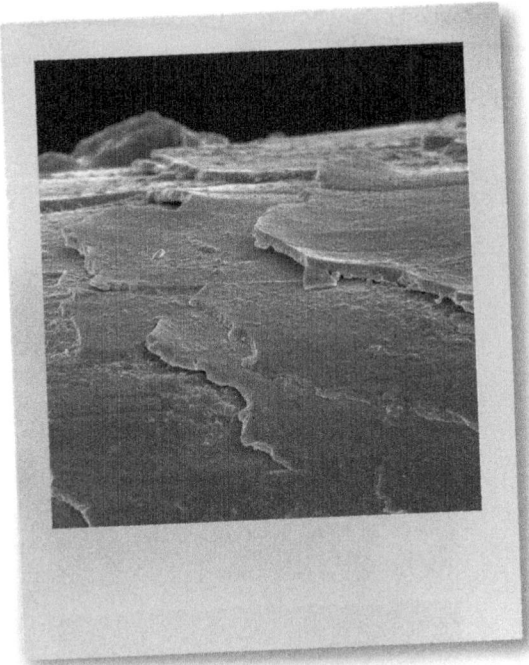

Figure 9: Colored scanning electron micrograph (SEM) of a shaft of negroid human hair. © SPL / Photo Researchers, Inc

Cuticle Structure

The cuticle can be further divided into five layers: epicuticle, A-layer, exocuticle, endocuticle and cuticular cell membrane complex (CMC). (1) (8)

Epicuticle

The outermost layer of the cuticle is known as the epicuticle. This super-thin membrane is rich in protein, fatty acids and lipids. There is evidence that the lipid content of the cuticle in black hair is less than in the hair of other races. This simply underscores the point that black hair requires dedicated moisturizing, lubricating and deep conditioning. (1)

A- Layer and Exocuticle

The cuticle's sulfur-rich A-layer is marked by extensive cystine cross-linking. This reinforced layer provides an element of strength and protects the innermost parts of the hair shaft from heat damage and other mechanical stressors. (1)

The exocuticle provides a second layer of defense against mechanical damage to the hair strand. This layer also features considerable cystine cross-linking, although not as generous as the cross-linking found in the A-layer. While not as strong as the A-layer, the exocuticle still offers great support to the cortex and constitutes roughly two thirds of the cuticle. (8)

The significant cross-linking found in the A-Layer and exocuticle makes them especially strong and resistant to attack from chemicals and other stressors.

Endocuticle

The endocuticle, the innermost cuticle layer, has a significantly lower natural sulfur content than the other four layers and therefore, fewer cross-links to provide strength to the hair fiber. It is the weakest cuticle layer. Fewer cross-links means that the endocuticle is highly porous and that water penetrates easily. In fact, the endocuticle is the only layer that swells and expands when exposed to water. As the endocuticle swells, the other layers lift away from the cortex of the fiber to allow materials to enter the shaft.

Cuticular Cell Membrane Complex (CMC)

The CMC is a layer of natural lipid glue that binds the cuticle layers together and marries them to the cortex to reinforce and secure the entire hair fiber. (21)

Understanding Hair Bonds

Deep within the hair structure, cross-bonds and -linkages create a network of strength that reinforces the hair fiber and allows it to remain responsive to our styling whims. Three types of hair bonds exist within the hair fiber: hydrogen bonds, salt bonds and disulfide bonds. Collectively, these bonds are known as side bonds. Side bonds link chains of the hair's amino acids together, and each type of side bond contributes approximately 33 percent to the hair's overall hair strength. (7) (20)

Disulfide Bonds

Though not as prevalent in the cortex as other bonds, disulfide or sulfur bonding is perhaps the most significant type of bonding in black hair care. The more disulfide bonding that occurs in the fiber, the curlier and kinkier the hair. These bonds are strong and cannot be broken by water or heat manipulation. Only chemical agents can break these bonds. Disulfide bonds join together the sulfur atoms of two nearby cysteine amino acid chains. Chemical relaxers work primarily by disrupting disulfide bonds. After breaking disulfide linkages, relaxers "cap" the bonds so that they cannot reform again. This is why relaxers cannot be stripped or undone. (7) (20) (21) Once broken, disulfide bonds cannot be reformed.

Salt Bonds

Abundant throughout the cortex, salt bonds are another important hair bond. These bonds are broken by pH changes in the hair in both the acid or alkaline direction. Readjusting the hair's pH will reform and stabilize these bonds. Salt bonds are formed when the positive end of an amino acid chain links to another amino acid's negative end. (7) (20) (21)

Hydrogen Bonds

Hydrogen bonds are the most flexible bonds in hair care. They are easily broken in the presence of water and heat and are the primary bonds responsible for changing our hair's overall shape. When the hair has been wetted either by shampooing or simply in the presence of humidity, the water molecules introduced to the fiber move in and break up the hair's preset hydrogen bonds and form new ones. Hydrogen bonding allows our hair to change shape temporarily and produces a remarkably strong hold. Roller sets,

flat-ironed hair and twist-outs are examples of hydrogen-bond manipulation resulting in altered appearance of the hair. To achieve these curly styles, the hair usually is set on rollers or rods or in braids while wet. The hair is then held in this position until it dries. As the hair dries, hydrogen rebonding occurs, but in the new shape or orientation of the planned hairstyle. The hair will remain in this position until it is again presented with water, either through shampooing or in the presence of humid air. Hydrogen bonding is the reason why hair frizzes and curls fall and why we are able to manipulate our hair into a range of styles. (1) (7) (21) (22)

Although hydrogen bonds are considered a weak form of bonding, these bonds are still quite strong. The strength of these bonds is evident when we compare hair that has been set while dry to hair that has been set while wet. Wet-set hair always has crisper, more defined, longer-lasting curls than dry-set hair because the hydrogen bonding arrangement in dry hair is already fixed. When we wet our hair, these bonds are temporarily disrupted and we are able to take advantage of the hair's flexible hydrogen-bonding arrangement to re-style the hair with more definition.

Hair Growth Cycles and Stages

Each hair grows from its own follicle independently of the ones next to it. The average hair grows 1/4 to 1/2 inch per month from a hair follicle situated roughly 4 millimeters below the surface of the scalp. Because this monthly growth rate is an average, some of us may experience more or less growth than this each month. Dominant growth factors include the time of year, the part of the body from which a particular hair grows, and your personal hair practices, diet, age and genetics.

All hair goes through three specific phases in its lifetime: a growing phase (anagen), a resting phase (catagen) and a shedding stage (telogen). In a fourth phase, exogen, the hair follicle lies dormant for a time after shedding before starting a new anagen growing phase. Only 80 percent of hair, however, ever enters an exogen phase. The length of these phases is genetically predetermined and differs for various types of body hair. The average (anagen) growing phase lasts for four to seven years and may be as short as one year or as long as ten years. As we age, however, our anagen phases slowly begin to shorten. At any one point, more than 88 percent of our hair strands are in the anagen phase.

Table 2: Length of Growing Phases Chart

Body Region	Length of Anagen Growing phase
Arms, fingers, eyelashes	1-6 months
Legs	5-7 months
Scalp	1-10 years

Did You Know?

If all the hairs on your head grew and went through the three phases of the hair life cycle all at the same time, we would all go bald every 4-7 years once the hairs hit telogen phase! Luckily, things have worked out for the better with each hair doing its own thing in its own time. The cycling of the phases on a staggered individual schedule assures that we always have hair covering our heads.

During the catagen phase, hair simply takes a growth break and is preparing to be shed. This phase can last from four weeks to as long as four months, and at any given time approximately 1 percent of our hair is in this phase. The hair follicle stops producing melanin (color) in the catagen phase, which is why the roots of hairs eventually shed in the telogen phase appear white or clear.

During the telogen phase the hair naturally sheds. Right now, approximately 11 percent of your hairs are in the telogen phase waiting to either fall on their own or to be pulled out as a result of your styling routine. The greatest percentage of our hair is in telogen phase during the late summer or early fall months. The telogen hair stage can last for as long as four months. If a hair is simply yanked from the scalp before it has entered its natural shedding phase, a new hair will not emerge from the follicle for roughly 130 days.

Exogen is an optional hair phase that follows the shedding of hair from a follicle. It describes a latency period in which the follicle rests and prepares to enter a new growing or anagen phase. The exogen phase can last anywhere from five to seven months. As we age, our natural exogen periods begin to lengthen.

Hair Growth Factors

Understanding key hair-growth factors is important for establishing a solid hair-care regimen. Knowing the processes that are truly responsible for hair growth and maintenance will put you in a better position to evaluate hair care product claims and get the information you need to adapt your regimen over time. Having a fundamental understanding of hair growth limitations is also in order so that you can remain encouraged and set realistic, obtainable goals.

Hormones

Hormones, one of the primary drivers of hair growth, are powerful regulators of cell processes within the human body. As their levels in the human body fluctuate, hormones have the ability to lengthen or shorten hair growing and resting stages. A key example of how hormones can regulate hair growth cycles occurs during and after pregnancy. Pregnancy is marked by a surge in hormone activity to prepare the mother's body to give birth. This upswing in pregnancy hormone levels locks the hair into its anagen (growing) and catogen (resting) phases. What we end up seeing then is renewed thickness as hairs that were on schedule to shed are no longer able to do so. Once the baby is born, however, hormone levels take a nosedive over the following three to six months. Postpartum hormone levels abruptly send the hair into telogen phase, and massive shedding can take place, literally by the handful! Halting oral-contraceptive use triggers the same hair-shedding phenomenon.

Low estrogen levels have long been linked to premature hair thinning and hair loss, particularly during menopause. While hormone replacement therapy has been shown to prevent further hair loss, it can do nothing for hair that has already thinned out.

Hair cannot be separated from the body as a holistic unit. If the body is in trouble, such trouble is also often reflected in the hair. Key health factors such as irregularities in menstrual cycles or infertility also can point to hormonal issues that could be adversely affecting hair growth. Irregular cycles and infertility, for instance, could be indicators that excess androgen/testosterone production is creating a poor environment for hair growth.

Terminal Length

Terminal length is the longest length that any hair on your head can grow given your monthly hair growth rate and the length of your anagen (growing) phase. It is the length that your hair would reach if it were never cut, never broke and was allowed to simply grow freely without interruption. Once a hair has completed its growth period (and therefore reached its terminal length), it will shed naturally and be pushed out by a new, growing strand. This process repeats all over your head, for every single strand of hair, everyday—for your entire lifetime. Hair that has reached its terminal length tapers naturally into this position. Hair "hemlines" that

have reached terminal length are rarely blunt or even because each strand of hair is at a different point in its personal growth phase. Factor in hair breakage, and hairs rarely ever reach terminal length together.

Did You Know?

Terminal length measurements are more about time than length. Take a hair growth cycle that happens to be 4 years long. No matter how long your hair is at the 4 year mark, the follicles on that 4 year shed schedule will release hair. You could have either gained as much possible length as your growth rate will allow in 4 years, or you could have shaven it bald at 3 years and 355 days in. Either way, the hair in the 4 year follicle will shed.

All hair on your body is subject to predetermined genetic growth rates, resting phases and terminal lengths. Eyelashes, arm and leg hairs go into their resting phases a few months after the onset of growth. This is why these body hairs never get very long. Without terminal hair lengths (and some type of order to our hair growth), we'd be braiding and brushing our leg hair! (See Table 2)

It is very important to keep in mind that terminal length is not determined by the current length of your hair at any point. This is a common misconception. Occasionally, someone will say, "Well, my hair always grows to my shoulders and then stops. This must be my terminal length." Not so! Hair follicles always rest when their growing time frame has expired—which may correlate with a certain length when experienced over time. But, our hair does not stop growing *because it is a certain length*—it stops growing *after a certain time period has elapsed*. It is the length of this time period that is genetically determined, not the hair length itself. Our job, then, is to maximize growing opportunities (and prevent breakage) during each hair's four- to seven-year growth phase.

Since your genetically determined hair growth period dictates terminal length, the argument logically follows that, if left to grow undisturbed (with no breakage or cutting), your hair will correspond to a particular length measurement at that terminal length. Unfortunately, many of us have not grown our hair for long enough, under healthy conditions, to see our strands reach and maintain true terminal lengths. Some of us have old, damaged hair from our pre-healthy hair care days that will need to be shed or cut before our hair ever stands a chance of reaching terminal length. Still others of us prefer our hair to have neat hemlines, so frequent trimming keeps us from reaching our full length potential.

In order to determine genetic predisposition to short hair, you would need to examine the hair care practices of all the women in your family over the course of a few years. Unfortunately, years of bad or nonexistent information on black hair care have put many of us at a great disadvantage. Most black women have never experienced the luxury of achieving their terminal hair lengths—nor have they seen their mothers, aunts or sisters do it. The point of this whole hair journey is to break the cycle of doubt and find out our true hair potential, once and for all.

Discovering your terminal hair length will take considerable time. Unfortunately, it is virtually impossible to use your hair in its current state as a baseline for judging your terminal length potential. The hair you have on your head now has been growing for years, and this aging hair most likely has not received the best care before this point. Without knowing the age of each hair, where it is in the growth cycle and how much breakage it has encountered during its entire history, you cannot determine terminal length. For example, if your hair growth phase is four years long, but during the first three of those years you cut and simply did not care for your tresses at all, the chances of seeing your hair's full terminal length potential in the fourth and final year of the growth phase are highly unlikely.

If you find that you have not reached a reasonable hair length after years, or have reached what seems to be a plateau in an otherwise healthy hair care regimen—before you chalk your length up to genetics, a reevaluation of your regimen may be in order.

Did You Know?

The Dreadlocks Question

In discussions about length potential, you often hear folks bring up the fact that dreadlocks grow so long that they must be a testament to the great lengths that we can achieve. I believe in the potential of every black woman to grow their hair to amazing lengths, but dreadlocks are not a good example in this case. While it is true that dreadlocks can and do reach great lengths, there is also a catch. Dreadlocks are unique in that they do not represent true *"root to ends"* length. They are the accumulation of shed, broken, and growing hairs matted together. Imagine if all of the shed or broken hair you ever had in the span of a year or in a lifetime were woven together! You too would have hair well down your back. This is the science behind loc'ing. Those hairs that are dropped are "locked" into your locs.

Interestingly, there is a process by which locs can successfully be undone or unloc'd, preserving quite a bit of the hair's natural length. But much of the hair is still lost to the process at the end of the day, and waist length or floor length locs simply do not translate into waist length of floor length loose hair.

Chapter 2: Textured Hair Properties & Principles

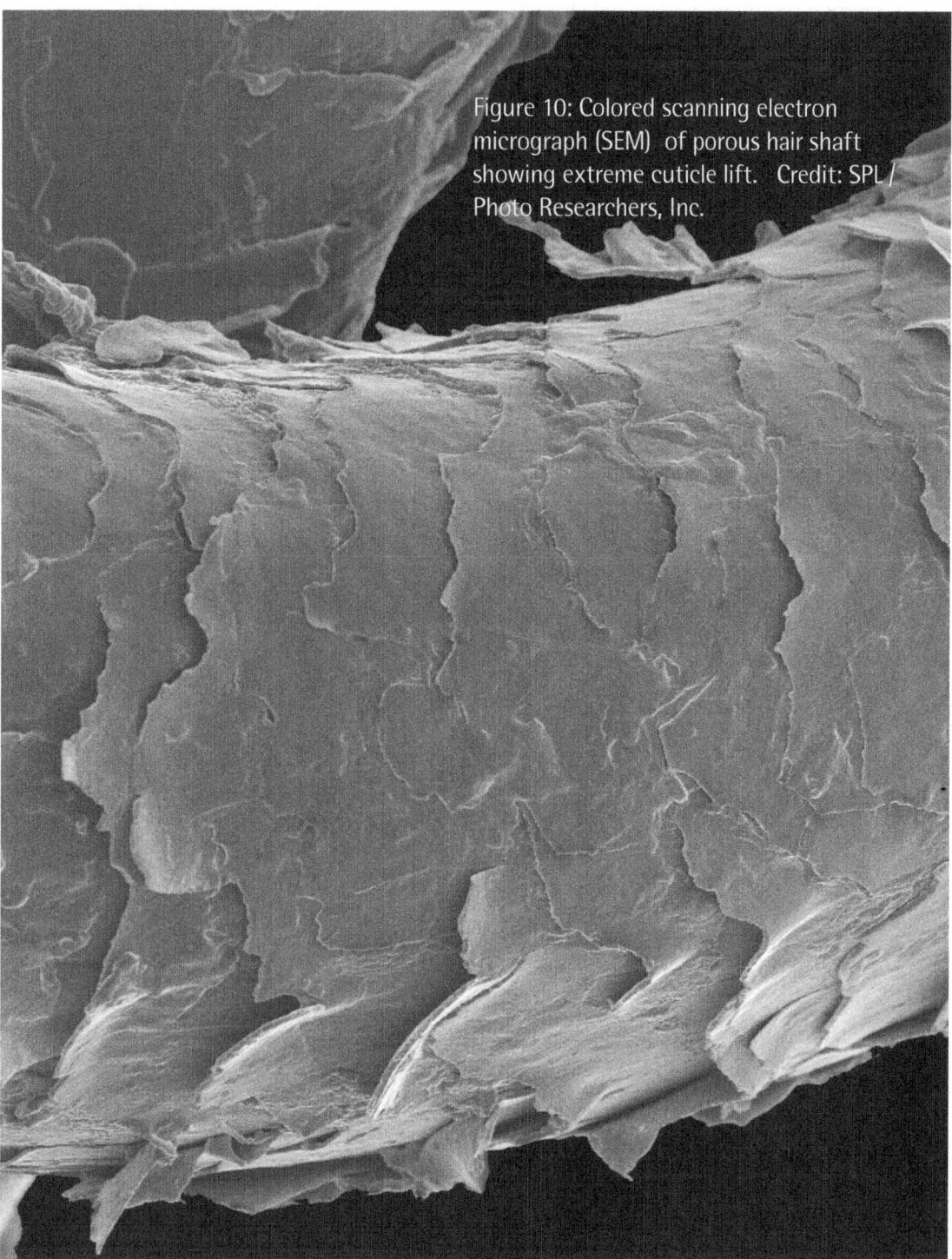

Figure 10: Colored scanning electron micrograph (SEM) of porous hair shaft showing extreme cuticle lift.   Credit: SPL / Photo Researchers, Inc.

Very few things are considered gospel in the world of healthy hair care. Nevertheless, the basic properties and principles that set the standard for healthy hair tend to remain the same across different heads of hair. All healthy hair has in common certain properties and characteristics. To understand these properly, we need to investigate black hair architecture, elasticity and porosity and how they each relate to healthy hair care. Our hair's robust infrastructure and properties are what enable these thin, threadlike fibers to endure a myriad of stressors over their lifetime. In order to successfully address your hair's needs as they arise, you must commit to developing an understanding of these basic hair properties and how they affect your hair. You must know what your hair *should be doing* and *how it should be feeling*—and to what degree.

Black Hair Architecture

There are two characteristic presentations of black hair: black hair in its natural state (not chemically straightened) and chemically-straightened black hair. In its natural state, black hair curls, twists, bends and kinks in a variety of interesting angles along the hair fiber. Very rarely is there perfect uniformity in the distribution of these curls and kinks. Kinks are given their character at the follicle level, with the shape of the hair follicle contributing significantly to the shape and appearance of the emerging hair fiber.

Kinky hair fibers are produced from elliptical or oval-shaped hair follicles in the scalp. (Caucasian and Asian hair fibers grow from round or circle-shaped hair follicles; these fibers tend to be slightly larger in diameter than black hair fibers and the follicles more densely distributed than black hair follicles.) Imagine the technique used to curl ribbons for gift wrapping. Typically, a piece of straight ribbon is held taut while a pair of scissors is held flat against one side of the ribbon. The ribbon is then pulled against the side of the scissors to produce a curl. In much the same way, our ovoid follicles flatten our hair fibers on one or both sides as they emerge from the scalp, creating an intense, unpredictable curl.

While Asian and Caucasian hair tends to be fairly uniform in thickness from the root to the end of the shaft, the shape and diameter of black hair shafts does not remain constant along the length of an individual strand. Black hair tends to flatten and decrease in diameter around its bends and twists—and fibers regularly make reversals in curl direction as we descend down the strand. (23) Even when black hair is chemically modified or straightened, this thinning of the fiber at points where the natural bends were located is still present and translates in the straightened hair fiber as an area of weakness. The bends and

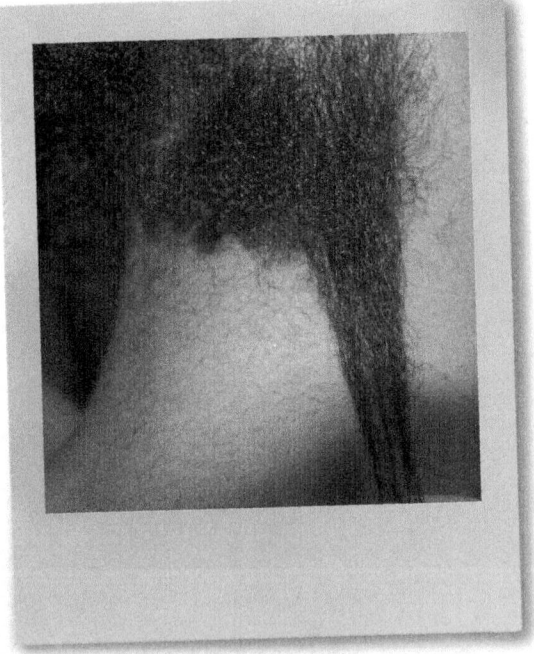

Figure 11: In its natural state, textured hair can shrink to half its stretched length or shorter.

changes in both direction of curl and diameter along a single strand make black hair fibers much more fragile than other hair types. Research has shown that the pulling force required to break a strand of black hair is less than the force required to break Caucasian or Asian strands. (23)

Gender and Textured Hair Thickness

Gender plays a role in the thickness of our individual fibers. Research has shown that in general, the hairs of black men tend to have larger diameters than that of black women. Larger-diameter hair shafts among men generally translate to more cuticle layers and coarser hair overall than their female counterparts. (21)

Shrinkage

In its natural state, black hair is prone to considerable fiber shrinkage (see figure 11). Natural hair's tendency to draw up tightly and hug the scalp when dry makes it appear much shorter than it truly is. This shrinkage is advantageous for some hair styles where compact shapes are desired (Afros and puffs). While shrinkage affects all curly-haired people to some extent, some textured hair types are more affected by hair shrinkage than others. Hair with a looser, wavier curl pattern may retain more of its natural length when going from wet to dry than naturally coiled or kinky hair. In fact, kinky natural hair may shrink to half its length or shorter; hair well below the shoulder, for instance, may shrink back to ear length. This shrinkage is normal and is simply a part of our hair's natural character.

Shine or Sheen?

Relaxed or natural, textured hair rarely shines outright. Rather, most healthy black hair types tend to have sheen and a matte appearance. Although shine is related to the ideal, flattened orientation of the cuticle layers, the inability to produce or maintain shine among some textured hair types is not always a reflection of poor condition (see figure 12).

Shine is a direct result of light bouncing from the hair's surface and being directed toward the eye. Tightly wound curls and intertwining coils, however, simply do not reflect light in the same manner that straighter hair shafts do. Because most black hair does not shine in the usual sense,

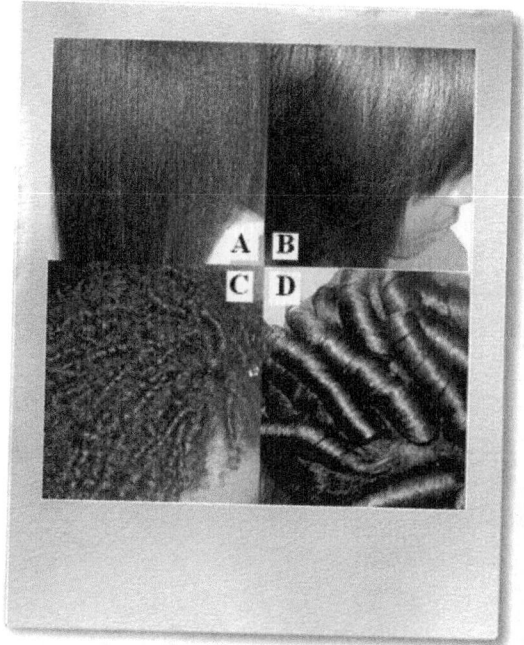

Figure 12: Healthy black hair rarely shines outright, although it may be in perfect condition. Photos A and C are examples of healthy hair sheen, Photos B and D are examples of shine. Most textured hair shines when it is straightened, oiled, or pulled taut.

unless aided by oils or serums, this hair may appear to be quite dry at first glance. Touching often reveals its true softness and health.

Hair is Mostly Protein

Since hair is mostly protein, its natural physical properties are related directly to the condition, organization and placement of these protein components within the fiber. Black hair's protein backbone is one of the most important features of the hair shaft. Even the slightest change in the hair's protein structure and components can significantly alter the hair's appearance and mechanical properties.

In its natural state, black hair is at its strongest and exhibits its greatest durability. A hair fiber's strength comes primarily from the extensive disulfide and protein cross-linking rampant throughout the hair's cortex. These disulfide links and bonds are some of the strongest bonds in hair

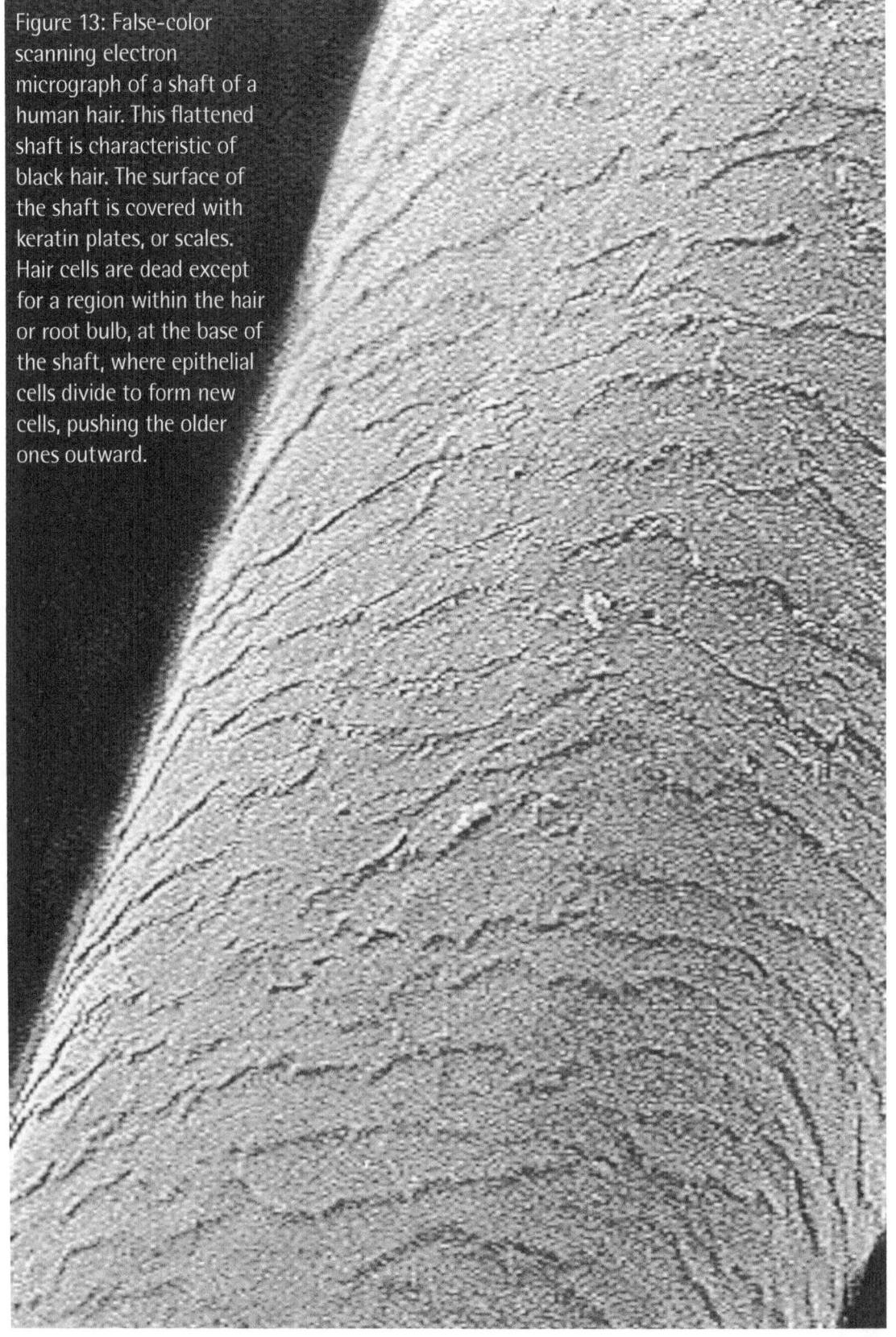

Figure 13: False-color scanning electron micrograph of a shaft of a human hair. This flattened shaft is characteristic of black hair. The surface of the shaft is covered with keratin plates, or scales. Hair cells are dead except for a region within the hair or root bulb, at the base of the shaft, where epithelial cells divide to form new cells, pushing the older ones outward.

care. When these bonds are altered through processes such as chemical relaxing, black hair loses its strength. Unprocessed, natural hair fibers are able to endure more stress than chemically relaxed fibers because the natural protein structure, the main factor in hair's strength, has not been compromised or changed. Properly maintained in its natural state, black hair is best able to thrive. To reach maximum lengths, however, natural hair must contend with its tendency to tangle and knot on itself, and the natural presence of unpredictable bends along the fiber that make it vulnerable to manipulation breakage.

Chemical relaxers work by exploiting many of the important linkages that give natural black hair its strength. Relaxing causes new permanent (but weaker) cross-linkages to be formed on newly straightened hair fibers. From a protein-structure and bond-loss standpoint, relaxing natural hair greatly weakens it. Despite this, there are some advantages to relaxing the hair.

Relaxed fibers are not as prone to manipulation breakage because the individual bends and kinks along the hair fiber have been chemically removed, making manipulation easier. Relaxing reduces the friction between individual hair fibers and decreases opportunities for breakage and tangling from kinking and knotting.

Unfortunately, chemically processing black hair opens the door to other types of hair breakage and damage. Steps must be taken to ensure that protein supplementation needs are met in chemically relaxed hair fibers to reduce the incidence of breakage from protein loss. Hair proteins have a strong affinity for water. The dynamics of the interrelationship between protein and water in the hair fiber make it absolutely essential that healthy hair care regimens address both the protein and water needs of the hair. When used as part of a balanced hair care regimen, protein and moisture-rich products greatly enhance the strength characteristics of chemically relaxed and natural hair.

When black hair, natural or relaxed, is maintained in a healthy manner, each may be grown out so that it wonderfully exhibits the best qualities of its type. All we must do is cater to the specific needs of each hair type to minimize its potential negatives.

Elasticity and Textured Fibers

Black hair fibers are elastic. When black hair is healthy, it is able to stretch and return to its original length many times over while resisting breakage. Elasticity is the stretching power that allows a comb to move through your hair without the fibers breaking from the contact and stress of pulling. Elasticity is what allows us to smooth and pull our hair back into a ponytail and perform other styling and grooming tasks as necessary.

The elasticity of the hair is extremely significant. Hair that is able to withstand tension and bounces back easily after extension with minimal breakage is said to have good elasticity. Without it, our hair would snap off left and right, even with very little tension placed upon it. Black hair's natural elasticity is exaggerated when the hair is wet because of the extensive hydrogen bonding and cross-linking that takes place throughout the hair fiber. When water or chemicals enter the cuticle and cortex, water molecules break and displace the existing hydrogen-bonding structure. The water molecules then institute a new temporary hydrogen-bonding arrangement in the fiber. When water molecules infiltrate our textured hair fibers, the hair can absorb up to 40 percent of its weight in water and lengthen by 40 to 50 percent of its normal dry length. This water absorption is why wet hair feels heavier than dried hair. Because wet hair is naturally more elastic than dry hair, it also appears—and often is—longer than dried hair. (1) (7)

A benefit of the enhanced elasticity of wet hair is the improved styling environment it affords textured hair. Moistening black hair prior to stretching or manipulating it reduces the chances of breaking it. (23) This reduced-breakage scenario is possible because adding moisture to the strands relaxes the hydrogen bonds in the cortex, so that the hair can be manipulated over a greater range of motion. Manipulating damp, moist hair is also preferable because wet hair returns to its original length after stretching faster than dry hair that has encountered the same level of tension. For black hair in particular, manipulating dampened hair eases the stress of combing and causes less breakage from friction than dry combing.

Our hair's elasticity is balanced and supported by its inner protein structure, and both characteristics work hand in hand to prevent premature breakage of the hair fiber. The proper elasticity, in conjunction with the proper protein structural properties, is needed if the hair is to resist breakage. (An in-depth discussion of protein/moisture balancing in healthy hair care will be covered in the chapters to follow.)

Hair Chemistry 101: Understanding pH Balance & Water Issues

Understanding pH Balance

Our hair is subject to the basic laws of chemistry. These laws govern its behavior, characteristics and appearance. Hair and product pH must be explored and regulated in order to maintain a healthy head of hair. Measuring pH has great utility for understanding the behavior of hair products on the strands and also assists in predicting the hair's response to these products. The function of pH in hair coloring, hair straightening and basic conditioning has been well established.

Very simply, pH is a measurement of ions in a water-based solution. Ions are charged particles that can either be positive or negative. When an ion is positive, it is known as a cation (cat-eye-on), and when negative, an ion is known as an anion (an-eye-on). Because the surface of our hair is slightly negative, hair responds well to cationic conditioning agents. Opposites attract!

The term *pH*, short for *potenz* hydrogen, translates directly from Danish as "hydrogen strength." The pH of a substance specifically indicates the amount of positive hydrogen cations (shown as $H+$) and negative hydroxide anions (shown as $OH-$) a solution contains. When the concentration of hydrogen ions is higher, a substance is considered acidic; if the concentration of hydroxide ions is higher, then the substance is alkaline or basic. (Because they are not water based and have neither $H+$ nor $OH-$ components, products such as oils and alcohols do not have a pH.) (7)

The pH scale ranges from 0 to 14, and at the center of this scale lies the neutral pH of 7. Pure

Product/Item	PH	Hair Effects
	0	Hair is dissolved and disintegrates completely.
	1	
Lemon Juice	2	Hair cuticle tightens and contracts. As cuticle scales close, hair porosity decreases and shine is enhanced.
Apple Cider Vinegar	3	
Hair Conditioners, Aloe Vera	4	
Hair and Skin	4.5- 5.5	Hair is normal. Normal shine and luster.
Black Coffee	5.5- 6	Hair begins to swell, and cuticles begin to lift. As pH increases, the shaft incurs an increased amount of damage. Lipids are lost from the hair.
Pure Water	7	
Blood, Semi-Permanent Hair color	8	
Baking Soda, Soaps	9	
Milk of Magnesia	10	
Relaxers		
Relaxers, Ammonia		
Relaxers	13	Hair begins to dissolve.
Relaxers	14	

Figure 14: Standard pH scale

water (H20) is an example of a substance with a neutral pH. Water is not neutral simply because it is neither acidic nor alkaline, but because it is both 50 percent acidic and 50 percent alkaline. It contains one positive and one negative ion (H+ and −OH). (7)

Acids

When a substance has a low pH reading of 0 to 6.9, it is considered acidic. Hair and skin are covered by a thin, slightly acidic film known as the acid mantle. Healthy hair and skin both have *acid mantles* with pHs in the 4 to 5.5 range. This acid mantle is more important for the skin where it acts as a barrier to viruses, bacteria and other undesirable contaminants that may try to enter the body. These contaminants, which are primarily alkaline, are neutralized by the body's protective acid mantle.

Maintaining the acid mantle is also very important for our hair. Hair responds to pH very distinctly. Low-pH substances affect the hair shaft by constricting the cuticle layers, causing them to lie flat and tightly against one another. In this state, with the cuticle closed tightly, the inner cortex of the hair strand is thoroughly protected. Tight and contracted cuticles also allow the individual hair strands to move freely past one another, and the uniform surface also better reflects light, creating sheen and shine. Neutralizing shampoos, conditioners, and natural substances such as lemon and apple cider vinegar fall into the acidic category.

Bases

A pH of 7.1 to 14 is considered basic, or alkaline. High-pH substances cause the hair's cuticle scales to lift and the hair shaft to swell and open. Your hair's reaction to plain water is an example of the effects of alkalinity. Although water is neutral, it is roughly 100 times more alkaline than our hair. Hair is acidic, but when water (which bears a higher pH of 7) interacts with the hair

shaft, the cuticles lift slightly in reaction to the water's more alkaline pH. (Relaxers and permanent hair colors also fall firmly into the alkaline/ basic category, with pH readings ranging from 10 to 13.) Lifted cuticles are responsible for tangly, dry-looking hair that does not shine, have sheen or hold moisture well. When the cuticle is lifted in this manner, the cortex is exposed, and the hair becomes weaker and more vulnerable. It is very important that the pH of hair be normalized, or returned to its normal 4 to 5.5 pH range, after using any alkaline product. Damage to the hair strand is often imminent if the cuticles are not returned to their normal, "closed" or tight position.

Regulation of pH Balance

Do It Yourself

Litmus paper is a special type of paper that changes colors as it reads the pH of the liquids you've submerged it in. The color change is immediate, and you should be able to measure the color change against a chart to find the pH level of the product you are testing. Litmus papers, or pH strips, are generally sold in drug stores.

Regulating product pH balance is important in a healthy hair care regimen. Great care must be taken to ensure that hair products used throughout the regimen contribute to restoring and maintaining the hair's natural acid balance. Because the hair must maintain its acidic pH mantle to remain healthy, products that keep the hair within its low pH range of 4 to 5.5 are ideal. When the hair's pH becomes too high or too low on the scale, the hair is always changed or damaged. Extremely high or low pH drastically affects the protein structure inside the cortex of your hair.

Keep in mind that pH ranges are logarithmic. This means that each increase in pH level represents a tenfold increase in the number of hydrogen ions. Thus, a jump in pH from 5 to 6 is not an increase in strength of one but, rather, an increase of ten times the strength. By the same token, a pH of 8 is 100 times more alkaline than a pH of 6. On the acidic end of the scale, a pH of 4 is ten times more acidic than a pH of 5. Avoid subjecting your strands to pH extremes for extended periods of time.

Shampoos and conditioners play an important role in regulating the hair's pH. Almost all shampoo and conditioner systems are pH balanced to normalize or keep the hair's pH within its normal, healthy acidic values. Shampoos are generally formulated at mildly acidic pHs (4-6), and conditioners tend to have even lower pHs (3.5-5). The decrease in pH as we move from shampoo to conditioner is intentional. The lower pH of the final product in the hair cleansing process—conditioner, helps to seal off the hair and constricts and smoothes the fiber to prevent moisture loss.

To keep product pHs within the proper range, it is preferable to use shampoos and conditioners from the same product line, which have been formulated to work together to achieve a particular pH balance. But using products from the same line often prevents the customization that is often needed to achieve other hair treatment goals, such as protein-and-moisture balancing. To ensure that your shampoo and conditioner products are maintaining your hair's acid balance, test the products (along with your tap water) with pH test strips. Water, and any water-based product, can be pH-tested quickly and inexpensively using kits that can be purchased from pharmacies or other retailers. Whenever possible, select shampoos, conditioners, and other hair products with pHs in the range of the hair's acid mantle: pH 4 to 5.5.

The pH Scale and Special Implications for Chemical Relaxing

For those of you who relax, understanding pH is particularly important. Relaxer chemicals are formulated in the alkaline pH range of 10 to

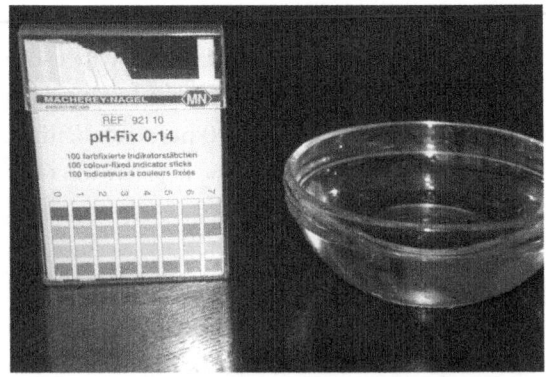

Figure 15: pH strips are used to help measure the acidity or alkalinity of various liquids and water-based products.

13, depending on the relaxer's strength. If your body chemistry is such that you have a naturally lower body pH (below 4 or 5), your relaxer may only take your hair to a pH of 8 or 9. A pH in this range will not effectively break down the bonds in your hair to allow you to obtain the desired straightened effect. If your scalp's sebum pH is naturally low, you may benefit from a relaxer with a greater strength—that is, one that bears a higher pH—to raise your hair to the proper pH range for effective relaxing. Washing your hair two days prior to relaxing may help the relaxer to take better. The shampoo will remove naturally acidic sebum residue from the scalp so that it does not affect the relaxer's ability to process.

Hard Water, Mineral Deposits and Textured Hair

Minerals are needed internally as part of a healthy, well balanced diet to support hair growth. Inside our bodies, minerals travel through the bloodstream and nourish hair follicles, enabling new hair cell regeneration. When deposited externally on the hair cuticle, however, minerals can cause breakage and dryness problems for black hair.

When water is hard, it is contaminated with dissolved minerals and metals such as calcium, magnesium, iron, copper, silica, lead and manganese. Hard water also has an increased -OH ion content, which makes it slightly more alkaline (pH= 8 +) than regular water with its neutral pH of 7. The minerals in hard water bind to the hair shaft during the course of normal shampooing and conditioning.

Hard water's elevated pH damages the hair shaft by causing it to swell and the cuticle layers to lift more than normal. Many of these minerals carry a positive charge and bind easily to the negatively charged hair shaft. Regular exposure to high-pH water and accumulation of stubborn mineral deposits on the hair shaft can lead to breakage and cause black hair to become unmanageable. Like stubborn oils, minerals have a drying effect on the outer hair cuticle because they coat the hair and prevent moisture from entering the shaft. The result is hard, dry, tangly, puffy, dull and strange-colored hair. The deposits also can build up on the scalp and cause a dandruff-like condition to arise.

Those who use no-lye relaxers must also contend with mineral buildup on the hair shaft. Like hard water, no-lye relaxers also leave mineral deposits on the cuticle that can dry out the hair if not treated promptly. Existing mineral deposits on the hair can also interfere with the success of other types of chemical products including lye-based relaxers and hair colors by affecting their ability to enter the shaft.

Hair Porosity

Porosity refers to the hair's ability, or inability, to absorb water or chemicals into the cortex. All hair is naturally porous and permeable to water, but the degree of porosity usually varies by the individual and the condition and shape of the hair's cuticle layers. When your hair faces a traumatic styling event such as chemical relaxing or permanent coloring, its protein structure is attacked and its protective cuticle shielding becomes tattered and torn. Hair in this condition is said to be porous. (8)

To better understand porosity, it is helpful to think of hair like a wooden fence. When the fence is new, it is able to shield the yard it surrounds. It can stand up to rain, sun, all of the elements—you name it. As it ages, the wood in the fence begins to soften, and the fence's once protective barrier can be breached. Over time, holes may appear in the fence or some planks may be missing in places. The fence has become porous. Our hair functions just like the fence. As it ages, the hair's protective cuticle layers begin to crack, peel and lift away. This change in the cuticle's presentation and shape makes the hair less able to absorb and hold the moisture it once could. Older hair is more porous, or has higher porosity, than newer hair. Porosity increases as we move from the roots to the ends of the hair because this represents age progression along the fiber.

Hair with low or poor porosity does not readily absorb moisture and resists chemical treatments. Such hair is generally quite healthy and has not been exposed to cuticle-degrading treatments. In low-porosity hair, the cuticle imbrications—or ridges along the hair shaft are tightly closed—just as they are when the hair first emerges from the hair follicle. The regular assault of daily living, chemical processes and styling manipulation, however, eventually causes the cuticle scales to lift and lose their tightness over time. Black hair tends to have low porosity naturally and is usually less porous than Caucasian or Asian hair types unless it has been chemically processed. For most people, it is ideal to have hair somewhere in the middle of the two extremes of porosity: hair with good porosity that retains moisture well and also accepts chemical treatments like coloring or relaxing if desired.

The hair's pH and porosity characteristics are intimately connected. Low-pH products and styling treatments reduce the hair's porosity by constricting the cuticle and causing it to tighten.

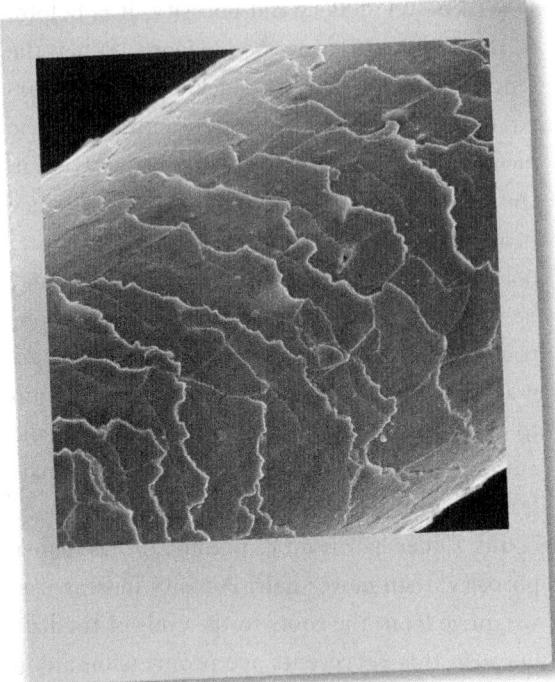

Figure 16: Colored Scanning Electron Micrograph (SEM) of the surface of a shaft of human hair. Cuticle imbrications are tight and fiber exhibits low porosity. Compare to lifted cuticles on damaged strand in Figure 10.

High-pH products have the opposite effect and increase the hair's porosity by swelling and lifting the cuticle scales.

Porosity Problems

High porosity is caused by anything that degrades or in any way changes the cuticle including excessive mechanical abuse from heat-styling tools, the sun, chemical relaxers and colors, and the use of sulfate-rich stripping shampoos. The more damage the cuticle has endured, the greater the hair's porosity—and the more water or moisture it tends to absorb. You're probably thinking, "Well, if my hair is dry, high moisture absorption is great, right?" Well, not quite. The down side of this high level of absorption is the high level of moisture loss that results from it. Highly porous hair absorbs more water when wet but loses even more as it dries. When it is

fully dried, porous hair feels swollen, puffy and rough to the touch due to the lifted, damaged cuticle layers which have instigated an inherent moisture deficiency.

Keeping this type of hair moisturized is a feat as it tends to continuously soak in moisture without ever actually feeling moisturized. Such hair is chronically dry and will not stay moisturized unless proper measures are taken to correct the issue.

Porosity Implications for the Relaxed and Color Treated

Relaxers and permanent hair color treatments use alkaline chemicals and/or heat to force open the cuticle layers so that they may reach the inner cortex. The cuticle layers do eventually close on their own, but never back to pre-treatment levels. If the damage is repeated too often (back-to-back coloring, too-frequent relaxing, heat abuse), the cuticle layers may never fully close. For this reason, relaxed, heat-abused and colored hair types have an inherently increased porosity. The prevailing problem with porous hair is the issue of raised cuticles. If you can close the cuticle layers, even a little, you will resolve a majority of your porosity issues. Because low pH products and treatments bring about cuticle closure, some porosity problems can be temporarily resolved by applying a low pH solution or product. A weekly acidic rinse with apple cider vinegar, a low-pH shampoo or even a simple cleansing with a neutralizing shampoo can help correct a porosity problem and help tighten and close the cuticle layers.

Checking for Porosity

It is best to measure your hair's porosity level on freshly cleaned and dried hair. Gently grasp a clump of your hair between your index finger and thumb, and slowly slide your fingers along the length of the strand, from the tips up toward the scalp. If you feel "bumps" or an overall un-

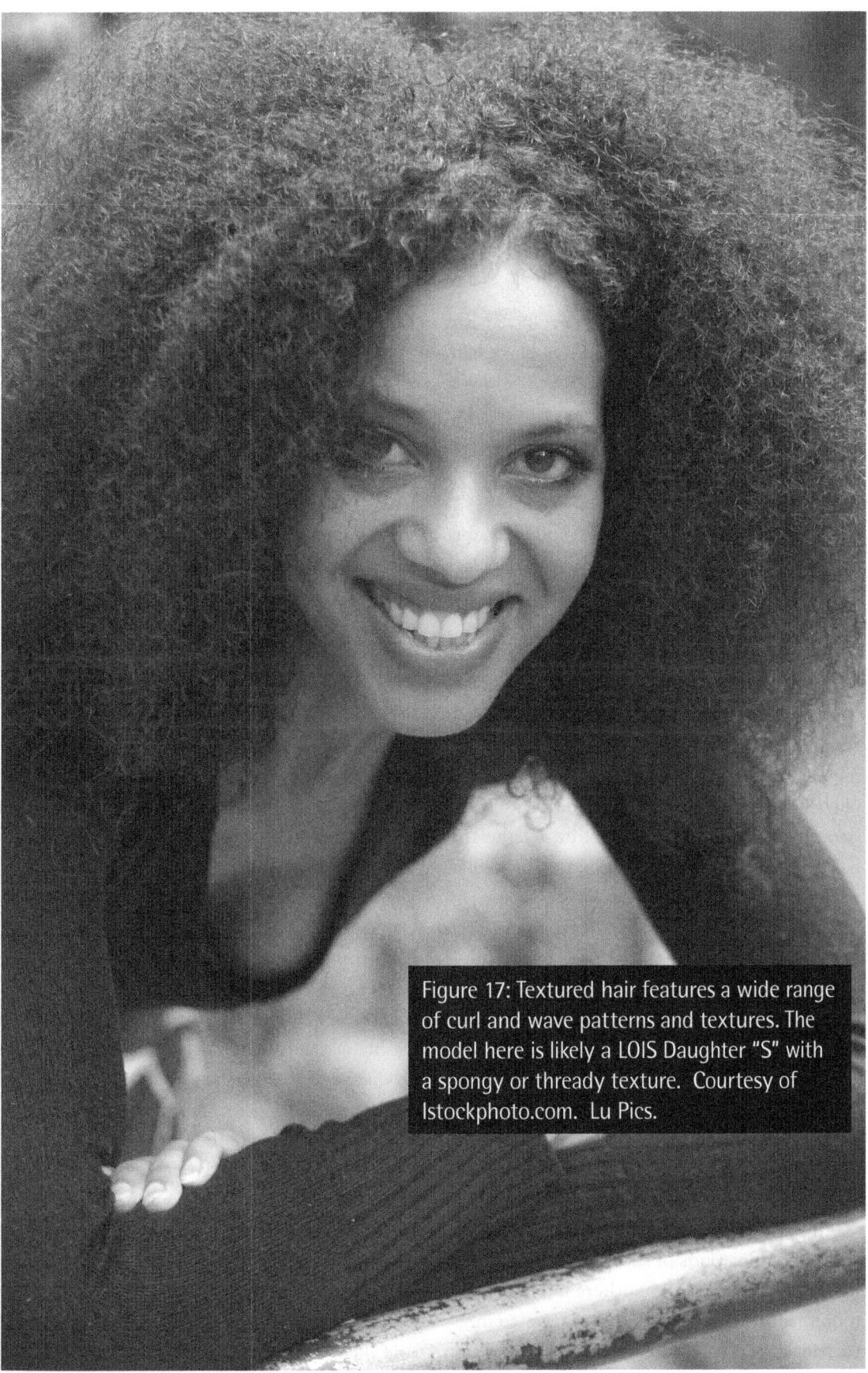

Figure 17: Textured hair features a wide range of curl and wave patterns and textures. The model here is likely a LOIS Daughter "S" with a spongy or thready texture. Courtesy of Istockphoto.com. Lu Pics.

even texture as you proceed up the shaft, your cuticles are not flat and your hair is slightly porous. Most individuals who have relaxed or color-treated their hair will find that their strands exhibit some degree of porosity. Hair that "wets" easily as you prepare it for shampooing is typically porous.

Now that you know the important healthy hair indicators and characteristics of black hair, you can begin to combat the number one threat to healthy textured tresses everywhere: hair breakage.

Textured Hair Typing

Hair-typing techniques are another way to explore various characteristics common to black hair fibers. Unfortunately, this topic can become a touchy subject for many women of color because of the deep-seated, historical and emotional issues it often brings to the fore. Those familiar with the "good hair/ bad hair" stereotypes that exist in our community already have been exposed to hair typing in its crudest and perhaps cruelest form. The old belief system, which has been deeply, subconsciously internalized by many of us, tells us that hair textures with tighter coils and sharper bends are inferior to silkier, looser, wavier textures. This form of hair typing is problematic on many levels and negatively affects the progressive movement of unity and thought in our communities. We must understand that no matter our hair type, we ALL have "good hair" as long as it is healthy and well maintained. The only "bad hair" to be had, whether relaxed or natural, is hair that is not thriving and is weak and/or damaged.

Why Type Our Hair At All?

It is important to understand your hair type and the implications of such a hair type. Some hair types are drier than others by nature and require more pampering and concentrated moisturizing efforts to maintain an optimal condition

of health. Hair typing is also a flexible guideline for comparing products—and the hair's reaction to products—between individuals with similar hair types. As you are learning to type your hair, remember that no two heads of hair are alike, and many different hair types may exist on one head.

The LOIS System©*

Over the years, several hair-type classification systems have been created. Unfortunately, the process of breaking hair down into any type of categorized system can end up alienating many people whose hair types fall into the in-between areas. The broad grouping of textured hair by the alpha-numeric typing system made popular years ago does not fairly represent the wide range of hair types and textures that must fit into the textured category. Of all the hair-typing systems in use, the one that I feel best addresses and embraces the wide variety of textured hair types is the LOIS System©. This letter-based system considers the actual bends, coils and kinks of individual hair strands and places them within more focused contexts of strand density, texture, sheen and shine for more accurate typing.

Using the LOIS System©
Examine your Hair Strands and Find Your Pattern

You should perform the LOIS assessment on freshly washed and air-dried hair with no extra products added. Hair should be rinsed in cold water for 5 minutes prior to drying in order to ensure proper sealing of the hair cuticle. This sealing will allow you to make the texture and sheen determinations for your hair type. Hair typing should be done on your natural, non-chemically treated hair texture.

---

* Generously shared courtesy of www.ourhair.net. Copyright 2006.

To begin the typing process, select a single strand of the most common type of hair on your head. The bends, kinks and coils of your hair will resemble one or more of the letters of the LOIS system: L, O, I or S.

- L - If the hair has all bends, right angles and folds with little to no curvature, then you are daughter L.
- O - If the strand is rolled up into the shape of one or several zeros like a spiral, then you are daughter O.
- I - If the hair lies mostly flat with no distinctive curves or bends, you are daughter I.
- S - If the strand looks like a wavy line with hills and valleys then you are daughter S.

You may have a combination of the LOIS letters, with one type usually being dominant. If you cannot determine a dominant letter type among your strands, then combine the letters to make a LOIS combination. Example: LO, IL or OS.

Find Your Texture

The LOIS System© also includes the texture of your hair as one of its hair-type classifiers. These classifiers assess your hair's overall shine, sheen, feel and response to wetting. Shine, for instance, is defined in the LOIS System© as a sharp reflection of light, and sheen as a dull reflection of light. Shine is a stronger, glossier, more consistent reflection of light. Sheen is a duller, softer glimmer that is more scattered throughout the hair. In essence, sheen is scattered shine.

If your hair is:
- Thready—Your hair has low to moderate natural sheen, with high shine when the hair is held taut (as in a braid). Frizz is low among thready hair types. Hair wets easily, but dries out quickly.
- Wiry—Your hair has a sparkly natural sheen, with low shine and low frizz. Water beads up or bounces off wiry hair strands, and it may take time before these strands feel fully wet.
- Cottony—Your hair has low natural sheen, but can produce high shine when the hair is held taut. This hair type is prone to high frizz. It absorbs water quickly, but takes time to feel thoroughly wet.
- Spongy—Your hair has high sheen, low shine and a compacted-looking frizz. It tends to absorb water before it gets thoroughly wet.
- Silky—Your hair has low sheen and very high shine. Your frizz potential varies, and your hair easily wets in water.

Find Your Strand Size

A strand of frayed thread is about the thickness of a medium-sized strand of human hair. If your strand is larger than this, then your hair is thick. If your strand is smaller than this, your hair is fine.

Determine your Overall Hair Density

Although the LOIS System© does not include a measurement of overall hair density, this hair-type classifier is also important to know. Changes in overall hair density may be indicative of health problems or hormonal changes. Hair density and strand size are not necessarily related to one another. You may have a head full of fine strands that are densely packed together, or thick strands that are sparsely arranged upon your head. The thickness of your hair is determined best by the diameter of your ponytail when your hair is dry.

If your ponytail, encircled by your thumb and forefinger, has a diameter larger than a quarter, your hair is considered thick. If the diameter of your ponytail is smaller than a quarter but larger than a nickel, your hair is considered normal. If the diameter of your ponytail is smaller than a nickel, your hair is considered fine.

Special Implications for Various Hair Types and Textures

Hair Types

L -type hair is perhaps the most fragile. The sharp, angular bending of this hair type means that a distinct potential breakage point lurks at each bend. The bends may be spaced irregularly, making the hair appear to have very little curl definition. The closer the bends, the more textured the hair will feel and the tighter this hair will draw up as it dries. L-types require lots of moisturizing attention, especially when the L-pattern is tightly arranged.

For I-types, the traditional kinks and curves associated with other LOIS curl patterns are not a concern. I-types tend to lie flatly against the scalp and are usually more breakage-resistant fibers overall. I-types often shine and reflect considerably more light than either L, O, or S hair types.

If L-type combines with I-type hair on the same head, great care should be taken to avoid damage from heavy manipulation or extended periods of moisture deficiency. We often see LI combinations at the relaxer/new growth hair boundary.

Types O and S are very similar types but differ in the way their curves are arranged. In O-types, the curls loop back onto themselves. In S-types, the loops are naturally stretched out. An O-type can see what an S-type would look like by simply pulling an O-type curl out a little. The tighter the curves, the more O and S hair types will draw up as they dry. These two hair types are easier to moisturize than L-types, but as with all textured hair, moisture retention is hard to come by.

Hair Texture Types

Our textured hair is moisture deficient by its very nature, regardless of the hair type. Intensive conditioning efforts are needed to keep our hair soft, pliable and supple—especially if the hair is a type L or LI combination, or some other hair type that has been chemically relaxed or colored. For those who are relaxed, remember that although your hair has been chemically straightened and the natural texture permanently

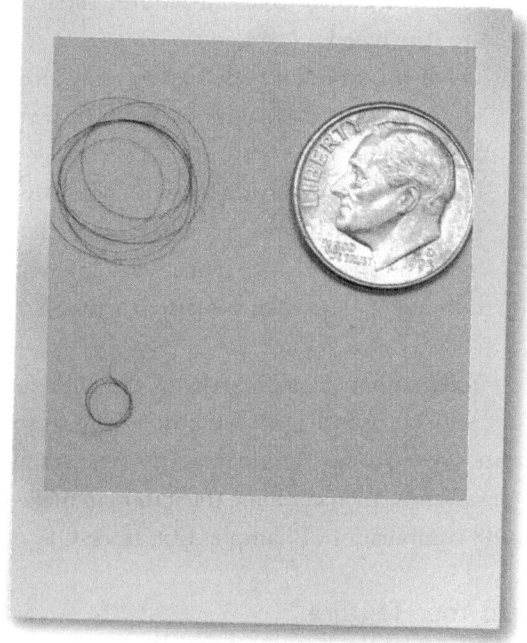

Figure 18: LOIS "O" curls can vary in size from tight coffee stirrer Os to large, loopy curls. The LOIS system focuses on total strand shape, and does not differentiate between curl/coil size.

altered, our hair still tends to exhibit many of the qualities it naturally exhibited before processing. Wiry natural hair tends to translate into straight, yet somewhat wiry relaxed hair, etc. Hair evidently does not forget itself, despite chemical treatment.

Thready

Thready hair can be considered porous because of its willingness to accept moisture and its tendency to lose it just as easily. Thready hair benefits from low-pH moisturizing deep conditioners. The benefits of moisturizing and sealing needed for just about all types of textured

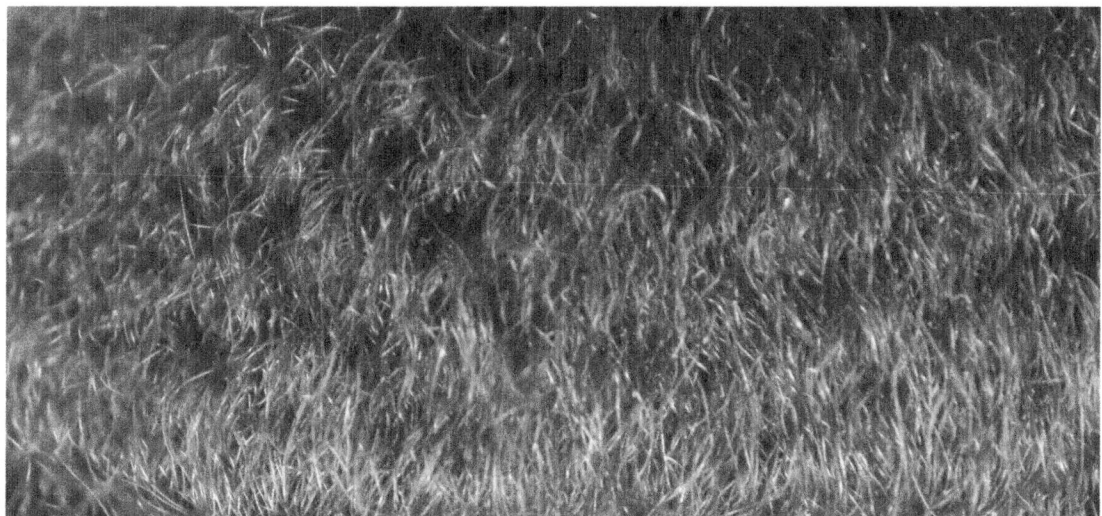

Figure 19: This wiry/coarse hair is an example of a tightly curled Daughter S with perhaps some Daughter L.

Wiry/Coarse

Wiry hair typically has an external structure in which the cuticle layers naturally lie flat and are oriented tightly against one another. These hairs are usually thicker and coarser individually, because they tend to have more cuticle layers. Occasionally, when the other texture types—thready, cottony, silky and other finer-stranded types of natural or relaxed hair—encounter dryness, they are mistakenly called coarse or wiry. Hair coarseness is a measure of the hair

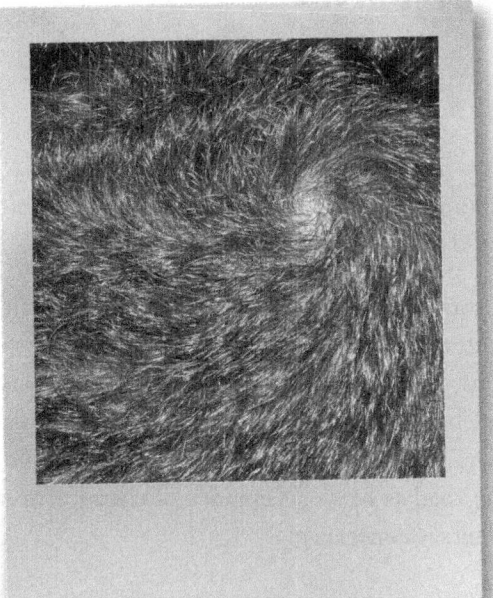

Figure 20: OS coarse hair type cut short.

hair make perhaps the most dramatic difference to this hair type. If proper measures are taken to keep the cuticle flat and smooth, thready hair will retain moisture more readily and sheen/shine can be enhanced naturally. Because of its high porosity, thready hair readily accepts chemical treatments.

Figure 21: Very tightly coiled, thready hair with irregular S and L combined (zigzag) pattern.

fiber's cuticle thickness and overall diameter, not its texture or moisture content. Hair can be coarse whether it is straight (Asian/Caucasian), curly or kinky.

In wiry hair, the cuticle layers work extra hard to keep materials from passing in and out of the hair shaft. Because of the strong quality of wiry hair's cuticle layers, this hair type is generally resistant to chemical processes and breakage. Wiry hair does not absorb water or hair products very well. Humidity does not quickly revert or frizz this type of hair in its natural or straightened state. Wiry and coarse hair types are some of the easiest hair types to grow long—relaxed or natural—because they are so resistant to daily breakage.

Cottony/Spongy

The qualities of cottony and spongy hair types are similar and fall somewhere between those of wiry and thready hair types. They dif-

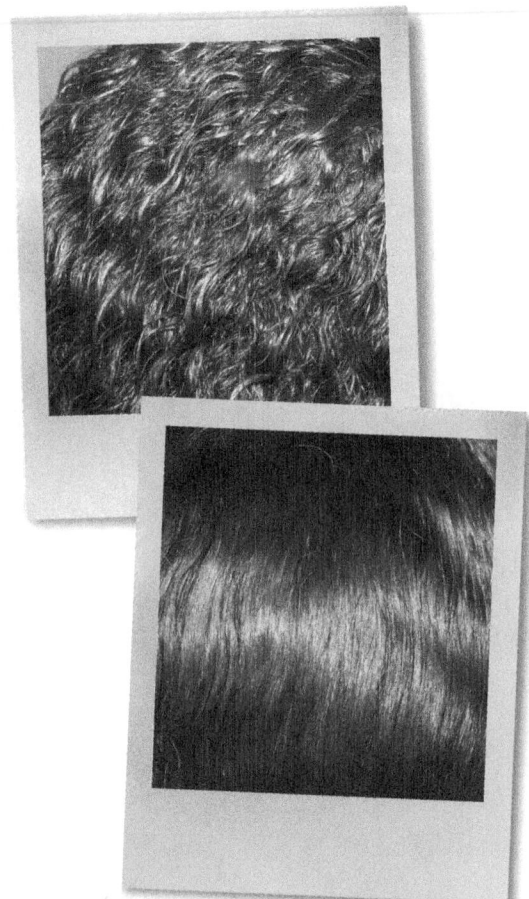

Figure 23: Silky hair types demonstrating both I and S curl patterns.

absorb moisture better than wiry hair, healthy cottony and spongy hair types are not very porous. Accepting the moisture they are given takes much longer for these hair types than for thready hair. These hair types also fall in the middle of the road as far as acceptance of chemical treatments is concerned.

Silky

Silky hair is perhaps the easiest to moisturize and keep moisturized. When healthy, it displays a flattened, highly reflective cuticle surface, which accounts for its high-octane shine. Silky hair usually is finer than wiry or cottony types as it typically has fewer cuticle layers. Humidity in the air can result in great frizz for some individuals with this hair type.

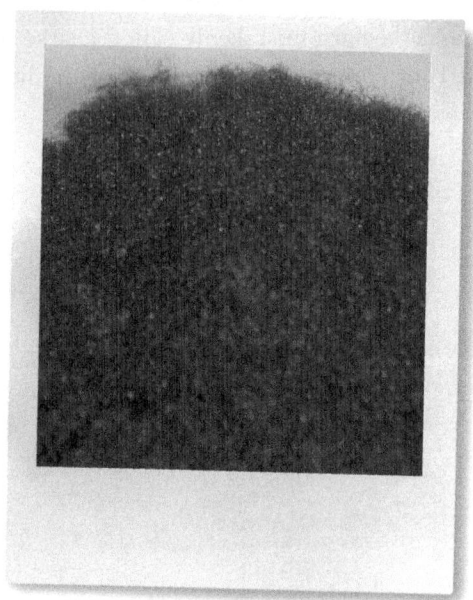

Figure 22: Tightly coiled, cottony hair.

fer in that cottony hair often appears drier than spongy hair when dried because it has low natural sheen. Although cottony and spongy hair types

unit 2

Healthy Hair Management

Chapter 3: Understanding Hair Growth and Damage for Healthier Hair Care

Effective hair care regimen building is an important, necessary step in the healthy hair care process. Because most of your hair care regimen will be carried out at home, it is imperative that you understand the basic hair care products, practices and methods that drive successful hair care regimens and encourage healthier hair growth.

When you ask most people about how our hair grows, they'll tell you correctly that our hair grows from our hair follicles which are situated within the scalp. Indeed, the first and most commonly understood step in the hair growth process is simply the emergence of new hair from the scalp. However, a secondary requirement for hair growth is often absent from these types of discussions: retention. Without retention, no visible length progress can be seen, although the scalp is continuing to push out new hair every day.

Black hair growth occurs via this two-step process: hair emergence at the roots and hair retention along the length and ends of the hair. Hair emergence is an unconscious, biological response to living. In healthy individuals, the hair emergence process occurs naturally—day after day, month after month, year after year—independent of external hair care practices. Length retention, however, is strongly dependent on personal hair care methods and requires concentrated efforts to sustain. When hair emerges from the scalp but is not preserved at the ends of the hair fiber, then no hair growth will be visible, no matter how fast or how much the hair grows out from the scalp. Hair growth will simply appear to be stagnant, although new hair is always emerging from the scalp.

Hair emergence can be seen as a constant, while length retention is the variable that we can manipulate. When emergence and retention are out of sync—that is, if retention is poor—hair length and thickness may remain unchanged over time or incur net losses. We see retention problems occur all the time when we perform touch-up chemical relaxer services and fail to see any growth from one relaxer to the next. New-growth hair emerges without incident every month, but because the length added through this new growth is not preserved at the ends, the newly emerged hair does not translate as growth. From one relaxer touch-up to the next, the hair appears not to have grown at all.

The Shoulder-Length Plateau

The fragility of textured hair has resulted in a widespread length plateau in black hair care. The default length for a vast majority of our population is several inches above or just below shoulder length. This shoulder-length phenomenon is most prevalent among those who wear their textured hair relaxed.

It is as if we have a black hair care neglect threshold. Approximately 18 to 24 months' growth, or shoulder length, marks the point where an individual who has no particular regimen for her hair, can expect her tresses to remain almost indefinitely. Twelve inches (and generally much shorter in the nape) is our average length—our hair growth plateau, if you will. If the average

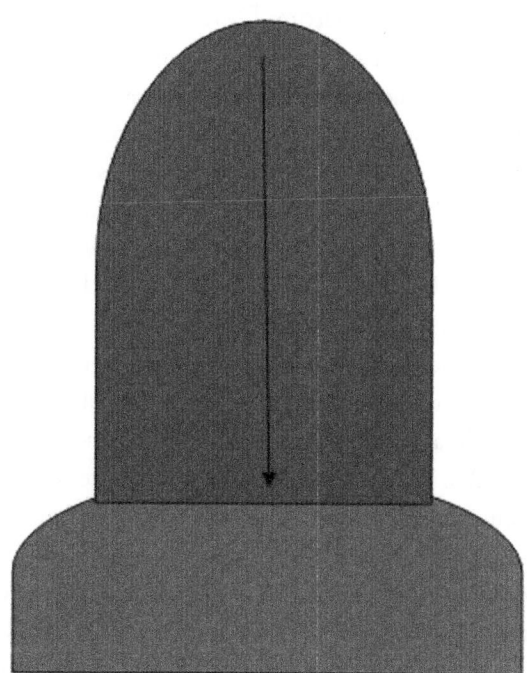

Figure 24: The Shoulder-Length Plateau, give or take a few inches above or below, is where most textured hair length falls.

person simply shampoos and conditions when she feels like it, plays around with color and heat, and stays away from other obviously destructive styling methods, this is the length she can expect to achieve. Of course, a few of us routinely defy the norm, practically ignore our hair and can virtually sit on it—but for a large subset of us, the two-year rule is quite valid. Achieving lengths longer than those 12 inches, for most of us, takes a change in attitude and perception about our hair. Making this change requires an exploration of new techniques for care and an abandonment of old ways of thinking about black hair. Poor hair retention along the length of the fiber is often due to several key categories of hair damage.

Understanding Common Causes of Hair Damage

No matter how well we take care of our textured hair, we are certain to come face to face with one type of damage or another. The con-

dition of your hair can be affected by chemical processes, the physical stress of daily styling and maintenance, environmental factors and nutritional deficiencies. Relaxers, permanent colors, aggressive combing and wet brushing all can land you in hair trouble. Your health also plays a great role in the condition of your hair as it grows from your scalp. An in-depth understanding of the major sources of hair damage is the first step toward achieving healthier hair.

Chemical Damage

Much of the damage textured hair experiences is a result of chemical processing. All permanent chemical alterations, no matter how well executed, render some degree of internal degradation to the hair fiber. Once chemicals are applied, the internal structure of the hair is changed forever and cannot be returned to its original state. Relaxers, texturizers, curly perms and permanent hair colors are all chemical-damage culprits. The amount of damage done to the hair fiber depends greatly on the knowledge and experience of the individual performing the process, and the frequency with which the process takes place. A working knowledge of the chemical structure of hair, and how topical chemical applications affect it, is extremely important for minimizing damage potential. These chemical alterations are discussed in detail in Units 3.

Physical Damage

The second major cause of hair damage to textured tresses is physical manipulation of the hair fiber. Physical damage comes from excessive manipulation, tension and handling of the hair. The use of heat-producing appliances aggravates this damage. Frequently brushing and wrapping the hair around the head to set a straight style, wearing braids that are too tight, or simply sliding a rough hair pin through the hair can all contribute to physical hair damage. Blow dryers, flat irons, rubber bands and poorly made hair ornaments are additional physical hair damage culprits. Even shampooing and conditioning in a manner that encourages the hair to tangle can lead to physical damage.

Environmental Damage

Environmental factors can also stress the hair. Ultraviolet sun rays and temperature extremes are the more obvious environmental obstacles to conquer for those seeking healthier black hair. Pollutants present in the atmosphere and water can fade hair colors and disturb the internal moisture balance of the strands. Heavily chlorinated swimming pool water, ocean water and hard water (with high concentrations of dissolved minerals) are common environmental inhibitors of ultimate hair health.

Nutritional/Dietary Deficiencies

Dietary or nutritional deficiencies can have a negative effect on the hair before it ever emerges from the scalp. The proper balance of vitamins and minerals is crucial to a healthy scalp and head of hair. Thyroid disorders, anemia, smoking, crash or restrictive-food-group dieting and a myriad of other factors contribute to the overall quality of textured hair.

When hair emergence and retention finally complement one another over a period of weeks, months and years, however, hair will demonstrate a visible increase in length. So how do we reduce hair damage and preserve the ends of the hair so that our tresses have the opportunity to increase in length over time? We build a solid hair care regimen that protects against damage and breakage through strategic product selection and other maintenance techniques.

Chapter 4: What's Your Hair Care Regimen?

Breakage reductions sustained over the course of several months or years make it possible to achieve noticeable increases in length as well as health results with black hair. To achieve maximum hair health and growth, the top goal of any healthy hair-care intervention should be achieving reduced hair fiber breakage and damage in nearly every aspect of your hair's daily care. Unfortunately, many of us subscribe to hair care regimens that are not designed to deliver health or even good looks beyond the moment. We care for our hair the best we know how and just hope that we'll stumble upon a magical idea, product or stylist who can fix all of our hair problems. Because we understand very little about what separates good hair care from bad hair care, we'll try just about everything. Most of us don't have a foundation. We don't have information, and we don't have a plan.

As we begin to explore the idea of actively managing our hair for the optimal appearance of health and vitality, it is important to consider how our current hair practices are either supporting or hurting our hair goals. Consider the cases of Myra and Pam:

Myra held clumps of hair in her hands. Her hair was shedding and falling everywhere, filling her combs and brushes with auburn-colored strands. Her products were simple. She'd been using the same shampoo and conditioner for black hair since she was a teenager, and it had always seemed to work okay. But Myra's hair was broken off badly on the left side from years of braids, and her temples were beginning to show stress as well from the wigs she was wearing to change up her style. She had always done her own relaxers to what she thought had been perfection every four to six weeks. Her hair was always extra smooth and straight. She was also a big fan of hair weaves and had wigs to suit every style. But more than anything, Myra's primary vice was hair coloring. She'd been everything from Fire Engine Red to Platinum Blonde to a strange Hunting Dog Brown color. Several weeks before her latest relaxer, she had her hair professionally colored—but apparently, her hair could not handle this degree of stress. She slicked her hair down and threw on her Tina wig. Her hair was no longer the mid-back length hair of her twenties. She was now thirty-eight, with thinning, damaged hair barely brushing her shoulders.

Pam, on the other hand, figured her hair was normal. She did not chemically relax her hair, and it was very thick. Her hair was just below shoulder length when pressed, and she'd worn her hair in the same puff style and picked-out Afro since she had graduated from high school five years ago. The clincher was that Pam was not cutting her hair to this length. In fact, she had rarely cut her hair at all in those post-school years! She washed it when she felt it was dirty, usually every two to three weeks with whatever shampoo her roommate had on hand. She used heat only occasionally, usually following her washes and perhaps a few sessions in between. Still, Pam's hair, like Myra's, never grew to any length past her shoulders. What was happening here?

Neither Myra nor Pam had a plan or strategy for their hair care. Neither gave attention to hydrating or deep conditioning their hair, despite their chemical use and stressful styling routines. Where one over-manipulated her hair, the other matched her in sheer neglect! Certainly, neither regimen was successful. On first meeting them, Myra and Pam may seem extreme, but the truth is, they are everywhere. You may recognize Myra and Pam in the people you know, or perhaps you see a little bit of yourself in each of them! The lesson to be learned here is that everyone follows a hair care regimen whether they have decided consciously to do so or not. Even the lack of an organized regimen constitutes a regimen. Whether product selection occurs randomly or in an organized, deliberate manner, these regimens affect your hair.

On the opposite end of the hair care spectrum is Kayla.

Kayla's hair was amazing. Several months ago, she had her hair cut into a chin-length bob to get rid of some of the damage she had sustained earlier from a permanent color. At this time, Kayla decided to begin a new hair care regimen. She began washing and conditioning her hair once a week and moisturizing and sealing her hair daily with oil. She put away her heat appliances and saved them for special occasions. She was transitioning her hair out of a relaxer and wore her hair in cute, curly rod sets and braid-out styles to get her through the difficult months. Her hard work paid off. Here it was, nearly four months later, and her hair had already improved greatly in thickness and new length.

Kayla's case demonstrates the power of re-evaluating a hair care regimen to correct for damaging hair practices. Kayla consciously chose a very different regimen from either Pam or Myra. When Kayla damaged her hair with color, she took action. She removed the damage quickly, increased her moisture conditioning and revamped her styling routine. Such effective regimen building is the heart of healthy hair care for all textured tresses.

Healthy Hair Care Regimen Building

In general, black hair care regimens can be classified in three broad categories:

- recessive-maintenance regimens
- basic-maintenance regimens
- healthy hair care regimens

Throughout our lives, and as our hair goals change, we may move in and out of one regimen type or another—sometimes purposefully, and at other times, without realizing it. The type of regimen you need to follow depends entirely upon your goals—and your success with any regimen is determined by your ability to make the required adjustments needed to satisfy the regimen. In the

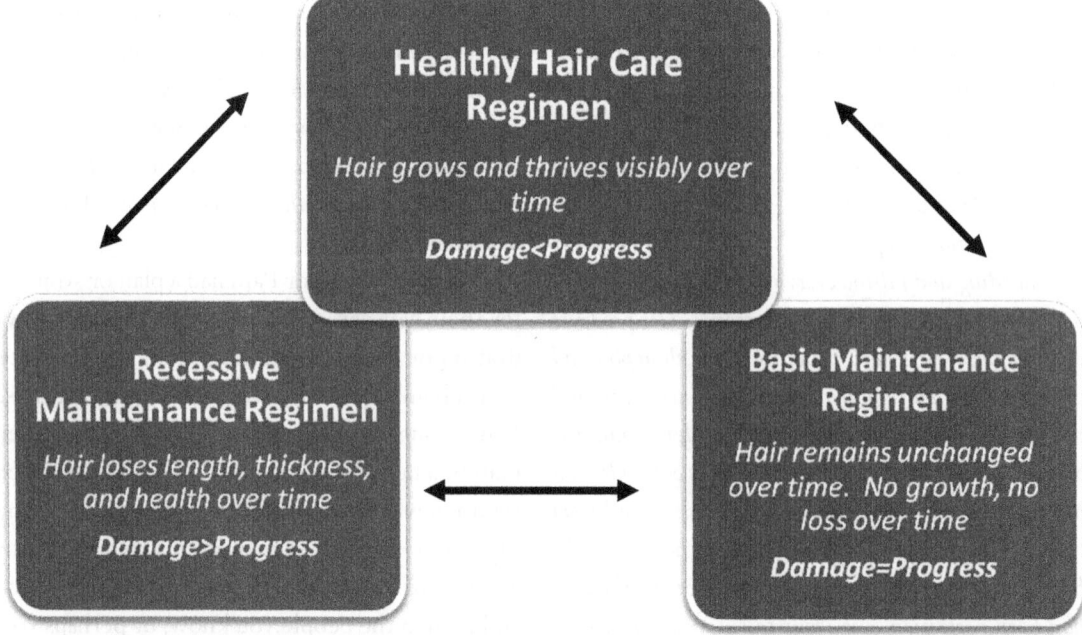

Figure 25: The three basic types of Hair Care Regimens

following pages, you will learn the principles and techniques needed to successfully build your own healthy hair care regimen.

Recessive-Maintenance Regimens

Myra's regimen, for example, is the type of regimen that is desired by no one but is subconsciously adopted by many: the recessive-maintenance hair care regimen.

In recessive-maintenance regimens, the rate of hair damage surpasses the rate of hair progress. Recessive-maintenance regimens typically involve:

- Poor product selection and incorrect product use.
- Extended periods of time between hair cleansings.
- No moisture sources/excessive use of protein products.
- Daily heat use.
- Rough handling of the hair.
- Color abuse: bleaching, multiple spins around the color wheel from one color to the next, too frequent coloring and/ or coloring hair already in poor condition.
- Excessive relaxing (less than six to eight weeks between applications).
- Improper neutralizing of relaxer chemicals.
- Weave and extension abuse.
- Excessive trimming due to damage.

Myra's routine is a classic example of a recessive-maintenance regimen in which a series of bad hair-care experiences begins to take a toll on the hair over a period of time. People who adopt recessive-maintenance regimens know that heat isn't great for their hair, but they use it weekly. They know that relaxing and coloring can cause damage, but they double-process their hair anyway. They know that their hair must be handled gently, but they snatch combs through it. They know many things, but their execution is poor and far from systematic, perhaps due to lack of time, money or interest. Hair, however, can only take so much!

Thinning, balding or losing length over time are central features of this type of regimen. Regular hair-unfriendly practices such as relaxing, coloring, heat abuse and inordinate styling manipulation contribute significantly to the fall of the hair and leave less and less hair to work with as the years progress. Hair health and growth soon become recessive. Enter the frustrated black woman with thinned, damaged hair wondering where the thick head of hair she had just a few years prior has gone!

Recessive-maintenance regimens never seem to yield the growth results we are looking to achieve, simply because these regimens tend to stress hair care techniques that provide temporary beauty without regard for the damage inflicted by the processes often needed to achieve these fashionable looks.

Basic-Maintenance Regimens

Similarly, Pam's regimen, a basic-maintenance regimen, is the type that frequently "just happens" in the course of a busy life. Lacking knowledge and perhaps great interest, hair choices are often made by default in this type of hair-care regimen.

Basic-maintenance regimens are similar to recessive-maintenance regimens in both practice and philosophy. Many regimens begin as basic-maintenance routines and later become recessive due to a lack of hair care knowledge and intervention. The single difference between basic and recessive maintenance is that in a basic maintenance regimen, the hair is being maintained just above the point of faltering. Basic-maintenance routines are regimens in which the rate of hair damage equals the rate of hair progress.

Hallmarks of a basic-maintenance regimen include:

- Hit-or-miss product selection and often incorrect product use.
- Very few moisture sources and/or greases and oils substituting for moisturizers.
- Infrequent hair cleansing and conditioning.
- Protein sources used in excess.
- Direct heat used for daily styling (or more than once per week).
- High-manipulation styling with no protection of the hair shaft or ends.
- Moderate relaxer use, every eight to ten weeks.
- Hair-coloring abuse.
- Infrequent hair trimming or abundant hair trimming that is not in sync with the hair's growth rate.

Basic-maintenance regimens are the average hair-care regimen. These are the very regimens that keep many women stuck at the shoulder-length growth plateau for years and years. Basic-maintenance regimens are often the result of no defined regimen at all—or of a poorly constructed one. Fortunately, hair is quite resilient and can be maintained with this level of disinterest at a decent length for a good period of time. Followers of basic-maintenance regimens depend on the natural strength of their hair fibers to forgive a multitude of hair faults and make up for their poor hair care. In both basic and recessive-maintenance regimens, movement and shine are often mistaken for health.

Healthy Hair Care Regimens

The recessive- and basic-maintenance regimens that Myra and Pam followed contrast starkly with healthy hair care regimens like the one that Kayla eventually adopted.

In a healthy hair care regimen, hair progress surpasses the rate of hair damage such that *hair grown in becomes hair retained at the ends*. In

this type of regimen, improvements in health and length can be seen and documented from month to month and year to year. This type of hair care regimen is the gold standard in which hair simply thrives.

Healthy hair care regimens promote one or more of these basic principles:

- Carefully planned and strategic product selection.
- Optimal moisture levels maintained within the strands.
- Moisture sources balanced with adequate protein sources.
- Protection of hair shaft and ends from heat and physical damage.
- Low-manipulation hair styling.
- Natural hair— with no chemical processes. Or, chemicals administered no more than every ten to twelve weeks.
- Diet and body maintained at peak levels.

Healthy hair care regimens ensure that hair emergence and retention complement one another over an extended period of time by reducing the hair's exposure to outside damage. Keep in mind that long hair is always old hair. As black hair ages and gains length, extra care must be taken to keep the ends from breaking. In fact, hair strands naturally have fewer protective cuticle layers at the ends because natural weathering of the hair fiber has stripped many of those layers away. As new growth pushes out, creating new length, the oldest parts of the hair need additional support to withstand day-to-day stressors.

In the approximately eighteen to twenty-four months of a shoulder-length strand's life, for example, the bottommost ends of the hair have been subjected to repeated combing, brushing, twisting, shampooing, conditioning, heat styling and other hair traumas. The condition of the cuticle at shoulder length is simply not as robust as during the time when the same cuticle was protecting our hair in its first few inches as new growth. This older hair must receive adequate moisture and protein supplementation because it has lost most of its natural protein and moisture to normal wear and tear over the years. Without strategic care, the hair will begin to dry out and eventually break.

Hair must also be detangled and combed differently as it grows out and the ends age. The same combing techniques used with success at shoulder-length cannot be easily translated at midback or waist lengths. For natural hair, lengthier tresses mean greater opportunities for single-strand knotting and greater coil entanglement in general. A considerable time investment is required to maintain textured hair, relaxed or natural, at greater lengths. Healthy hair care regimens must easily evolve to account for changes in the length and strength of the hair fiber.

Making the Healthy Hair Investment

Regimen building takes considerable time and effort. Some individuals believe that a single product (or combination of products) is all that is required to get their hair healthy and growing strong. Not surprisingly, these people often do not find or maintain the level of progress they are seeking for the long term. People who are on the lookout for quick fixes will find themselves sorely disappointed in the hair care game, where time is everything. The one commodity, the common factor, that all people with healthy, long hair share—whether black, white, relaxed, natural, young or old—is the time investment they have made in their hair.

Keys to Responsible Regimen Building

What Is Protective Styling?

When most people think of protective styling, they think of hairstyles. Although the way we choose to present our hair is a major component of the method, protective styling involves much more than simply styling the hair. Protective styling is a comprehensive strategy for hair protection. It is a series of deliberate actions that, committed to habit and taken all together, reduce breakage and stress upon textured hair fibers. Protective styling is a way of understanding our hair that translates into a certain way of selecting and using products, a certain way of shampooing, conditioning, styling and handling the hair, and finally, a certain attitude toward and approach to chemical treatments.

Healthy hair care regimens are successful because they take on this holistic view of protective styling. In this multifaceted approach to black hair care, ends preservation occurs through a systematic protective approach that emphasizes proper product selection, an overall reduction in hairstyling manipulation, and effective protein and moisture balancing to keep breakage at bay.

Remember, in hair care, there is often more than one way to get from Point A to Point B successfully. The same applies to regimen building. While no two healthy hair care regimens are the same, most tend to have several basic things in common. Most include good strategies for product selection and for balancing protein and moisture sources in the regimen. Many also tend to be very simple, low-manipulation regimens. You must always use your own discretion when putting together a hair care regimen. What is tolerable for your hair may not work well for another person's hair. Experimentation is key!

Having Your Cake, and Eating It Too?

Of course, you can still enjoy your hair while growing it and improving its health. With the proper knowledge and precautions, healthy hair can be achieved while adopting practices (even the not-so-healthy practices) from all three types of hair care regimens discussed. Keep in mind, however, that the more practices you draw from a particular regimen type, the more your hair will display the characteristics associated with that regimen. The degree to which you allow yourself to borrow from or delve into any regimen type will influence your overall hair success. For example, you may follow a healthy hair care regimen but choose to color-treat your hair with a permanent dye (a characteristic typical of both basic- and recessive-maintenance regimens). You can still achieve a healthy, growing head of hair if you diligently practice the other supporting tenets of a healthy hair care regimen.

Trade-offs are common in successful regimen building. For example, infrequent conditioning and a lack of effective protein/moisture balancing tends to lead to poor hair outcomes. If, however, this infrequent conditioning is traded off with a low-heat or very-low-maintenance styling regimen in which hair is simply left alone (braided, for example), hair still may thrive quite well.

Simply stated, the common growth denominator for every single person with long, healthy hair is time. The waiting element of growing and improving hair health cannot be avoided. Time cannot be bottled or purchased on the shelf.

Black women, in particular, must be sensitive to the fact that, on average, our hair grows slightly slower than that of other races. It also grows in a manner that requires unique care. This means that our time investment for achieving longer lengths must be greater, and our hair care must be more concentrated, dedicated and diligent. Finally, we must also understand that some types of healthy hair progress will become apparent before others. For example, improvements in thickness and pliability can be observed weeks, even months before noticeable improvements in length. Progress takes time. Your hair is a worthwhile investment and a journey. If you are diligent, the reward is sweet.

Let's explore healthy hair care regimen building in greater detail, beginning with proper product selection. Next, we will round out the discussion with protein and moisture balancing techniques for breakage correction. Finally, we will discuss low-manipulation hair handling and styling techniques and total body wellness for healthy hair care.

Chapter 5: Hair Product Selection Basics

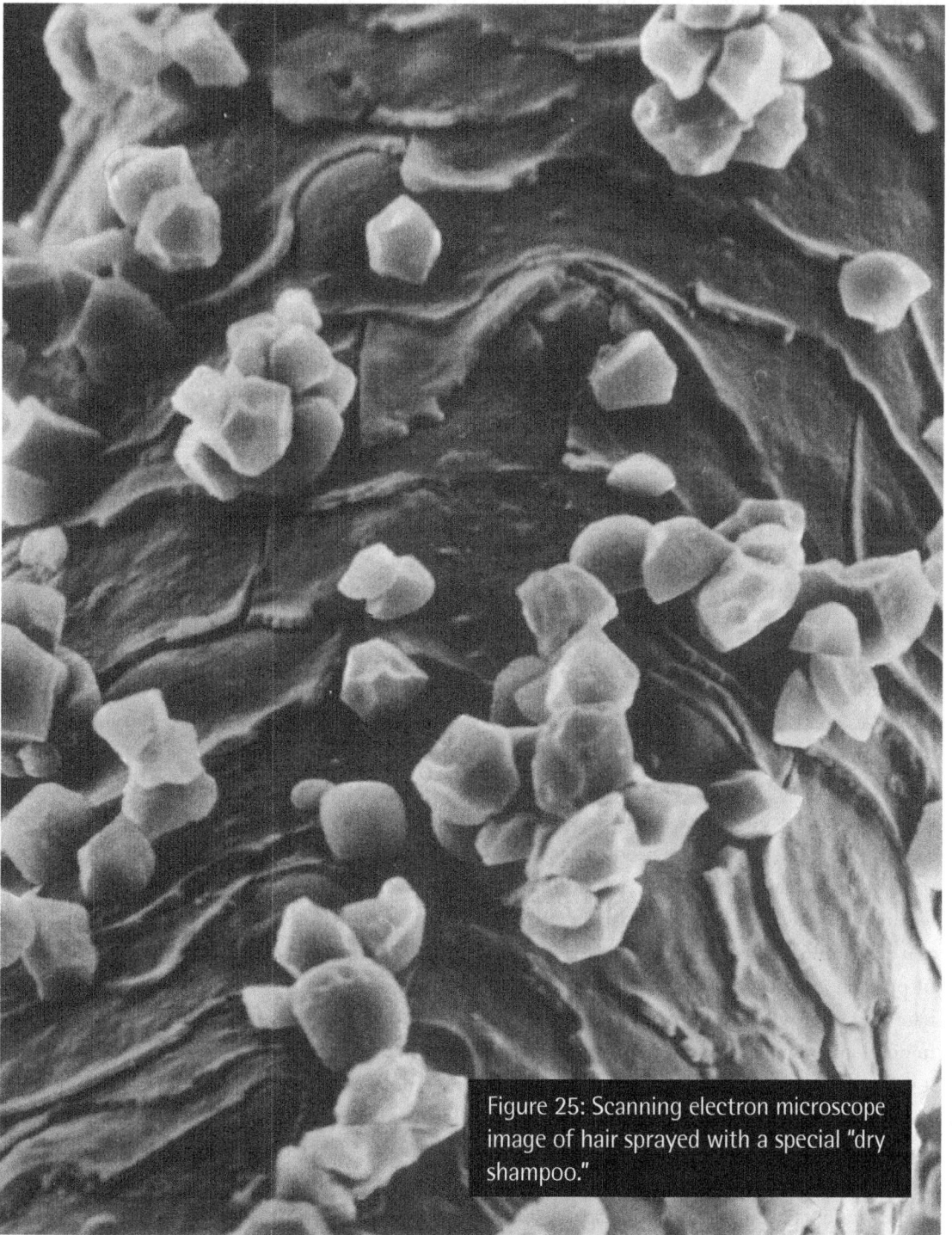

Figure 25: Scanning electron microscope image of hair sprayed with a special "dry shampoo."

I always think back to an encounter I had in elementary school with my best friend, Jennifer. I remember asking her why her hair grew while mine did not. Nine-year old Jenny didn't have the answer to that question, but that did not stop her from trying to help out a dear friend. The next day, she arrived at school with a backpack full of her hair products and wanted to give them all to me! You cannot imagine the joy I felt! I thought, *Wow! Now my hair is going to grow and be just like hers!* I now had my hands on her Holy Grail! Her products! I eagerly washed and washed and conditioned my hair every day with those precious products. But much to my disappointment (and I am sure Jenny shared the frustration), our little product swap had no effect on my hair. It was not that the products did not work; it was simply our lack of understanding about black hair needs that caused our experiment to fail. We did not understand how products must complement each other and work together to benefit the hair.

Let's take a closer look at the various types of products used in a healthy hair care regimen. Ingredients-label reading will take on a central role in this chapter as we develop our product understanding. Most shampoos, conditioners and moisturizers are not simply natural concoctions of berries and flowers. Many hair products contain complex chemicals to make the formulas less runny, more fragrant, and more pearlescent or foamy. As you become more label savvy, you will be better able to evaluate hair products and compare product claims against reality. Additionally, learning how to dissect product labels will help you determine the protein and moisture strength of products before you ever use them on your hair. Not only will this improve your efficiency in developing an appropriate hair care regimen, it will save you lots of money.

Quality hair care products combined with the proper hair care techniques can make a difference in the overall quality of our hair. When these products are used in a hair care regimen

as part of a basic protein and moisture balancing strategy, hair will always reach its greatest potential. But because today's hair care market is so saturated with products to meet consumers' needs, separating the good products from the bad ones can be difficult.

Your Hair Product Arsenal

Shampooing and conditioning are processes often taken for granted in most healthy hair care regimens. In addition to the healthy hair foundation that quality shampoos and conditioners provide, ancillary hair products such as leave-in conditioners, water-based moisturizers, oils and serums also help round out healthy hair regimens. These products help support our styles and keep our hair looking polished and well put together.

Even if no other hair products are used, shampoos and conditioners are almost always a part of an individual's hair product arsenal. Shampoos and conditioners are the foundations of your healthy hair care regimen. Selecting the right shampoo and conditioning formulas for your textured hair type is imperative if growth results are to be realized. Shampoos and conditioners not only cleanse the hair, they support the overall cosmetic integrity of our hair fibers. The moisturizer you select also makes a large contribution to your hair's cosmetic appearance. Without a doubt, oils reign supreme in black hair care and are supported by generations of strong tradition. By contrast, the importance of water and hydration in black hair care has only recently garnered much-deserved attention.

You will find a detailed list of product recommendations toward the end of this unit. Do keep in mind that new products enter and older products exit the market on a continuous basis, so the products listed in the Regimen Builder should not be considered the entire range of your product options.

Textured Hair Cleansing Basics
The Power of Frequent Hydration

Textured hair thrives in high-moisture environments. Regular shampooing and conditioning sessions allow us to fully supply this need for moisture. Frequent cleansing greatly improves the hair's moisture content because water is encouraged to bind within the hair shaft each time. Ideally, textured hair should be hydrated (by shampooing/rinsing) and conditioned once per week. Extra hydrating and conditioning may be necessary in the early stages of starting a healthy hair care regimen. In the first few critical months of regimen building, engaging the hair by hydrating and conditioning every three to four days can help to restore the hair's moisture balance quickly.

Does Water Dry Out the Hair?

Black hair desperately needs moisture and hydration more than any other hair type. Unfortunately, generations of old wives' tales have told us, "Water is bad" and "Water dries out our hair"—neither of which happens to be true. This unfortunate line of thinking places water and moisture in an antagonistic relationship with our hair and scalp. As a testament to the strength of misinformation given a platform, many of us still do not take advantage of weekly cleansing and conditioning as a critical step in healthy hair maintenance. How can water, nature's primary moisturizer, dry the hair out?

The question we should probably ask is: How is it that some people *do seem to experience dryness* when they shampoo and condition their hair weekly? The answer is: Dry scalp and hair come from using products that are not suited for frequent use or are improperly designed for textured hair. The products that are typically expected to suit the unique moisture needs of the black community are 1) oily, silicone-heavy coating conditioners, moisturizers and greases and 2) harsh stripping shampoos that are intended to remove those oily conditioners, moisturizers and greases. Unfortunately, none of these types of products works to support proper moisturization of our scalps and hair fibers. Using them frequently will certainly dry out our hair.

Squeaky-clean hair is not a goal in black hair care. Proper cleansing can be achieved with gentle shampoo formulas or even with shampoo-less hair care regimens. Stripping shampoo products produce bare, unprotected hair fibers that become prone to dryness, cracking, splitting and breakage over time. The moisture stakes are high for black hair. We need properly lubricated fibers to help us retain internal moisture and reduce frictional forces between our hair fibers. Unfortunately, many commercial black shampoo formulas strip the hair of its natural oils and leave the hair feeling squeaky clean. If this stripped-clean state is not addressed with application of a proper conditioner with humectants and light emollients, the hair will begin to feel dry.

Just as squeaky-clean hair is not a goal in black hair care, oily, weighed-down hair is not a goal either. Inadequate moisturizers, pomades and conditioners that load the cuticles down with silicones and oils rather than infuse true moisture into the fiber—also leave the hair feeling dry. These formulas make the hair look nice immediately after use, but never actually support the true, longer term needs of the fiber.

Under these conditions, frequent shampooing and conditioning become a battle. Without adequate sources of true moisture and products to support effective hair hydration, we end up with dry, parched hair. The market offers an abundance of sealants and moisture-barrier products, as well as shampoo products to remove the barriers, but very few black hair-care products work to infuse water into the fiber. This is why we perceive "dryness" when we attempt to regularly hydrate our hair.

Hair Proteins Love Water

Our hair loves water. Black hair thrives when it is maintained in a high-moisture, hydration-focused environment. The proteins that make up our hair are attracted to water, and water is incorporated extensively into our hair's natural bonding structure. Hair proteins even seek out water in the air around us! But daily wear and tear causes us to lose much of our hair's natural moisture to the air and to treatments like blow drying and flat ironing that work by quickly evaporating the hair's moisture in order to flatten and straighten the hair fiber. Sometimes water never makes it into our hair fibers because it is blocked by layers of oils and silicone coatings. Regular misting, wetting, and conditioning keep the hair's elasticity within normal ranges and reduce breakage when the hair is manipulated.

Daily Cleansing

While regular cleansing benefits black hair, daily cleansing, particularly for lengthier black hair, may not be optimal. A great deal of manipulation is required to detangle and handle longer hair. Daily misting and sealing is a great, healthy hair alternative.

Shampoo Basics

Shampoos are the single most purchased hair product, accounting for roughly 50 percent of market sales. A shampoo's cleansing ability is perhaps the factor by which it is most closely scrutinized. Various degrees of cleansing ability, or product lift, are available in today's shampoos. Take a stroll down the shampoo aisle in your local store, and you will find shampoo options in every color imaginable and for every hair ailment known to man. There are shampoos for preserving color-treated hair, for

thickening the hair, fighting head lice and treating dandruff. Some are formulated to strip the hair of oils, and others are designed to put oils back in. There are clarifying shampoos, chelating shampoos—you name it, and most likely, you will find it!

Deconstructing Shampoo: What's In There?

Shampoos are composed of 40 to 70 percent water. They also contain surfactants (cleansing agents), thickeners, proteins, foam boosters and other ingredients. Shampoo formulas, like hair, are somewhat acidic but are formulated at a slightly higher pH than conditioners to lift the cuticles and help remove product buildup from the hair. Here's a rundown of common shampoo ingredients and how they work on the hair:

Cleansing Ingredients

The most distinguishing feature of a shampoo is its cleansing ability, which is primarily determined by its surfactant content. Surfactants—or *surface acting ingredients*—are cleansing agents designed to remove impurities such as dust, dirt, oil and other debris from the hair. Detergents are a special group of surfactants with superior cleansing abilities. Other surfactants aren't strong enough to cleanse the hair well but serve best as foam boosters or thickeners in the shampoo formula. Typical shampoo formulas contain 15 to 40 percent detergent surfactants by weight or volume, and many formulas feature multiple surfactants. Surfactants are attracted to both oil and water, and are divided into categories based on their particular ionic charge.

Surfactants can be anionic (negatively charged), cationic (positively charged), nonionic (no charge) or amphoteric (charge changes according to the pH level of the product (see Figure 26). Hair carries a net negative charge, so most surfactants also are designed to be negatively charged. Because "like repels like" in the chemical world, these negatively charged anionic surfactants are the best cleansers since they are not attracted to hair and cannot bind to it. Instead, they attract the positively charged oils along the surface of the cuticle, which then rinse cleanly from the hair—perhaps a bit too cleanly. Because black hair tends to lack full coverage of natural oils (sebum) along much of the fiber due to its regular bends and kinks, these shampoo surfactants tend to have an overall drying and stripping effect on the fiber.

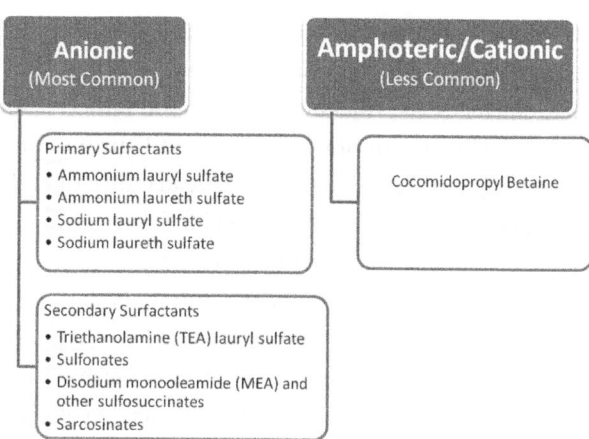

Figure 26: Common Shampoo Surfactants

Sulfates and Other Cleansers

Sulfates are surfactants commonly used in today's shampoo formulas to lift product residues from the hair and scalp. Sulfate-based ingredients are easy to spot in the ingredients list since they always contain some version of the word *sulfate*. If you check the shampoo bottles in your home, you'll find that nearly all of them contain sulfates, as do the vast majority of shampoos on the market. If you have ever shampooed your hair or brushed your teeth, you have used sulfates.

Sulfates are harsh detergents that vary in terms of their stripping power. Ammonium lauryl and laureth sulfates (ALS) are harshest and tend to be the best cleansers, followed by sodium lauryl and laureth sulfates (SLS) respectively. TEA laureth sulfate and sodium myreth sulfate are gentler sulfate detergents.

Despite the proliferation of sulfates in the hair care market, textured hair rarely performs or responds well to large amounts of sulfate-based ingredients in cleansing formulas. Sulfate shampoos literally strip the hair, removing not only undesirable product buildup but also the desirable natural oils that black hair needs to remain supple. With weekly use, these harsh detergents can deplete black hair of its vital moisture balance and cause the hair and scalp to feel dry and rough.

Keep in mind that although sulfate surfactants can detract from the moisturizing capabilities of shampoo, the mere presence of a surfactant or sulfate in a formula is not cause to give up entirely on what you believe to be a good shampoo. It is an indication, however, that depending on such a shampoo for moisture may be less than ideal, especially if used weekly or even more frequently. Cocamidopropyl betaine is a popular secondary surfactant in sulfate-free shampoos and is better for use on black hair. As sulfate-free shampoos become more popular on the market, watch out for "sulfate-free" look-alikes that contain familiar sulfate names but aren't the standard ALS and SLS sulfates. These shampoos may be even more stripping than regular shampoos because the detergents in the formula are often bundled with two or three other detergent ingredients. Detergent bundling can lead to shampoos that are still too strong and still manage to strip black hair, despite being "sulfate free."

Foam Boosters

Common Foam Boosters

- Cocomidapropyl betaine
- Cocamidapropyl hydroxysultaine
- Lauramide oxide
- Lauramide diethanolamine (DEA)
- Cocamide diethanolamine (DEA)
- Cocamide monoethanolamine (MEA)

Figure 27: Common Foam Boosters

Lathering ability is an important feature of shampoos. Foam boosters are a class of surfactant that enhances the thickness of shampoo lather. One benefit of superior lathering and foaming is (see Figure 27) the enhanced spreadability of shampoo product throughout the hair. There are three prominent classes of foam boosters: fatty acid alkanolamides, betaines and amide oxides. Although manufacturers repeatedly tell us that strong lather is not an indication of good cleansing ability, it is certainly one of the features most of us consider when looking for a great shampoo, and there is a good reason for this. Lather is formed when surfactant molecules surround air molecules rather than oil molecules. When detergent surfactants first come in contact with the dirt and oils in our hair, lathering is minimal. As the shampoo lifts oils, dirt and other products from the hair, lathering ability picks up again as the surfactant molecules combine with air. Strong lathering is an indication that the hair is clean and that no products or debris are present to reduce the lather. This is why the lather produced by a first application of shampoo tends to be less foamy than the lather produced with a second application. In addition, lather makes shampoo products easier to work through tightly coiled hair, reducing the need for manipulation (and therefore the potential for tangling) during the shampoo process.

Conditioning Agents

Today's shampoos now often contain conditioning ingredients to balance their cleansing and stripping abilities. Popular conditioning ingredients include silicones, quaternary compounds, light proteins and fatty acids. These agents are reviewed in detail in the section on conditioner products.

Selecting a Shampoo

Because black hair encompasses such a vast category of textures and types that may respond differently to products, there is no one shampoo formula that is "perfect" for black hair. Furthermore, shampoos of different strengths are often required to achieve various styling goals. For the purposes of this discussion, there are three main types of shampoos: moisturizing, clarifying and chelating.

Moisturizing Shampoos

Black hair should be presented with adequate moisture supplementation at every turn. Of the thousands upon thousands of shampoos and conditioners on the market, very few are gentle enough for regular use on textured tresses. Our hair already naturally falls on the dry end of the moisture spectrum; therefore, using a shampoo that removes the little moisture we are able to retain naturally further devastates the moisture balance within the hair shaft. Moisturizing shampoos, especially those that are sulfate-free, will cleanse the hair gently without stripping it bare of natural oils. These shampoos are best to use on black hair for weekly light-duty cleansing. A list of safe, recommended sulfate- free shampoos is provided in the Regimen Builder.

Moisturizing? Or Coating?

The term *moisturizing* has become more of a marketing term than anything else these days. It is always necessary to differentiate between true moisture and oils masquerading as moisture sources. Many black hair products on the market are loaded with cheap oils such as petroleum, petrolatum and mineral oil to give the illusion that they moisturize textured fibers. In the absence of truly moisturizing ingredients, however, the best that oil-rich products can do is temporarily give black hair the appearance of good health. The regular use of these oily products, unfortunately, can lead to problematic issues with chronic dryness. These products coat black hair and give it a temporary shine and sheen, but this "manufactured" shine is cosmetic and provides no actual moisture benefit to the hair shaft. The mere appearance of moisturization is not enough to support and grow textured tresses.

Oils and moisturizers must never be confused or used interchangeably to combat dryness. Oils work to form an impenetrable barrier so that moisture contained within a strand stays there. The problem with oils is that any moisture that might attempt to enter the strand is kept out after they are applied. If the hair already feels dry, the last thing you want to do is create a barrier to moisture! Oils can mix with other oils but can never form important hydrogen bonds within the hair. In fact, oils by their nature can only repel water. If water is not being cross-linked and bound within the hair shaft, then no moisturization is taking place. It is as simple as that. Make sure that you are truly moisturizing your hair and not simply coating it with artificial shine. Subsequent chapters discuss how the coating action of oils can be used to support your vital moisturization efforts, but oils must never be used as or confused with the moisture source!

Clarifying Shampoos

Because our hair craves moisture, gentle shampoos must be used on a regular basis. There are times, however, when product buildup can be a major problem in black hair care because of the heavy oils, pomades, greases and gels we tend to use. If you find that your moisturizing shampoo no longer effectively removes buildup, it is time to break routine and use a clarifying shampoo. Clarifying shampoos are specially formulated to lift heavy product residues from the hair fiber. While sulfate-free moisturizing shampoos are great for gentle weekly cleansings, excessively stubborn products and debris may put up a fight and require stronger sulfate-based cleansers for removal.

You'll know that product buildup is a problem for your hair when you experience any of the following:

- Your shampoo is not lathering as well or seems to not be working in general.
- Your hair and scalp feel coated.
- Your hair feels limp and flat, with less body and movement.
- You are getting unexplainable hair breakage, despite balancing protein and moisture in your regimen.

Product buildup can be quite problematic. When you cut out sulfates, there is a trade-off between gaining moisture enrichment from the gentler shampoo and retaining its product-lift and -removal capabilities. With product buildup, stubborn debris may linger on the hair shaft and leave the hair with a coated feeling. Other hair products in the regimen may seem to lose their effectiveness (i.e., shampoos won't lather, conditioners feel like they are just sitting on the hair) when product buildup affects the hair's cuticles. When people say that hair "gets used to" certain products over time, they are usually referring unknowingly to the ineffectiveness of products when there is product buildup. Product buildup on the shaft is also a leading cause of ambiguous hair breakage that cannot be explained by protein or moisture imbalances.

Clarifying shampoos are particularly useful for cleansing black hair that routinely has heavy oils, gels, serums and greases applied between regular shampooings. Acetic acid, EDTA, sodium citrate and trisodium phosphate are common ingredients in clarifying shampoo formulas. These ingredients are deep cleansers, degreasers, chelators (mineral-deposit removers) and pH balancers. Clarifying shampoos are best used once monthly as maintenance shampoos to lift the buildup from the strands that most gentle, moisturizing shampoos and other hair care products may be leaving behind. Some sulfate-based shampoos are strong enough to be considered full-fledged clarifying shampoos on black hair—even if these shampoo formulas claim to be moisturizing.

Clarifying shampoos are usually clear product formulas because they lack the cloud-colored, opaque ingredients that typically add softness to the hair. These shampoos often leave the hair with a squeaky-clean feeling, something that black hair isn't able to tolerate on a consistent basis. That squeaky-clean feeling means that the natural oils that keep the hair pliable and supple have been stripped away, leaving the cuticle open and the hair shaft vulnerable to dryness and damage. For this reason, clarifying shampoos only need to be used once in every four to six weeks unless you are a heavy user of oils, serums, gels and greases.

Any Sulfate Shampoo Can Clarify

Although there are shampoos specifically formulated to clarify the hair, any regular shampoo that contains either ALS or SLS can work very well on textured hair for light clarifying purposes. These shampoos tend to be gentler than a true clarifier but are able to remove the bulk of leftover product. When product buildup is removed, the hair's cuticles can reflect light at a higher rate. Increased light reflection across the hair's surface increases the hair's natural shine or sheen. Monthly clarifying is a necessary part of any healthy hair care regimen and will give the hair a clean start each month. While clarifying refreshes the hair, doing so more than once or twice a month may result in extra-dry hair.

Chelating Shampoos

Clarifying and chelating (pronounced kee-lating) shampoos are two types of cleansers that are often confused. The two are similar in that both deeply clean the hair and remove product buildup, however, there are notable differences. Like simple product residues and oils, minerals that are dissolved in our water also bind to the hair shaft. The bonds that minerals make with the hair, however, are stronger than those made by products, dirt and oils. Mineral bonds with

the hair fiber are chemical bonds that cannot be removed with the simple surfactants found in moisturizing and clarifying shampoos.

A specially-formulated chelating shampoo is required to remove mineral deposits from the hair. The ingredients in chelating shampoos chemically bind to hard-water minerals and help to lift them away. Although many clarifying shampoos are quite stripping, remember that they are surface-acting and simply remove oil and product buildup that is superficially covering the cuticle. Chelating shampoos work on a deeper level, affecting the hair's bonding structure. Chelators bind to dulling mineral deposits on the hair shaft and remove them in the lather. The ingredient EDTA (ethylenediaminetetra acetic acid) is a common chelating ingredient that latches on to minerals and removes them as the hair is rinsed. Sodium citrate and trisodium phosphate are other common ingredients in chelating shampoo formulas.

> **Common Chelating Ingredients**
> - Disodium EDTA
> - EDTA
> - HEDTA
> - Oxalic acid
> - Potassium Citrate
> - Sodium Citrate
> - Sodium Oxalate
> - TEA-EDTA
> - Tetrasodium EDTA
> - Trisodium EDTA
> - Trisodium HEDTA

Chelating shampoos are potent and best for those who live in hard-water areas, where dulling metal ions are present in the water. The minerals in hard water react with shampoo detergents and create stubborn films that block shampoos' ability to produce a big, foamy lather. Like hard-water mineral deposits, conditioners also carry a positive charge and are attracted to the cuticle's negative charge. Because the presence of positively charged minerals along the cuticle changes the outer charge and chemistry of the hair shaft, conditioners must compete with hard-water minerals for placement along the cuticle. With fewer places to bind along the now positively charged hair shaft, conditioners are unable to attach to the shaft and condition the hair effectively. The chlorine that is often added to hard water also has negative effects on black hair.

Is My Water Hard?

When your water is hard, you certainly know it. Review the hard-water checklist (see Figure 28). If you've answered yes to any of the questions, then you may have a hard-water problem. According to the United States Geological Survey, areas with the softest water (with fewest dissolved minerals) are parts of New England, the South Atlantic-Gulf States, the Pacific Northwest and Hawaii. Moderately hard waters exist in Tennessee, the Great Lakes area and the Pacific Northwest regions of the United States. Hard to very hard waters can be found in Texas, New Mexico, Kansas, Arizona and southern California.

When Should I Chelate?

Despite their high levels of potency, chelating shampoos do have an important place in your regimen. One of the telltale signs of a hard-water problem is breakage that will just not end, no matter what. Hard-water-damaged black hair simply does not respond to anything but feels like it needs everything. For instance, it may feel weighed down (needs to be clarified), like coarse hay (needs moisture), and gummy or limp (needs protein)—all at once, in some cases. Hard-water-damaged hair is truly ambiguous.

When you notice moisturizers and oils sitting on your hair without really being absorbed, it may be time to clarify or chelate. Limp, lifeless hair, shampoos that just don't lather, and conditioners that no longer condition may also be indications that your hair is burdened with product or mineral buildup. If you ever experience unexplained hair breakage that does not respond to the treatments listed in the Protein and Moisture Balancing chapter (Chapter 6), you may need to chelate your hair to remove stubborn mineral buildup.

Chelating shampoos are also often used just prior to salon chemical services because of their ability to go deep down into the hair fiber and free up hair bonds that have been interfered with by unwanted mineral deposits. With minerals removed and hair bonds free, chemical processes can work smoothly and take properly.

Because chelating shampoos can be extremely drying, it is best to use them in moderation. With black hair, diligent deep conditioning must always follow the use of chelators.

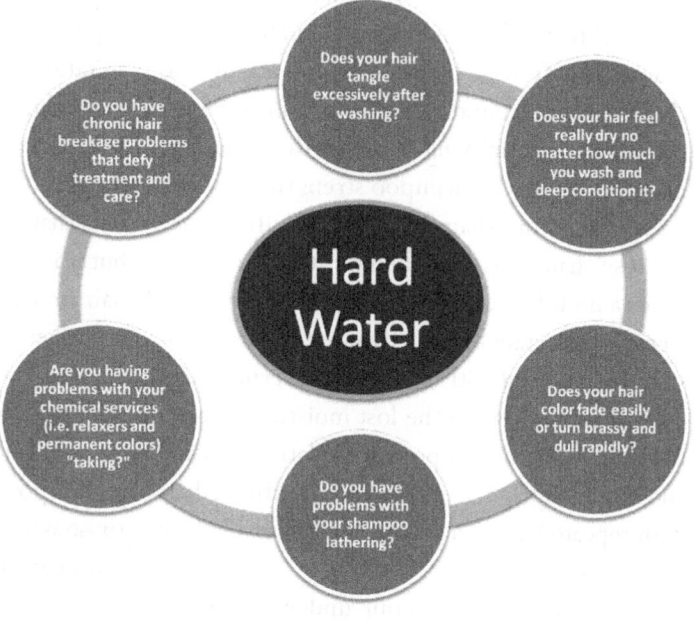

Figure 28: Hard Water Diagnosis Chart

Filters: Another Solution for Hard Water

If you live in a hard-water area, finding a permanent solution to your hard-water problem may be necessary to avoid stressing the hair with stripping shampoos. For roughly $70 to $100, you can buy a portable water filter that attaches to your shower head and filters out dirt and metals (including chlorine) coming through the tap. Minerals and salts, however, cannot be filtered out. More expensive whole-home water-softening units are also available and can improve the quality of your water. These units convert the mineral ions in hard water into less harmful sodium ions. Because they purify all of the water feeding into a home, these permanent plumbing fixtures may cost several hundred dollars.

Chelating vs. Clarifying

Chelating shampoos are much more potent than clarifiers because they work below the surface of the hair shaft. Frequent use of both types of strong shampoos can cause black hair to become extremely dry and brittle, and may lead to dandruff from a lack of moisture and hydration. Always clarify your hair before you attempt to chelate. If your buildup problem cannot be resolved in two clarifying sessions, then you may need to step up the shampoo strength and work with a chelating shampoo. Like clarifiers, use of these shampoos should be limited to once or twice a month because of their potency. It is extremely important that clarifying or chelating sessions be followed with a good moisturizing deep conditioner to return the lost moisture balance to the hair. Both shampoos are relatively strong and can compromise our fragile, textured hair with repeated use and inadequate follow-on deep conditioning.

As science improves our understanding of cleansing processes, gentler varieties of chelating and clarifying shampoo products that are acceptable for more regular use are hitting the market. Examples of these products can be found in the Regimen Builder's shampoo section. However, if you find these shampoos to be drying and continue to have chronic issues with hard water, purchasing a water-softener or water-filtration system may benefit your hair in the long run. After cleansing the hair with a good moisturizing shampoo, a thorough conditioning session should always follow.

No-Shampoo Shampooing Methods

Shampooing is not the only method by which textured hair may be cleansed. No-shampoo methods are growing in popularity among some segments of our population. The desire to reduce the use of synthetic cleansers including sulfates has propelled the "no-poo" revolution in hair care. There are several popular methods of shampoo-less cleansing.

Water-Only Method

The water-only method is as simple as it sounds. With this method, the hair is simply rinsed with water, and no shampoo products are applied. Cleansing takes place primarily through agitation from finger massage and gentle squeezing and manipulation of the hair under the force of warm water. This method may prove difficult for those who use heavy oils and styling products that occasionally build up on the hair shaft, but it is great for those who wear short, natural hair or who work out and simply need a quick, refresher rinse.

Baking Soda Cleansing

Baking soda, or sodium bicarbonate, has gained popularity as a natural cleansing agent for those who do not wish to use standard shampoo. For shampooing, a few tablespoons of baking soda are generally diluted in water and applied to the hair in much the same manner as a regular shampoo. The result is often soft, fluffy, clean hair. Unfortunately, some natural products are not necessarily ideal for textured hair, although they may feel good and can improve the fiber's cosmetic appearance. Abrasion is one factor to consider when using baking soda as a cleanser. Baking soda is a gritty, abrasive material almost like fine sand. Its grittiness is very damaging to black hair and can scratch and abrade the hair cuticle.

The pH of baking soda is also another factor to consider. Baking soda measures in at a moderately high alkaline pH of 9—the same pH as a weak chemical relaxer. Alkaline pHs always disturb the flattened orientation of the hair cuticle and cause the hair fiber to swell. Hair fiber swelling is a normal part of the cleansing process. Pure water (pH 7) is more alkaline than our acidic hair fibers and water produces a natural swelling action in the fiber. However, baking-soda hair washing increases the amount of hair swelling by significantly increasing the pH environment of your cleansing session. This swelling (and eventual contraction) weakens the hair fiber over time.

Conditioner Washing

Another popular shampoo-less method of hair cleansing that many find useful is conditioner washing, sometimes referred to as co-washing, or conditioner-only washing. Please see the discussion in the conditioner section for a full explanation of the benefits of this cleansing method.

Conditioner Basics

The conditioner you select is perhaps the single most important element in your regimen. We demand a lot from our hair, and conditioner products are what make (or break) a healthy hair care regimen. Conditioners restore moisture lost to the shampooing process and improve the hair's manageability. Because they are meant to adhere to the hair's cuticle and produce long-

lasting effects that remain after rinsing, conditioners play the most critical role in maintaining the hair's protein/moisture balance. Conditioners are important because they are specifically formulated to help us achieve one of the two healthy hair characteristics: strength or softness. Although conditioners are usually formulated to both strengthen and soften the hair, they almost always tend to be better at one than the other.

Conditioners are the products charged with working on the surface of the hair to improve its look, feel and texture. The conditioning step is when key cuticle elements are addressed and reinforced in the hair. It goes without saying that damaged hair reaps the greatest benefit from conditioning. Because damaged hair has more negatively charged binding sites along its protein structure than healthy hair, positively charged conditioners are able to bind more intently to these needy strands. Despite the fact that damage to the hair fiber is always cumulative and can never be permanently repaired, hair can be conditioned in ways that temporarily bond split ends, fill in missing material along the cuticle and add a layer of protection against further assault.

Deconstructing Conditioners: What's In There?

Conditioners are water-based, low-pH products that are added to the hair after shampooing to smooth and soften the hair cuticle. Conditioner products tend to contain much less water than shampoos and often contain a wide range of cuticle-enveloping ingredients. Conditioners are cationic (positively charged) and contain humectants, moisturizers, oils and small amounts of proteins to improve the overall quality of the hair. A conditioner's ability to condition the hair is largely dependent on the pH of the hair, the hair's general condition and the size of the conditioner's various molecules. Higher-pH damaged hair more readily binds with conditioner because hair in this state bears a strong negative charge that attracts positively charged conditioners. The positive charge of the conditioner neutralizes damaged hair's strong negative charge. This neutralization of oppositional charges allows the cuticle's scales to lie flat. Like conditioners, healthy hair carries a positive charge. When matched with a positively charged conditioner, healthy hair tends to resist the conditioning product.

Cationic Conditioning Agents

The two main types of cationic conditioning agents used in black hair care are cationic surfactants and cationic polymers (see Figure 29). These cationic ingredients work together to improve the hair's shine, sheen and pliability.

Cationic Surfactants

Cationic surfactants are the static fighters in most product formulas. Cationic surfactant ingredients are typically amines (nitrogen-based organic compounds) combined with fatty acids. When label reading, you can indentify cationic surfactants by their fatty acid chains (denoted by the common prefixes found in Figure 30).

These ingredients deposit themselves on the shaft very minimally and leave very little residue behind upon rinsing. Because they do not deposit well and rinse very cleanly, cationic surfactants tend to be used more in conditioning or moisturizing shampoos than in conditioners.

Cationic Polymers

In conditioners, cationic polymers are more desirable and important than cationic surfactants because of the expectation that conditioning will contribute shine, bounce and softness that will remain long after hair rinsing. Cationic polymers are especially popular additions to black hair-care conditioner formulas. These polymers, often added to thicken the consistency of the conditioning product itself, also add structure and thickness to the hair. Cationic polymers improve manageability and even reinforce existing curl patterns in natural hair. Polysaccharides and proteins make up the largest group of natural cationic polymers. The polysaccharides commonly used in conditioners are chitin, cellulose and cellulose derivatives such as hydroxyethyl cellulose.

Occasionally, various hair-product ingredients undergo quaternization, a chemical process that enhances their hair-binding abilities. Quaternization of polysaccharides and proteins enables them to adhere exceptionally well to the cuticle scales. Quaternized compounds form light, clear films on the cuticle. Of these poly-

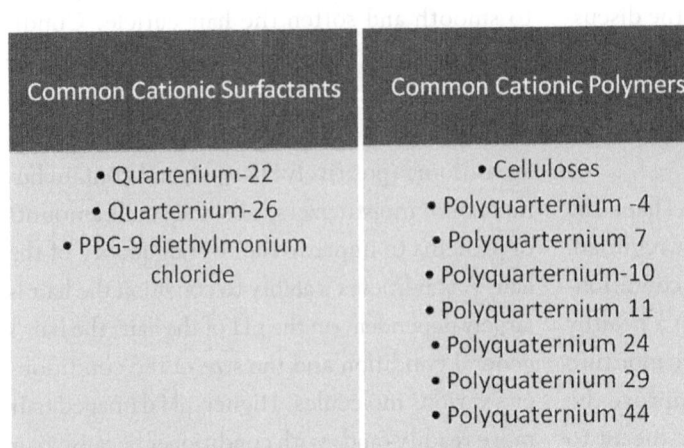

Common Cationic Surfactants	Common Cationic Polymers
• Quartenium-22 • Quarternium-26 • PPG-9 diethylmonium chloride	• Celluloses • Polyquarternium -4 • Polyquarternium 7 • Polyquarternium-10 • Polyquarternium 11 • Polyquaternium 24 • Polyquaternium 29 • Polyquaternium 44

Figure 29: Cationic Surfactants and Polymers

Common Conditioner Fatty Acid Prefixes

• Lauric/Lauryl
• Myristic/Myristyl
• Palmitic
• Stearic/Stearyl
• Oleic/Oleyl
• Linoleic
• Cetyl
• Behenyl

Figure 30: Common Conditioner Fatty Acids

mers, polyquaternium compounds are the most commonly used in conditioners. Polyquaternium 4 and 24, for instance, are both quaternized varieties of cellulose. The polyquaternium umbrella covers more than thirty-seven different compounds, and as science progresses, the number of polyquaternium compounds will only grow.

Silicones

Conditioners, especially those formulated for dry, coarse or curly hair, often contain cationic silicone-based ingredients to smooth the hair fibers. Silicones, commonly referred to as "cones" on Internet hair forums, coat the hair shaft in a thin, breathable layer of protection that allows the strands to move freely and easily past one another. These products are easily identified by their common word endings: *-cone*, *-conol*, *-col* and *-xane*.

Silicones generally have a lighter feel on the hair than oils, but can be more difficult to wash away. These ingredients are used primarily to improve wet combing and enhance shine. Lighter-weight silicones are sometimes used in black hair shampoos to provide a brief slippery feel to the hair before conditioner is introduced. These easy-to-rinse silicones often contain the abbreviations PPG or PEG before their formal names. Heavier, more substantial silicones such as dimethicone are found in conditioners, where it is important that the materials remain on the hair shaft after rinsing. Silicones may be great for improving manageability and reducing hair breakage during wet combing, but problems can arise when silicones are allowed to build up on the hair shaft. Silicone-burdened hair has a heavy, coated feel to it, and its straw-like dryness makes it prone to breakage. When silicones build up on the hair shaft, they can begin to mimic traditional oils (see Lipids, Emollients and Oils, below). They seal and coat the hair shaft, preventing moisture from getting through to where it is needed.

Water solubility is the largest determining factor in whether a particular silicone ingredient will cause buildup issues on the hair shaft. Water-soluble silicones dissolve or break apart readily in water, so they are less of a threat. Water-insoluble silicones, however, create waterproof barriers on the hair that are difficult to rinse away without an active shampoo detergent. These stubborn silicones cling to the hair and begin accumulating, use after use (see Figure 31). When silicones have been quaternized, they adhere even more tenaciously to the hair shaft and are more difficult to remove. These silicones tend to be strong humidity blockers and great shine boosters. Some water-insoluble silicones, such as cyclomethicone and PEG-modified dimethicone, are fairly easy to remove with a gentle, sulfate-free shampoo and light agitation from showerhead pressure or massaging. (1) (24)

A. Removed Easily with Water	B. Slightly more difficult to remove with water	C. Stubborm. Requires detergent/surfactant to remove
•Dimethicone copolyol	•Cyclomethicone	•Dimethicone
•PEG/PPG silicones	•Cyclopentasiloxane,	•Dimethiconol
• Lauryl methicone copolyol	•Trimethylsilylamodimethicone,	•Behenoxy Dimethicone
• Hydroxypropyl Polysiloxane	•Trimethylsiloxysilicates	•Phenyl Trimethicone
	•PEG-modified dimethicone	•Simethicone
	•Dimethicone copolyol	•Trimethicone
		•Polydimethysiloxane

Figure 31: Silicone Solubility Table

Lipids, Emollients and Oils

The next group of related conditioning agents consists of lipids, emollients and oils. Lipids are found naturally within the hair fiber and in the hair's sebum. These lipids provide conditioning for the fiber but are often lost over the course of day-to-day styling and manipulation. The lipid group includes water-repelling ingredients such as natural fats (triglycerides), waxes, ceramides and oils. (1) The common prefixes used to distinguish these ingredients are listed in Figure 29. In many high quality conditioner formulas, these fats are used in the place of cheaper oils such as mineral oil and petrolatum. (7) This group of lightweight emollients delivers extremely breathable films to the hair shaft without the heaviness and greasiness of oils. (8)

Low-Molecular-Weight Conditioning Ingredients

Panthenol, also known as pro-vitamin B5 or Panthenoic acid, is an ingredient whose small molecular size allows it to deeply penetrate the hair's cuticle layers. Panthenol is water soluble and is a common ingredient in quality conditioners. In fact, one of America's favorite hair care lines, Pantene, is named in its honor. Panthenol is a humectants: an agent that absorbs moisture from the surrounding air and pulls it to the hair.

Selecting a Conditioner

Our hair, perhaps more than any other type, needs sufficient conditioning on a regular basis. It is very important that we invest in quality conditioners. While conditioners cannot undo the years of trauma a single hair will experience in its lifetime, a solid conditioner can slow the deterioration process. There are several types of conditioners on the market that are suitable for black hair and address our primary need for moisture. On our quest to achieve healthier black hair, the wide variety of hair conditioners can lead to some confusion about which types should be used and when. Some conditioners are intended for daily use and others for weekly use. Some specialized formulas may be designed for monthly use.

Many conditioner products give very little information about how long they should be left on the hair fiber, and the time spent with conditioner generally varies from user to user, depending on their goals. As a baseline, the best advice for textured hair is to leave conditioner on the hair for ten to fifteen minutes, or until you begin to feel the hair soften a bit. For some curly-textured hair types, leaving conditioner on the hair without rinsing until the next wash improves manageability and brings out the best curls. If hair dryness and frizziness are major problems after shampooing and conditioning your hair, consider allowing a small amount of your "rinse-out" conditioner to remain in the hair after rinsing for additional control and sleekness. This technique also works better on thicker-textured hair types such as coarse relaxed hair, transitioning hair or fully natural, very curly hair. Note that leaving heavier conditioners in the hair without rinsing may lead to scalp itchiness for some. Those with fine hair may find that their hair feels weighed down and greasy if the wrong conditioners are used and left in. Remember, leaving conditioner on the hair for long periods of time does not increase a product's actual conditioning power but rather supports detangling, manageability and post-wash frizz.

Instant Conditioners

Instant conditioners are thin and lotion-like. These watery products generally are best suited for those with fine or oily hair, and are the best "rinse-out" conditioners to leave in. Instant conditioner formulas rinse from the hair easily and cleanly. Because of their high water content and the large molecular size of their ingredients, these conditioners only coat the outer parts of the hair shaft and do not deep condition well. Instant conditioners are not suitable for weekly deep conditioning since they wear off soon after the shampooing/conditioning session. A thicker conditioner product is required to really nourish the hair strands during the week and keep the hair supple for an extended period of time.

One of the most common conditioner mistakes for those of us with kinky-textured hair is using a lightweight instant conditioner as a weekly deep conditioner. Using instant conditioners for deep conditioning may eventually take a toll on the hair. Instant conditioners are best suited for individuals with fine hair who require a conditioner formula that does not deposit cationic substances too heavily on the fiber. They are also great for daily washers, those who work out and those who conditioner wash their hair. Bargain-basement conditioners that can be purchased for around a dollar are common examples of these water-rich, light instant conditioners.

Cream-Rinse Conditioners

Cream-rinse conditioners are generally used as a final rinse and, like instant conditioners, they are often left on the hair shaft for less than three to five minutes. Cream-rinse conditioners contain a considerable amount of cationic and shaft-smoothing ingredients such as silicones, oils and emollients, all of which support hair detangling. These conditioners also work well for protecting the hair against damage from heat styling that may follow a shampoo and conditioning session.

Deep Conditioners

Deep conditioners contain a concentrated mixture of cationic, moisture-boosting elements and proteins to both reinforce the hair cuticle and impart moisture to the strand. The proteins in the formula ensure that the hair retains the moisture it receives and secures it deep within the fiber to support the hair until the next deep-conditioning treatment. Heat is often used with deep conditioners to ensure the best penetration of moisture, and cuticle adhesion of protein molecules and other cationic substances. Deep conditioners should be used weekly on damaged hair and hair that is just beginning a new healthy hair care regimen. Once hair regains its strength, deep conditioning frequency then becomes a matter of personal choice. Those with relatively healthy hair may choose to deep condition weekly or every two to four weeks as needed.

Moisturizing Conditioners

Moisturizing conditioners work to increase the moisture content of the hair and improve its elasticity. These products smooth the cuticle and soften the hair, improving its manageability and eliminating frizz. Moisturizing conditioners contain a high percentage of cationic surfactants and polymers, which boost the moisture content of the hair shaft and reduce and neutralize the negative charges along the strand.

Protein Conditioners

Protein-based conditioners may range in protein content from extremely light to much heavier protein concentrations. Nearly all conditioners contain at least some protein. These conditioners temporarily rebuild the cuticle layer of the hair shaft by filling in areas of weakness along the strand and often contain very few additional conditioning agents. The molecules in basic protein conditioners are too large to fully penetrate the hair shaft; therefore, the hair retains the strengthening properties of these protein conditioners for about seven to ten days (or roughly one to three shampooings). The strengthening effect of protein conditioners depends on the level of hair-shaft damage and the frequency of use. Because these proteins are superficially deposited (surface acting), the introduction of water with each shampooing loosens the protein's hold on the hair shaft.

Protein-rich conditioners with a high degree of protein concentration are called protein reconstructors. The main difference between basic protein conditioners and protein reconstructor formulas lies in the size, type, and concentration of protein molecules in the product. Unlike protein reconstructors, regular protein conditioners tend to have a greater moisturizing element to complement their protein characteristics. In fact, many formulas actually add to the moisture levels in your hair by binding with the moisture already present and repairing weak spots in the hair's cuticle. These basic protein-conditioning formulas generally do not require a secondary deep-conditioning moisture treatment to replenish the moisture within the strands. Furthermore, at the lowest protein concentrations, such conditioners typically do not create wild swings in our hair's protein/moisture balance unless they are the only conditioning products used. Black hair in its natural state, however, may be more sensitive to proteins in conditioners than relaxed and/or color-treated hair types.

Protein Reconstructors/Treatments

Protein reconstructors offer more concentrated levels of protein than regular protein-based conditioners. These treatments are often more intensive and tend to require heat during the application for maximum penetration or adherence of the protein molecules. Since these treatments work deeply to penetrate and rebuild the hair shaft from within, their results are more dramatic and longer lasting than those of protein-based conditioners. The effects of the most highly potent protein treatments are so dramatic that they continue to work and remain on the hair for four to six weeks. The

strengthening effect of protein reconstructors always depends on the level of hair damage and the frequency of shampooing.

Much of the protein in these products is hydrolyzed, meaning it has been broken down into smaller components and is the correct molecular size to be absorbed into the cuticle. Since these types of protein products need to penetrate the hair shaft in order to be effective, they work better on hair that is already extremely porous and damaged. Hair with its own sound cuticle and protein structure will not readily accept the extra protein molecules, but will instead allow the protein molecules to build up on the outside of the hair shaft. The frequent use of these potent proteins on hair that has already satisfied its protein requirement results in over-rigid, dry hair that breaks easily at the slightest touch.

Because the sole purpose of protein reconstructors is to increase tensile strength and add additional structure to the hair strand, the conditioning properties of these products are minimal. Reconstructors must be followed up with an additional moisturizing deep-conditioning treatment to restore the hair's proper elasticity and prevent hair breakage.

Leave-In Conditioners

Leave-in conditioners come in the form of both creams and liquids, and some are dually formulated as detangling products. Creamy leave-ins are best for those with thick, coarse hair, while sprays often suffice for those with finer hair types. Most leave-ins with a creamy consistency are also great as water-based moisturizers. They are also excellent for those with fine hair who cannot use heavier water-based moisturizers and want to simply work with a lighter product. Leave-in sprays and mists are great for touching up and reinvigorating natural hair curls and coils throughout the day. Spray-based products are also superior moisture boosters for relaxed, braided, sewn-in or twisted hair.

When selecting a leave-in conditioner for your hair, always choose one that addresses your hair's moisture or protein needs at the time of use. If your hair is in need of more protein, opt for a protein-based leave-in conditioner. If your hair desperately needs moisture, choose a moisturizing leave-in conditioner. Having two dedicated products for this purpose—one for moisture and one for protein—is a good idea. See the Regimen Builder for product references and ideas.

Conditioner Washing

Conditioner washing is a moisture-boosting method that skips the shampoo stage of hair cleansing and uses conditioner only. The hair is simply rinsed with warm water and "washed" with a light conditioner. Conditioner washing is a good option for children, who require gentle products, and for people who work out and require regular hair and scalp cleansing that does not lead to dryness. Conditioner washing can work well for both natural and relaxed hair types, although the technique is considerably more popular among those with natural hair.

Hair can be effectively cleansed using this method because today's instant and lightweight conditioners often contain gentle cleansers in their formulations. Formulas of this type do not deposit heavy conditioning films on the hair and therefore rinse relatively cleanly. Conditioner washing can continue effectively for lengthy periods of time if regular use of other hair products in the regimen—moisturizers and oils, for example—remains light to moderate. Conditioner-washing success greatly depends on the type of conditioner selected. Again, lightweight, watery-type conditioners are preferable.

Implications of Conditioner Washing

The greatest obstacle to conditioner washing is managing potential product buildup. Because no shampoo is used, weekly products can begin to build up on the hair shaft, even when using a light conditioner with water-soluble silicones. Buildup will worsen if heavy, daily moisturizers containing silicones or heavy oils are used. If an inappropriate conditioner is used for cleansing, or if weekly product use is too heavy to sustain frequent conditioner washing, the hair may begin to refuse moisture and other treatments. Such moisture refusal can result in hair breakage. Occasional clarifying (once or twice each month) with shampoo while actively following a shampoo-free regimen may prove beneficial for managing buildup from conditioner-only washing.

Water-Based Moisturizing Basics

In addition to regular deep conditioning with quality conditioner products, other sources of external moisture supplementation are a must for healthy black hair. Maintaining appropriate levels of moisture in textured hair fibers, however, is one of the most pressing challenges in black hair care. The lack of adequate moisture retention is one of the leading causes of hair breakage within the black hair community. Product manufacturers have spent countless research and development dollars on new formulations designed to meet the extraordinary moisture demand in our hair care. Despite advancements in our understanding of the way our hair responds to water, the proper techniques for moisturizing black tresses continue to remain a commonly misunderstood part of many black hair care regimens. Moisturizers generally come in the form of light sprays, creams, custards, pastes and puddings. Sprays work well for those with fine hair or braided hair styles, while heavier creams and custards are generally best for those with thicker, coarser hair.

What is Moisture?

Moisturization, or hydration, is a primary characteristic of water. Water is the universal moisturizer. Good moisturizers will always contain water as a first ingredient. But water is always on the move, and as a result, the hair's moisture levels are always in a state of flux. Water's tendency to rapidly enter and exit the hair's cuticle and cortex means that hair cannot be maintained in a moisturized state for prolonged periods with water alone. Moisturizing formulas often contain humectants and blended emollients and oils to draw additional moisture to your hair and keep it there.

Did You Know?

Hydro= Water
Phobic= Fear/Fearing

Hydrophobic= **"water fearing"** or lacking affinity for water.
Merriam Webster

The primary action of moisturizers is twofold. Moisturizers support the hair's infrastructure by replenishing internal water and other essential elements that have been lost naturally to the surrounding dry air and processes such as heat styling, chemical processing and coloring. Next, carefully blended emollients and oil ingredients support and restore the hair and skin's lipid-rich outer layer to prevent the escape of this moisture back into the surrounding environment.

The idea that oils moisturize the hair goes way back into antiquity. Lengthy debates continue in the real world and online about this very topic. Product manufacturers have not helped the issue by continuing to refer to the petroleum, petrolatum, and mineral oil–based greases, creams, lotions, pomades and even conditioners that they produce as "moisturizers." In black hair care, in particular, oils and greases have taken a prominent role and often overshadow or stand in the place of water as a moisturizer.

The confusion arises because oils and moisturizers do have some similarities. Like true moisturizers, oils and greases do soften, nourish, add shine and increase the hair's pliability. However, they are not moisturizers.

Greases and oils are hydrophobic substances, meaning they repel water chemically. The old saying, "Oil and water do not mix," holds true, literally. Oils are unable to bind to water, and hair products that contain both oils and water require special blending ingredients called emulsifiers to keep the mixture from separating.

Finally, the ability of certain types of oil to penetrate the hair shaft does not confer moisturizing ability. Penetration does not equal moisturization. Where full-fledged greases and petroleum jelly–type products provide a clear external barrier to moisture, some lighter oils are more flexible in their chemistry and provide moisture-barrier benefits beyond the superficial cuticle layers.

Water-Based Moisturizers: What's In There?

Water forms the base of any effective moisturizing product, but a host of other ingredients work together with water to provide a moisture benefit to the strands. Humectants, emollients and occlusive ingredients play an important role in moisturizing the hair.

Humectants

Humectants draw moisture from the surrounding air and bring it to the hair or skin. On the scalp, humectants also draw moisture from the deeper skin layers up to the stratum corneum, the uppermost scalp skin layer. One of the most effective humectants found in black hair products is glycerin. Other common humectant ingredients in products designed for our hair include NaPCA (sodium pyrrolidone carboxylic acid [PCA], or simply sodium PCA), panthenol, urea, propylene glycol, sorbitol, sodium lactate and some hydrolyzed proteins. Keep in mind that while the presence of humectants in a moisturizer is highly desirable, products with high, concentrated volumes of humectants can leave the hair with a sticky or tacky, coated feel if applied too heavily.

Some suggest that the use of certain humectants, particularly glycerin, in the colder, winter months (or during periods of low atmospheric humidity) causes the humectants to actually draw moisture away from the hair. The reasoning is that without atmospheric moisture to draw in, glycerin and other humectants may seek out the next best source of moisture and begin to pull moisture from the hair back into the environment. Used on its own, glycerin and other humectants can draw moisture from the hair and skin, but when used as part of a larger water-based mixture, glycerin molecules support hair moisturization by utilizing the water inherent in the product or mixture to saturate and stabilize itself. To combat winter dryness, always use humectants as part of a balanced, water-based mixture, and seal sources of water-based moisture with a heavier oil or butter product to prevent moisture-escape into the surrounding environment. If humectant-rich products continue to present a dryness concern for your tresses, opt for moisture products that do not contain them in large concentrations and have them listed farther down in the ingredients list.

Emollients

Emollients are lubricating, film-producing ingredients that fill in cracks along the cuticle surface. Emollients can be water or oil-based and are used in products to help smooth and seal the hair fiber. Emollients include fatty alcohols like cetyl alcohol and ceramides.

Occlusive Agents

Occlusive agents are exactly what they sound like: product ingredients that occlude or block the entry and exit of water through the cuticle. These ingredients, when present in high concentrations, contribute to the greasy feel of some moisturizing products. Common occlusive ingredients include petrolatum, mineral oil, waxes, other oils and silicones. These ingredients are primarily responsi-

ble for the shine moisturizers give, but, the price for shine with these products, unfortunately, is the heavy film they leave on the hair fiber. When occlusive ingredients build up on black hair and scalps, moisture is unable to enter the hair shaft or reach the scalp skin, creating a cycle of dryness. To remedy this problem, many consumers simply pile on more of the offending product, which continues the cycle of dryness.

Petrolatum is the worst offender and creates the strongest moisture barrier. Lanolin, mineral oil and silicones follow petrolatum in strength in that exact order. Research has shown that the film petrolatum leaves behind blocks more than 98 percent of the moisture entering or exiting the skin and hair shaft. Petrolatum is therefore an excellent moisture retainer for both skin and hair, but it prevents external moisturizing efforts from taking effect. Petrolatum is difficult to remove from the strands without harsh, sulfate-based cleansers. Its use as a scalp protectant during chemical relaxing is a testament to the ruggedness of the barrier it forms on hair. The seal created by petrolatum is near absolute.

Selecting a Water-Based Moisturizer

Selecting a moisturizer is perhaps the most challenging part of the regimen-building process. It is very important to make sure that the moisturizer you are using is indeed a moisturizer. In most product formulations, the first three or four ingredients set the tone for the nature and quality of the hair product. Because there can be no moisture delivery without water, water is always listed as a first ingredient in moisturizing products. Black hair moisturizers should contain very few occlusive ingredients such as petrolatum, mineral oil, or lanolin oil. These product fillers deposit heavy films on the hair with regular use. These ingredients offer no intrinsic moisture benefit outside of sealing the hair for better moisture retention, because the large molecules that make up these sealants are unable to effectively penetrate the hair shaft. Trapped on the outside of the hair strand, these oily ingredients merely coat the hair, repelling potential sources of moisture and giving the fiber a temporary shine. This temporary shine and sheen are commonly mistaken for moisture!

Unfortunately, heavy occlusive oils are pervasive in black hair moisturizing products and sometimes immediately follow water in the ingredients list. These oils, in particular mineral oil, are extremely difficult to avoid. The higher up in the ingredients list these oils are found, the higher their concentration in the hair product and the more influence they have on moisture delivery and repulsion. Salon-quality and organic products tend to far outpace their drugstore counterparts in effective moisture delivery and avoidance of these occlusive agents.

If you have difficulty finding water-based moisturizers that do not contain mineral oil and other heavy, shaft-coating oils, opt for moisturizing products that contain these oils closer to the bottom of the ingredients list. As a rule of thumb, these sealants should never be listed in the top five ingredients of any moisturizer you use. A top-five listing means that these ingredients make up the bulk of the formulation and ultimately will work against your moisturizing efforts. Occasionally, you will find a product that contains mineral oil and still works well for your hair. Always use caution, however, when introducing these kinds of products into your regimen.

Of the two moisturizers listed below:

SUPER Moisturizer A: **Water, Petrolatum, Mineral Oil, Glycerine, Panthenol...**

AND

SUPER Moisturizer B: **Water, Glycerin, Cetearyl Alcohol, Panthenol, Coconut oil,...**

Moisturizer B is preferable, and the much better moisturizer!

When Should I Moisturize My Hair?

You should get in the habit of moisturizing your hair several times per week or whenever your hair feels dried out by the surrounding air. Daily moisturizing can be extremely important for those who are just starting out with their healthy hair regimens and for some with natural hair. Having to apply a moisturizer product multiple times throughout the day, on the other hand, also can be an indication that either the product is not a true moisturizer or that there is damage to the hair cuticle. If you find that you have to apply moisturizer to your hair several times in one day, you may be dealing with a porosity issue. Your cuticles may be damaged and releasing moisture just as fast as you are putting it there. Those who follow a dedicated deep-conditioning regimen often find that their hair's daily moisture requirements drop significantly, and that they are able to go an average of three to four days or longer between moisturizing touch-ups.

The best times to apply moisturizing products are just before bed, prior to combing or manipulating the hair, before outdoor activities and after you've rinsed out a conditioner or leave-in conditioner during your normal shampoo/conditioner regimen. Focus all moisturizing efforts on the ends of your tresses, where the hair is oldest and trauma and damage are most concentrated.

Moisturizing the hair before bed is particularly beneficial. Tying your moisturized hair up at night reduces friction to the fibers from rubbing that might occur from your late-night tossing and turning. This will also give you a fresh, moisturized start in the morning. If you go to bed with dry, parched hair, you will wake up with even drier hair. Although it is preferable to first moisturize and then oil the hair as part of your night routine, simply applying an oil lubricant to the hair to reduce friction between the strands at night can also be beneficial. This is the simple science behind those "grow-your-hair" night caps and bonnets often advertised in stores. These satin bonnets usually come with some sort of oil product that is applied to the hair each night. These products work because they reduce friction between the hair fibers. The oil product lubricates and smoothes the cuticles, and the satin bonnet protects the hair from cotton pillowcases which helps reduce hair breakage.

Moisturizing the hair before heading outside for prolonged outdoor activities, especially in the hot summer and bitter cold months, is also a wise practice. Extreme temperatures can deplete moisture down to zero, leaving your hair a dry, brittle mess.

A water-based moisturizer may follow a leave-in conditioner in your normal washing routine or, depending on the moisturizing product, replace a leave-in conditioner altogether. For those with fine hair, leave-in conditioners often work well as water-based moisturizers.

Sealing in Moisture

Although hair naturally contains moisture, and we are able to supply moisture externally to support the hair fiber, our hair remains naturally porous to a certain degree. Keeping the moisture securely within the hair shaft can be a difficult task. Moisture from supplemental moisturizing products easily passes into the hair shaft but may pass out just as easily. Stabilization of internal moisture levels requires external oil-layering support.

Effective Product Layering

Moisturizing success is all in the order in which you apply your products. Oils are hydrophobic or "water-fearing" substances that repel moisture. If you use oils without a moisturizer or before one, the oil will deter moisture from entering the hair strand and lead to eventual dryness. The key is to lock moisture within the strands with the help of an oil or butter. A light

coating of oil on top of your moisturizer product will help seal the moisture inside and prevent outside humidity from frizzing the hair. This specific method of layering products (see Figure 33) enhances optimal moisture absorption and retention because moisture is introduced to the hair fiber first and is then locked into place with an oil. If your hair isn't properly moisturized before the barrier goes on, you can expect dryness.

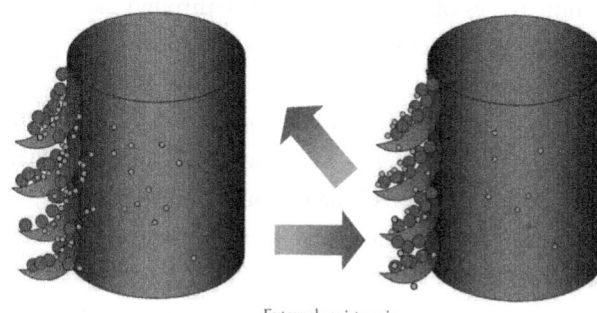

Oil and Moisture Product Layering Technique

● = Oil molecule • = Water molecule

Strand A   External moisture is primarily deflected from the hair shaft   Strand B

Figure 33: Moisturizing Product layering technique. Blue dots represent moisture, red dots represent an oil product. "Strand A" demonstrates effective product layering where a moisture based product is introduced to the shaft and is "locked" into the fiber by an oil barrier. Strand B shows incorrect layering where oil blocks the entry of water into the hair fiber.

How Long Does Hair Remain Moisturized after It Is Sealed?

Applying oils to the hair and scalp will coat them and trap the moisture that is inside the hair on the inside and keep any moisture that is outside the hair on the outside. The sealing effects of most oils, however, are only temporary. The length of time hair remains moisturized depends on a variety of factors including the hair's level of porosity, the weather, the type of moisturizer used, the type of oil used and your hairstyle. Highly porous hair will feel dry faster than hair with low porosity, and natural hair may simply look and feel drier because of its highly textured kinks and coils. Hot, arid climates dry out hair faster than temperate or humid climates. Additionally, some moisturizers have more effective humectants and emollients than others, and protective styles also prevent hair from drying out better than other styles.

In many cases, the seals we create with oils are not 100 percent complete and still allow some minute traces of moisture to diffuse through the barrier. An obvious correlation exists between the consistency of the oil and the oil seal it creates on the hair shaft. Heavier oils tend to seal the hair strand better and for longer periods of time than lighter oils. Shampooing, daily wear and tear, and exposure to air and the elements can break down and dry out oil seals.

Water-Based vs. Oil-Based Moisturizers

There may be times when oils and oil-based moisturizers are preferable to water-based moisturizers for maintaining hair in a particular style. For example, for naturals who press or straighten their hair, or anyone who sets their hair, water-based moisturizers will always cause the hair to revert. The high water content of water-based moisturizers breaks and reestablishes the hydrogen bonds that pressing and setting temporarily reorganizes or eliminates. A moisturizer with a higher synthetic oil or silicone content will better seal the hair against intrusion from external moisture and humidity in the surrounding air. While typically not as moisturizing as water-based products, oil-based products will resist introducing more moisture into the strands and serve as a barrier as well.

Oil and Butter Basics

Oils and butters have long had a prominent role in black hair care, and for good reason.

They are vitally important materials in hair-care in general and support a number of hair-product formulations. The word oil is a broad term that encompasses a wide range of solid and liquid materials including fatty alcohols, triglycerides, butters and oil-soluble silicones. Oils and butters enhance the shine, softness and flexibility of textured hair fibers. Some oils even offer sensory benefits and healing properties for the user. For centuries, our ancestors relied on oils and butters of various kinds to keep their textured tresses looking great, and their utility and implications for healthy black hair care continue to be immense.

Synthetic Oils
Mineral Oil and Petrolatum

Petroleum-based oils such as petrolatum and mineral oil (liquid petroleum)—along with silicones—comprise the synthetic oil group. Both mineral oil and petrolatum are by-products of the crude-oil refining process and are perhaps the most pervasive oils in black hair care. Because they are quite inexpensive, these oils are used in just about everything from cosmetics to baby-care products. (Baby oil is 100 percent mineral oil.) These oils provide the skin and hair with amazing softness and shine, and as barriers, they prevent the escape of moisture from the hair and skin.

Did You Know?
All traditional oils are technically natural, including mineral oil and petrolatum. They are both natural byproducts of the distillation of crude oil.

Since these oils' molecules are much too large for penetration, mineral oil and petrolatum simply form a film on the hair fiber. Because they are non-polar and extremely hydrophobic, these oils are unable to bind to the hair's keratin proteins.

Their excellent ability to repel moisture coupled with their inability to make real chemical contact with the hair fiber, makes them some of the most effective oils for sealing in moisture.

Silicone-based Serums/Glossifiers

Serums are finishing products that add shine, manageability and often layers of heat protection to the hair. These products contain silicone ingredients, such as dimethicone, that coat the hair strands and reduce friction between the cuticle scales of neighboring hairs. This reduction of friction allows the strands to slip past one another easily, greatly reducing tangling and improving manageability.

In general, serums behave like oils on the hair fiber. Like natural oils, silicone-based serums and gloss products should be used only after a moisturizer has been applied. They coat and seal the fiber, giving the hair incredible, long-lasting shine. Compared to oil films, serum films deposited on the strands are often lighter, produce a more brilliant shine, and are able to provide a stronger external moisture barrier with less product. Because serums are generally lighter than oils, they are the sealant of choice for those with frizz-prone hair or those who wear straight styles or roller sets.

Synthetic oils and serums coat the surface of the hair cuticle with little to no integration into the interior of the hair fiber. Silicone buildup, however, can cause extreme dryness and render attempts at moisturizing and deep conditioning the hair futile. Products with silicones should be regularly removed from the hair through frequent cleansing with a stronger shampoo, ideally a clarifier.

Synthetic oils far exceed the primary goal of preventing the evaporation of internal moisture from the strands, and most produce a nice, high-octane shine on textured tresses. But the best oils for black hair should exhibit beneficial characteristics other than simple barrier formation. Oil properties such as saturation and polarity play a major role in shaping key characteristics that are of great use to those of us with textured hair. These beneficial qualities are played up in natural oils, which make them preferable to synthetic oils in healthy hair care.

Natural Oils and Butters

Oils derived from plants, flowers, seeds and fruits are superior healthy hair care oils. They form light, semi-permeable films on the exterior of the hair cuticle to help seal in moisture. Depending on their chemistry, many of these oils quickly wear off from the hair's surface or actively penetrate the hair fiber over time to provide opportunities for re-moisturization of the fiber.

Hair butters are thick, semi-solid, wax-like products that offer an alternative texture to traditional oils. Butter products work well for those with hair types that require products with a bit more weightiness or have more difficulty staying moisturized. Natural butter products are extracted from plant seeds (i.e., shea butter) or made directly from other oils combined with a thickener (i.e., coffee butter). Butters are excellent sealants and protect the hair exceptionally well against moisture loss.

Essential Oils

Essential oils are plant-based oils with small molecules that evaporate quickly from the scalp skin. Their watery consistency and high price for tiny volumes make sealing the hair with these oils impractical. A list of common essential oils can be found in the Regimen Builder. These oils are commonly used in hair care for their sensory and scalp skin stimulating abilities. Always consult a physician prior to trying essential oils, especially if you are a woman who is pregnant or nursing.

Using Essential Oils

Essential oils are extremely potent. They should be used only three to four drops at a time, and must be diluted in a thicker oil prior to using on the scalp skin. This thicker oil is known as a carrier oil because it carries the essential oil and helps to spread it out over a larger coverage area. Proper dilution is the key. Too much carrier oil, and you risk drowning out the benefits of your essential oil. Generally, you need just enough carrier oil to prevent burning or irritation from the strong essential oil. Slowly add one drop of the essential oil at a time to the carrier oil, testing between drops to insure the proper dilution for your personal tolerance level is met. Two to three drops of essential oil diluted in about two tablespoons of carrier oil is a great starting mixture, which you can then adjust to your tastes. Warming your carrier oil beforehand will enhance your essential oil experience.

NOTE: To find essential oils and complementary carriers, check your local health foods store or visit essential oil vendors online.

Storage and Care

Essential oils keep for years. Keep your oils in a cool, dry place. Make sure the bottles are composed of a dark glass that does not allow sunlight to pass through. Sunlight denatures essential oils and causes them to lose their effectiveness and potency.

TIP
You can easily turn your everyday shampoo into a custom-made scalp-stimulating shampoo by adding a few drops of an essential oil such as peppermint or rosemary. Different oils serve different functions. Some have antiseptic qualities, while others have soothing or stimulating effects. You will look forward to your shampoo days with these great-smelling scalp-tingling oils. You may even add essential oils to the other products in your regimen such as leave-ins, moisturizers and conditioners.

Breaking Down Oils: Saturated and Unsaturated Oils

The terms *saturated* and *unsaturated* in relation to fats and oils are commonly discussed in nutrition circles, but interestingly, the saturated/unsaturated chemical distinction has meaning for black hair care as well. There are three common types of natural oils: saturated, monounsaturated and polyunsaturated.

Oils are commonly made up of combined saturated and unsaturated elements. Saturated oils are solids at room temperature and are able to penetrate hair strands more readily than unsaturated fats and oils because of the relative shapes of their molecules. Saturated structures produce straight-chain molecules that slip easily into hair fibers, while the highly-kinked or branched-chain molecules of unsaturated oils cannot get through. Polyunsaturated oils, or oils with multiple miss-

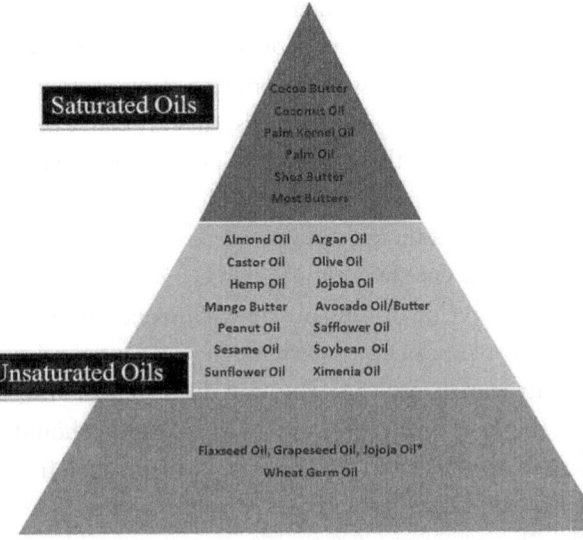

Figure 34: Oil and Butter Saturations. Remember most oils and butters contain elements of both saturated and non-saturated types. The dominant type is indicated in the pyramid chart.

ing bonds and kinks, have the greatest difficulty getting through the fiber. (25) These unsaturated oil molecules simply collect on the exterior of the hair fiber. The good news is that the lack of saturation does not always doom an oil to sit on the outside of the hair shaft. New research has shown that monounsaturated oils, or oils with only one kink in their molecular chain, can pass into the hair fiber with some ease. Most hair butters fall into the monounsaturated oil category.

Polar Hair Oils

When the atoms of any molecule are arranged such that one end of the molecule has a positive charge and the other end has a negative charge, the molecule is called a polar molecule. Water is an example of a polar molecule. Non-polar molecules do not have opposing charges at their ends. Oils can be classified as non-polar substances. Because polar and non-polar substances cannot readily mix, they repel one another. Although all oils are technically non-polar by design, some oils have small molecular regions that display seemingly polar characteristics. These non-polar oils have *polar regions.*

Polarity is a relative term, especially for oils that are non-polar by nature. On a sliding scale, some oils are simply more or less polar than other oils. Oils such as coconut oil, almond oil, sunflower seed oil, and castor oil are examples of oils with high relative polarity. Although these oils resemble non-polar oils chemically, polar oils contain acid groups that enhance their chemistry.

The polarity of a hair oil plays a role in the strength of the moisture barrier and seal it creates. Polar oils offer the most permeable oil seals. As sealants, they protect well against internal moisture exit and external moisture entry, but their polarity causes them to migrate into the hair fiber over time. This migration of polar oil molecules into the hair fiber causes the seal on the outer surface of the hair fiber to deteriorate. When this happens, the moisture seal is less ef-

fective, and external moisture can enter the shaft and cause the hair to frizz. Largely non-polar oils, namely mineral oil and petrolatum, create stronger, near-complete moisture barriers that can linger on the hair for long periods of time. Because their seals are near absolute, they provide the best protection against hair reversion and frizz. Polar oils, however, offer the greatest flexibility for black hair. These oils can be rinsed from the hair easily, and their migration into the hair strand allows the hair to be rewetted (remoisturized) and resealed without causing much buildup on the outer cuticle. Non-polar oils, which resist migration into the hair shaft, often need to be shampooed away before additional moisturizing and sealing can take place. Rewetting and reactivating these seals does very little for full-fiber moisturization and can lead to tacky buildup on the hair fiber.

A polar oil's acid groups are attracted to polar sites within our hair fiber. Our hair's polar keratin protein is the perfect match. Polar oils' attraction to the proteins deep within the hair fiber strengthens the hair's overall architecture and reinforces the hair shaft from within. Their migration into the hair fiber is largely dependent on their saturation level. Coconut oil is one of the few oils that is both a polar, and a completely saturated, straight-chain oil.

In addition to the strength and integrity that oil-protein binding confers, this binding is important for another reason. Oil-protein binding reduces the rate at which hair shafts are able to expand in the presence of water. This is a very important property for reducing the trauma that cleansing and conditioning sometimes inflict upon our hair. Here's how it works.

Polar Oils and Hygral Fatigue

Each time we shampoo and condition our hair, our hair shafts must expand to accommodate the additional water. When the hair dries, our hair contracts and returns to its normal size and state. The process of hair expansion in wet conditions and contraction under dry conditions is both stressful and damaging to the hair fiber over time. Damage to the hair fiber from repeated expansion and contraction is known as hygral fatigue. Black hair, which is more susceptible to damage and high porosity problems, tends to take in more water during the washing process than other types of hair. This causes our hair fibers to swell considerably when wet. Our hair fibers must then shrink back to their normal sizes during the drying process, but the cuticle can fray, split or crack as this happens. Damage may be especially pronounced when the hair cuticle rapidly contracts from a state of intense swelling (as in porous hair).

Researchers have discovered that using polar oils such as coconut as a pre-shampoo treatment can protect the fiber against hygral

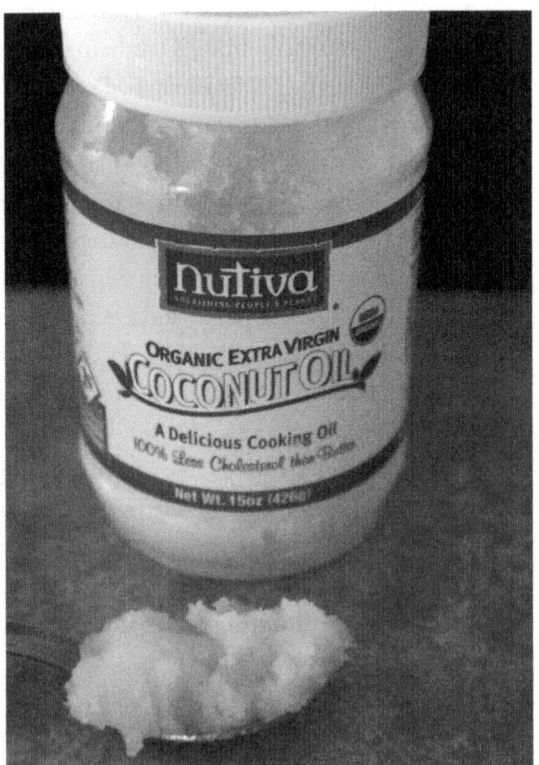

Figure 35: Coconut oil is one of the best hair oils for black hair because of its unique properties.

fatigue. (26) (27) When a straight-chained, polar oil is used on the hair as a pre-shampoo treatment, a small portion of the oil is absorbed into the hair fiber when the fiber naturally swells. Polar oils protect the hair by binding to the hair's inner proteins, which in turn reduces the protein's chemical ability to bind to water molecules. Swelling in reaction to water is kept to a minimum in the hair fiber, which experiences considerably less trauma as it naturally contracts to dry.

Which Oils are Best?

An ideal oil for black hair would have the following characteristics:

- Slight polarity to support protein reinforcement in the fiber.
- Capacity to form light, permeable films.
- High level of saturation.

Butters and natural oils seal in moisture and are much more suitable for healthy hair growing than synthetic, petroleum-derived oils. Polarity and the presence of saturated and monounsaturated fatty acids in plant- and seed-based oils and butters makes them superior to petrolatum and mineral oils, which have no affinity for our hair and do not penetrate well to reinforce the hair fiber. To date, research has shown that only polar oils with straight or minimally branched chemical chains are able to migrate deeply within the hair fiber. (26) (28)

There may be times when synthetic oils are preferable to natural ones. If you are wearing a certain hairstyle and the life of the set is dependent on keeping as much moisture away from the hair as possible, then heavier synthetic oils are preferable to condition and add shine to the style. Synthetic oils will prevent moisture entry more reliably than most natural oils. Synthetic oils will also linger on the hair shaft for longer periods of time and give longer-lasting coverage against moisture entry.

Saturated Vs. Unsaturated Oil Penetration

● = Unsaturated oil molecule   ○ = Water molecule   ● = Keratin Protein

Oils are "moisture blockers" that protect the strand against excessive moisture entry and exit. Without this barrier, moisture freely exits the hair.

Oil films vary in permeability. Saturated oils and butters create semi-permeable films on the hair which block the exit of moisture from the strand, but these seals are not as strong as synthetic and unsaturated oils. Saturated oils can partially migrate into the hair fiber, so their seals tend to "wear off" over time. Polar oils migrate into the fiber and bind with hair protein to strengthen the hair.

Normal Hair, No Oil Seal

Oil molecules migrate into the strand and bind to keratin protein in the hair. This prevents protein loss.

Strand A- Saturated (Polar) Oil Seal

Typical oil molecules are not attracted to keratin, and do not migrate into the fiber at appreciable levels

Strand B- Unsaturated Oil Seal

Figure 36: Saturated oils vs. unsaturated oils. Strand A shows a polar, saturated oil binding with protein in the hair shaft. Moisture is primarily blocked from entering and exiting the strand, but trace amounts of moisture are able to diffuse through the barrier. Strand B shows the standard action of oils on the hair, providing a tough barrier to moisture. No protein bonding occurs with typical, synthetic or largely non-polar oils.

Coconut Oil Benefits for Black Hair

The most popular polar oil in hair care is coconut oil. Solid at room temperature, coconut oil has been used for centuries by men and women the world over to improve the health of their skin and hair. Touted first in the West as a nutritional power food, coconut oil's benefits as a hair and skin enhancer have only recently gained popularity and traction in Western popular culture. In recent years, new research on this oil has given us valuable insight into its special benefits as both a protein reconstructor and a moisture sealant in hair care. Its polarity and straight-chain chemistry gives coconut oil particular advantages for those of us with textured hair types.

Coconut oil is a versatile, low-molecular-weight oil that effectively seals the hair and has a strong affinity for hair proteins not found in other hair oils. Coconut oil benefits black hair in two important ways. First, coconut oil's hydrophobic oil characteristics allow it to inhibit the penetration of water from the surrounding air and environment. Second, coconut oil is able to bind to the natural protein structure of the hair. This helps the hair retain its natural moisture content and reinforces the hair fiber, making it stronger. Coconut oil's ability to prevent protein loss and reduce hair porosity makes it valuable for those who chemically relax, regularly heat straighten or permanently color their hair. (26), (28)

Ancillary Hair Product Basics
Hair Gels

Hair gels are a popular styling product in the black community. These putty- and paste-like semi-solids help mold, sculpt and flatten textured tresses into a variety of sleek and defined curly styles. Despite their abilities to slick down or volumize hair on a whim, gels are often vilified hair products in the healthy hair care world. This backlash against hair gels is not without cause. Many commercial hair gels are simply too hard on fragile textured hair. When used regularly in a hair regimen, their mix of hard proteins and drying SD alcohols quickly depleted precious moisture and elasticity from the hair. Fortunately, there are a number of things you can do to increase the conditioning power of your hair gel.

First, only use gels on clean, conditioned hair. If you allow gels to accumulate on the hair fiber with oils and other styling products, you are creating a prime opportunity for dryness and hair breakage. Next, buffer the drying qualities of your hair gel by applying a moisturizer, oil or butter product to the hair prior to adding the gel. The moisture or lubricant buffer will sit under the gel and protect the hair fiber from contact with the gel's drying elements. Alternatively, you may combine your gel with a butter or oil before use to enhance its conditioning qualities and nourishing effect on the hair.

Never attempt to comb through or manipulate hard or dried gel. If you've used gel the day before, re-mist the hair to weaken the gel before attempting to detangle or style the hair. If you would simply like to refresh your gelled hairstyle, simply re-mist the hair with water to help it remember the hold, and then scrunch the hair for curl definition or tie it down briefly with a satin scarf to obtain a sleeker style.

Always use hair-friendly soft gels like Fantasia IC Polisher Gel with Sparkle-Lites, Ecostyler Gel or Kinky Curly Curling Custard. These gels have great hold but are much easier on textured hair. Avoid gel products that contain heavy proteins and harsh alcohol ingredients. These are most common in "quick-drying" protein gel formulas.

Heat Protectants

Heat protectants are used in healthy hair care regimens to slow heat transfer into the hair fiber and protect delicate strands from damage. These products come in a variety of forms including serums, creams, sprays and lotions. Silicones are common ingredients in heat protectants because they provide a slower rate of heat transfer from the heated appliance to the hair. Other common heat- protectant ingredients include silk amino acids and hydrolyzed wheat protein. Relaxed or fine hair types tend to do better with lotions and spray or mist-type heat protectants, while those with thicker, coarser strands often require creams and serums with a bit more weight.

Setting Lotions/Design Foams

Setting lotions and design foams are liquid, cream or foam-based styling products that are used to add structure, body, and hold to wet sets and blown-out, straightened styles. Setting lotions—similar to lightweight hair gels—generally dry the hair quickly and vary in moisturizing ability and hold. Depending on the formula, these lotions may require dilution prior to use on the hair.

Gel-Free Styling

If you would prefer to go gel-free but still want the option to wear sleek, slick styles, skip the gel and use the water-misting/satin-scarf method. First, mist your hair with water or a conditioning leave-in spray to soften the hair's hydrogen bonds and set your hair. Next, tie your moistened hair down with a scarf for five to ten minutes. Remove the scarf and enjoy your soft, sleek, gel-free tresses. For extra conditioning and hold, apply a hair butter to the hair after misting with the leave-in, and then tie the scarf down for control.

Chapter 6: Protein & Moisture Balancing Strategies for Breakage Correction and Defense

You've just learned about the basic roles of hair products and have made some initial product choices. Now it's time to learn about how to use those products and techniques strategically to solve hair problems. By far, the number one challenge facing those of us who are trying to achieve healthier hair is *chronic hair breakage*. Breakage is a common theme in recessive-maintenance and basic-maintenance hair regimens and it successfully keeps most of us with hair permanently cropped above our shoulders. It is like the haircut that you never asked for! Many times, hair breakage occurs so subtly that we don't perceive it—at least not initially. This form of chronic breakage is so slow and omnipresent that it may only be noticeable after some months and years have gone by.

In many hair care circles, protein conditioning is commonly called upon to fight every kind of hair breakage problem. Unfortunately, following this strategy often causes breakage issues to worsen. Instead, it's important to first understand that there are essentially two types of hair breakage. Each type must be handled differently.

Hair breakage is caused by protein and moisture imbalances in the hair fiber that are primarily brought on by patterns of improper product use and regular handling. Left unchecked, disturbances and irregularities in the hair's protein-moisture balance always lead to hair dryness and breakage. Unfortunately, as our styling choices have evolved over the years, our fragile hair's tendency toward breakage has only increased. Our hair is simply not equipped to handle the intense styling load of permanent hair coloring, high-tension weaving, heat styling and chemical relaxing on top of general cleansing, combing, and styling maintenance which naturally contribute to its demise.

Contrary to popular belief, there is no single product that can fight breakage alone, nor is there a product that can be used or applied across all breakage situations. Instead, we must employ a multi-product strategy to address the hair's needs. Every hair breakage scenario must be evaluated on its own merits and may require a different approach and product selection strategy to bring it under control. While it is impossible to completely rid the hair of breakage, when breakage levels are adequately *managed and controlled*, black hair thrives naturally.

Protein and Moisture Considerations Should Drive Product Choice

Establishing and maintaining an appropriate protein/moisture balance in the hair is vital to the success of any hair care regimen, and it is THE KEY to fighting hair breakage. Informed hair product selection is absolutely essential for making the protein and moisture balancing processes work. The right combination of products can make a major difference in the quality and appearance of textured hair.

Knowing the protein/moisture nature of products helps tremendously when it is time to rotate hair products in and out of a healthy hair care regimen. Some of us religiously use the same product line day in and day out without giving

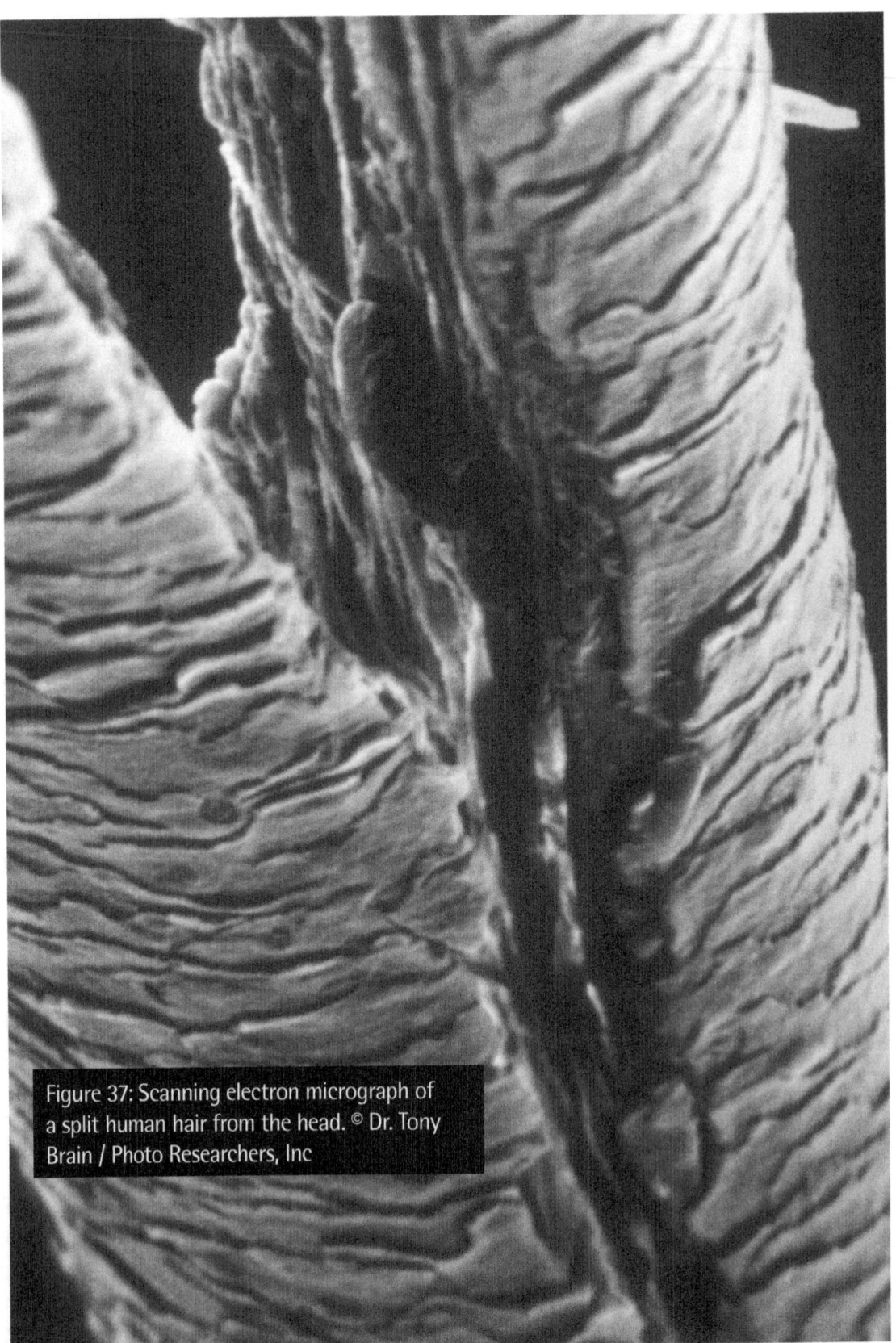

Figure 37: Scanning electron micrograph of a split human hair from the head. © Dr. Tony Brain / Photo Researchers, Inc

much thought to how the product is intended to work on the hair from a protein or moisture standpoint. Many of us select products based on word of mouth or what we have seen others use with amazing hair results. Unfortunately, these methods of hair product selection rarely work long term. If you aren't evaluating your products from the vantage point of protein versus moisture, you are not maximizing your hair products' potential.

Products: One Size Fits All?

Product selection is similar to purchasing the same gorgeous, designer dress that you saw your favorite celebrity wear on the red carpet. The dress hugs her curves and complements her skin tone flawlessly, but when you put the same dress on, the fit isn't as nice. In fact, it looks like a totally different dress! If your hair has one set of needs, but you choose hair care products based on what someone with different hair and different needs uses successfully, your hair will not respond well—even if the product you chose is of superior quality.

Understanding the Protein & Moisture Balancing Act

Protein and Moisture: The Cornerstones of Hair Care

Although a number of things can break hair fibers, black hair breakage tends to occur in two very basic forms: (Moisture Deficient) Protein-Induced hair breakage and (Protein Deficient) Moisture-Induced hair breakage. Both types of breakage stem from unbalanced, unresolved structural and elasticity conditions within the hair fiber. Here's how these imbalances affect the hair:

(Moisture Deficient) Protein-Induced Hair Breakage

Excess sun exposure, harsh shampoo products, heavy oil use and the overuse of styling techniques such as blow drying and flat ironing can all trigger moisture-deficiency in the hair. These stressors evaporate precious moisture from the hair strands or, in the case of oils, prevent the entry of moisture into the strands. The overutilization of protein-rich products such as protein conditioners, reconstructive treatments and hard gels also induces moisture deficiency. Hair in this state is usually hard, inelastic and rigid.

(Protein Deficient) Moisture-Induced Hair Breakage

Excess sun exposure and the overuse of styling techniques such as hair coloring and chemical relaxing are the chief culprits when it comes to protein-deficient hair. These stressors destroy the hair's natural protein structure. The overuse of rich, deep-conditioning treatments in a regimen (over-conditioning) that is not sufficiently balanced with protein-rebuilding products can also induce protein deficiency in hair. Hair in this state is often super-elastic or too soft, stretchy and may not hold curls or styles well.

Learning to effectively recognize the difference between protein-based and moisture-based breakage problems will help you to organize, or reorganize, your hair care regimen to effectively combat breakage issues as they arise. But the unique relationship that exists between protein and moisture within the hair strand is not simply a case of balancing one opposing force over the other. Rather, protein and moisture work together synergistically to produce a healthy head of hair. Neither can work well without the other. A heavy tendency or preference toward either protein or moisture in a hair care regimen, without a sufficient balance, always results in breakage. Hair damage that changes the hair's natural protein architecture, for instance, is almost always followed by some degree of moisture loss to the hair. Similarly, hair that is properly proteinated absorbs moisture more efficiently than hair with a shoddy protein structure because water molecules bind more easily to hair with a sound protein structure. When either the protein or moisture conditioning focus is lacking in a hair care regimen, the hair responds with breakage. Keeping the hair balanced between these two entities is vitally important to maintaining the condition of your hair.

Why Are We Breaking?

Breakage is the result of the hair's chemistry being thrown off balance. Growing out your hair, then, is a constant juggling act to maintain even protein and moisture balances within the hair fiber.

The vast majority of black hair breakage issues stem from simple overutilization of protein-rich products and the lack of real moisture sources in the regimen. Many of the products marketed to black hair product consumers are intensely protein-rich reconstructive treatments or oil-rich lubricating creams and conditioners—none of which contributes positively to the hair's moisture or hydration profile. The protein-rich products are in the marketplace because a majority of us chemically relax our hair and need the protein supplementation and replacement to rebuild our ravaged cuticles. We also need the oil-rich creams and conditioners to help reduce friction between the fibers and improve manageability. Because oils are not true sources of hair moisture, many of us are often shocked to find that we have very few real moisturizing products in our hair care regimens. Without a true hydration (water) component, our regimens are doomed to continue an endless cycle of dryness and breakage. Achieving the proper protein/moisture balance involves using the right combinations of protein and moisture-based products for your hair type at the right time. If many of us reconfigured our regimens to include real sources of moisture in place of oils, our hair would rehydrate and thrive!

Breaking Down Your Products

Your two biggest weapons against hair breakage will always be protein-based products and moisture-based products. Most hair products that you already own will fall into one of these two categories, and every product that you use tips your hair one way or the other on the protein/moisture balance scale. Whether your hair products are salon exclusive or yesterday's special from the grocery store, most can be classified as either moisture or protein based.

Hair products are either:

- protein reconstructing and rebuilding, **or**
- moisture replenishing and conditioning

Only non–water-based products such as oils, serums and relaxers fall outside the protein/moisture classification. These products are protein/moisture neutral. Understanding the difference between protein- and moisture-based products and what they do for your hair is the key to stopping breakage and achieving a healthier, more vibrant head of hair with increased length.

Using hair products that push your hair too far on either side of the protein/moisture-balance spectrum will always lead to hair breakage. Classifying the products you are using and developing a strategy to maintain a proper product balance is therefore extremely important. Breakage can be significantly minimized and managed by strategically alternating protein- and moisture-based products in your regimen.

Ingredients-Based Product Selection

The Science of Black Hair uses an "ingredients-based" approach to protein and moisture balancing. Although products in a particular line or brand are often designed to work with one another, there will never be one hair product or brand of products that can meet the entire scope of our hair needs 100 percent of the time. Product rotation is required, and to master product rotation, experimentation is key. An ingredients-focused regimen building strategy will always bring effective, high quality products into a regimen better than shopping by popular brands names alone.

Go ahead and grab your favorite products and take note of the labels.

The Ingredients List

As we discussed earlier, learning how to read a product ingredients list is an important skill that will enhance your healthy hair care efforts. Although many product labels seem to have been written by scientists for scientists, only a cursory understanding of these lists is needed to make a difference in the quality of your hair.

First, the ingredients list is usually a ranking of ingredients from highest to lowest concentration in the formula. As a rule of thumb, ingredients listed at the top of the list make up the bulk of the product, while ingredients found toward the end of the list are present in the product only in trace amounts. Knowing that most consumer-friendly product ingredients lists are presented in a top-down fashion can give you good information about whether a product will contribute to your hair's protein or moisture profile needs.

Occasionally, a manufacturer may present a product's ingredient information in alphabetical order—or attempt to play around a bit with the position of water and various trace ingredients in the list. This is why you should always take note of the placement of water in the list. In 99.9 percent of hair products that aren't greases, pomades, and serums, water will be the first ingredient. Occasionally, water will appear as one of the last ingredients in the list, and this is typically the work of a clever marketer and product manufacturer who has either alphabetized the list or floated the herbal ingredients in water. For example, you may see "aloe, rosemary extract, ginger root and thyme sprigs in spring water." In such a list, water is still the most plentiful ingredient percentage-wise, even though it comes last.

After the placement of water, the other things you want to look for in any product ingredients list are:

- the presence and variety of proteins,
- the presence of humectants or water-attracting ingredients, and
- the presence of emollients, oils and silicones.

Depending on the types of products you are reviewing, there may be other ingredients to track. For example, if you are considering a shampoo product, you should also check for a fourth type of ingredient: surfactants and/or detergents like sodium lauryl sulfate.

What To Check for in Protein Products

Almost all hair products contain some type of protein, but some contain more concentrated amounts of protein than others. Proteins in hair products comprise a vast ingredients category. The type of protein used in a hair care product will often give you a clue about the protein strength or protein richness of the product. Some proteins are better suited for reinforcing the hair's architecture, while others are better at supporting the hair's stretching and elastic characteristics. Because the proteins in hair products are fairly large substances relative to the naturally occurring components of hair, they are, for the most part, unable to penetrate the fiber and are largely surface-acting. Modern protein-rich deep conditioners often contain partially hydrolyzed proteins; this means that they have been broken down into low-molecular-weight amino acids that are more likely to bind strongly to the hair fiber. The smaller amino acids of these hydrolyzed proteins have longer-lasting effects on the hair fiber.

The major unknown with many of these products, however, is the percentage of protein in their composition. While its placement in the list gives us a clue about the strength of the protein in the product, we still cannot determine whether third place in line equals 40 percent or 4 percent of the total product composition. This is where experimentation with your hair will have to come into play.

When it comes to over-proteinating hair, the obvious culprits will be protein-reconstructor treatment products, volumizing shampoo and conditioner lines, most leave-in conditioners, setting lotions, gels, hair color rinses, thickening products, and other products that contain protein or hydrolyzed-protein-derived ingredients such as:

- amino acids (various)
- animal protein
- cholesterol
- collagen
- keratin
- milk protein
- panthenol
- soy protein
- wheat protein.

Hydrolyzed proteins tend to be the most aggressive types of proteins because they are small and concentrated. They can bind quickly to the tiny crevices in and around the cuticle scales.

What To Check for in Moisture Products

Water is by far the best moisturizing ingredient for black hair. Although many in our community still believe that water dries out the hair, this concept makes very little sense upon inspection. This old wives' tale, unfortunately, encourages many of us to hold off washing or wetting our hair for weeks and weeks at a time—often, to our detriment. Water alone simply cannot dry out the hair. Shampooing with harsh, sulfate detergent-rich shampoos is more likely the culprit. This aversion to the benefits of pure water for our hair, may be most responsible for the stagnant hair growth that is so common in the black community.

In addition to water, the universal moisturizer, humectants help to encourage moisture absorption in the hair fiber. These water-loving ingredients draw in moisture from the surrounding air to replenish and nourish the hair. Ceramides and emollients are another group of moisture-supporting ingredients that work by forming a breathable water barrier around the hair cuticle. These ingredients are lighter than traditional oils and help nourish the hair's cuticle. Examples of moisturizing ingredients include

alpha hydroxy acids
aqua
cetearyl alcohol
cetyl alcohol
glycerin(e)
glycerol
glyceryl triacetate
lactate
oleic acid
palmitic acid
polyquaternium
propylene glycol
pyrrolidine carboxylic acid
sodium PCA
sorbitol
stearic acid
stearyl alcohol
urea
water

Hair Evaluation Methodology

Shampooing and conditioning are significant hair maintenance steps that do more than simply clean the hair. These processes also provide important moisture and protein information about our hair fibers. Although healthy hair assessments can be performed on dry hair, determining the cause of hair breakage problems is often best determined on wet hair. When hair is wet, its strength and elasticity are amplified. The hair cleansing process enables us to quickly evaluate and address the condition of our hair and apply appropriate treatments to correct any deficiencies we may identify.

Wet Assessment: A Proven Strategy for Determining Causes of Breakage

Understanding the information your wet hair provides will help you keep your hair appropriately balanced between moisture and protein. Each shampoo and conditioning session is a prime opportunity for hair evaluation and problem correction. Hair can be manipulated and wet tested during the normal course of shampooing, conditioning and detangling hair. Thorough and frequent wet assessments will help you maintain your hair's health and condition.

Pay close attention to the way your hair feels when it is wet. Is it spongy? Hard? Stretchy? Fragile? Does it dry very quickly in the air? Does it take time to feel fully wet? Take the time to note any shed or broken hair strands that come about from your cleansing session. Consider the amount of fallen hair and the means by which the hair was lost. Were you shampooing too roughly? Was your hair tangling terribly? Were you combing it out too aggressively? These wet assessments are very important for identifying and treating hair dryness and breakage issues. Once you develop a baseline for how your hair should feel, you will be able to properly catch and diagnose any deviations from its normal, healthy feel.

The Difference between Shedding and Breakage

Before we move into solving hair breakage problems through wet assessment, we must make an important distinction between naturally shed hairs and truly broken hairs. You will encounter both types of strands as you deal with your hair. People often use the terms "shed" and "broken" interchangeably to describe any and all

What if you Cannot Wet Assess the Hair?

If your hair is braided or styled in a way that does not allow you to easily determine your protein or moisture needs, you will need to alternate the protein and moisture on a weekly or bi-weekly schedule as preventive maintenance. Always lean on the side of moisture when in doubt. Breakage or problems from over-conditioning with moisture are easier to correct than problems from over-conditioning with protein. Spray your hair daily with a moisturizing spray for three days and alternate with a protein spray daily for two. The technique is three days on moisture, two days on protein alternating in that manner.

hair that falls from the scalp. The major difference between hair shedding and hair breakage is that hair shedding is a natural process that takes place regardless of the quality of your hair care. Light shedding should be viewed as a sign of a healthy, normally functioning scalp. Breakage, on the other hand, is caused by damage, stress or deficiencies in the hair fiber.

Hair shedding is a response to hormonal signaling in the body and is largely dependent on the hair's natural growth phase, which you'll remember moves naturally from growth, to rest and to fall before starting all over again. Only hair that has reached the end of its growing cycle falls from the scalp with its tiny, white "root" attached. Remember, this bulbous part of the hair is not the actual root (or follicle), which is secured deep within your scalp, but rather the base of the hair strand that originates in the scalp. This so-called root is white because hair stops producing melanin (color) at the point in its growth cycle just before it is programmed to fall. If a hair does not possess this white bulb, then it is not a naturally shed hair but a broken one.

Shed hairs also tend to be longer than broken hairs, which are generally short pieces of varying lengths. If your hair is relaxed, your shed hair will generally have curly new growth present on the root end.

What Can I Do about Shedding?

Because shedding is a natural, internal process, it may not respond to topical or external treatments. Similarly, shedding is not easily solved by protein- or moisture-balancing treatments because it has nothing to do with the hair shaft itself but is a response to hormonal influences on the hair follicle. Our hair naturally cycles in and out of seasonal shedding phases, which may last for days or even weeks in some individuals. A healthy head of hair may shed as many as fifty to one hundred hairs per day. (7) Some individuals shed much less. You should be concerned only if your shedding rate suddenly increases to a rate that was uncommon for you previously or if the shedding seems to be prolonged over a period of several weeks or months without cause.

Shedding naturally increases during certain points in our lives. For example, women who have recently given birth generally experience postpartum shedding. After giving birth,

Why is My Hair Shedding?
- Styling methods that place stress on the follicles
- Birth control/menstrual cycles/menopause
- Pregnancy
- Heredity—runs in the family
- Crash dieting/ low protein diets
- High fever as a prevailing symptom
- Anemia
- Thyroid disorders
- Certain medications, major surgeries and chemotherapy

a woman's shedding rate may increase dramatically for several months in response to a steep decline in her hormone levels that occurs after the baby is delivered. The profuse shedding ceases only when her normal pre-baby hormone levels return.

If your shedding seems to have increased significantly or you are concerned that your shedding may be medically-related, consult a medical professional.

What Is Balanced, Healthy Hair?

Balanced

Your wet hair feels strong, stretches slightly and returns to its original length with no breakage.

Balanced, healthy hair is very resilient. Its protein strength and elastic moisture characteristics are well balanced within the fiber. The hair feels great, moves well and has amazing luster. Depending on the individual's hair type, it will either have great shine or sheen. Although balanced, healthy black hair (like all hair) is weaker when wet, it will not break unless unusual stress is applied to it through aggressive handling, combing or detangling. Healthy protein and moisture-balanced hair feels soft and supple yet strong, whether wet or dry.

Organization Is Great, but... Flexibility Is the Key!

The protein/moisture balance is very personal and it varies by the individual. Your job is to keep your hair balanced in the middle of your protein/moisture spectrum, which can be quite a feat! Flexibility will be your best aid in maintaining a proper balance. Unfortunately, when many people begin to put a regimen together, they schedule everything and essentially put their hair on a calendar. This method is difficult to keep up, and it rarely works in the long term. Hair is very fickle and its needs change daily. You simply have to follow it as it leads you.

So, back to wet assessment! If you are experiencing hair breakage, the way your hair feels and breaks while it is wet will give you an indication of whether more protein or moisture supplementation is required to regain the proper balance. You can use the sample product regimens that follow in the sections below to improve your hair's con-

dition and curb breakage issues. These regimens are totally flexible! You may use the products in the Regimen Builder to complete each sample regimen, or if you do not own these products, you can simply gauge the products you currently own by analyzing their ingredients lists to determine where they would fit into these regimens.

Recognizing Moisture Deficiencies
Low Moisture Hair Breakage

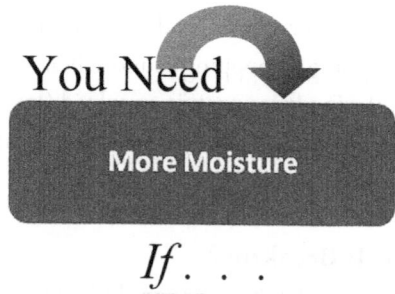

You Need

More Moisture

If . . .

Your wet hair feels rough, hard and tangly. Hair does not stretch much before breaking

Low moisture hair care regimens are the most common source of breakage in black hair care. Hair that is not treated regularly with moisturizing deep-conditioning treatments, and hair that is cleansed less than once weekly with moisturizing products is a prime candidate for moisture deficiency breakage. Regimens that feature regular heat styling and daily products such as greases, pomades, alcohol-based hair gels and holding sprays also tend to fall into this breakage category.

Occasionally, the overuse of protein-based products such as "hair repair" and reconstructor treatments is to blame for low moisture hair breakage. This condition is often referred to as "protein overload" in Internet hair care circles. Because proteins bind very strongly to the hair's cuticle and cortex in an effort to strengthen the fiber, this form of hair breakage can take the longest time to correct and bring under control.

Protein binding is marked in extremely damaged, stressed or porous hair. When there is too much protein working in a regimen, the bound protein must be freed from the cuticle by subsequent wettings/washings. This process can take several wash cycles to complete.

Hair that suffers from moisture-deficiency breakage is super fragile but looks and feels rough and tough. Hair in this condition is often stiff because, without moisture, it lacks natural elasticity. Moisture-deficient hair breaks easily and snaps most often into tiny, short pieces. This form of breakage tends to produce an audible snapping or popping sound when it occurs. Hair suffering from protein overload/low moisture also may take time to feel thoroughly wet when it is cleansed.

Why Is It Breaking?

Breakage from moisture deficiency occurs when the hair is not receiving enough hydration on a daily or weekly basis. The hair's moisture level could be negatively affected by heat styling or chemical processes, for example. Hair products may be largely lubricants and oils which reduces the net moisture contribution through product usage. Or an individual with this type of breakage may not be hydrating her hair often enough from within (water intake) and without (regular moisturizing deep-conditioning/daily water-based moisturizer). In relative terms, the hair is receiving more conditioning and treatment from protein sources than from moisture sources.

Protein-rich products support the cuticle by filling up broken spaces and adding structure to the entire length of the hair strand. Unfortunately, cuticle repair can go into overdrive through overuse of products, resulting in increased hair breakage. Adding too much structure to the hair fiber makes it rigid and reduces its elastic properties, leaving it brittle and prone to breakage. When you give your hair more protein than is needed to maintain a healthy balance, you will experience hair breakage from protein overload.

I often hear from women who say, "Well, I don't use protein reconstructors. How could I be getting breakage from protein overload?" The answer is, while you may not be doing protein treatments or using specific damage-repair reconstructors, you may be using other products such as leave-in conditioners, gels or moisturizers that are protein heavy relative to the moisturizing products in your regimen.

How Much Is Too Much Protein?

We are all different, and our hair's protein needs will vary from individual to individual. From chemical relaxing, bleaching and coloring, some of us have lost more of the natural protein in our strands than others and therefore require personalized levels of protein replacement. Given the variance in protein needs across the board, there is no right or wrong amount of protein supplementation needed in a hair care regimen. You should always note how your hair feels after using your protein-rich products, whether these are moisturizers, leave-ins or specific treatments. If you notice that your hair has become harder, more rigid and less pliable, and that it subsequently begins breaking more easily—you need to alternate to a more moisturizing, less protein-heavy product regimen. This will increase the moisture levels in your hair and reinstate your hair's natural elasticity and moisture balance.

Recognizing Protein Deficiencies
Low Protein Hair Breakage

Low protein hair breakage tends to come more often from processes that actively destroy the hair's natural protein—chemical processing, permanent coloring, excessive heat use and severe sun damage—than from simple overutilization of moisture-rich products. These processes cause damage to the hair cuticle that increases porosity. Therefore, the source of the dryness in this

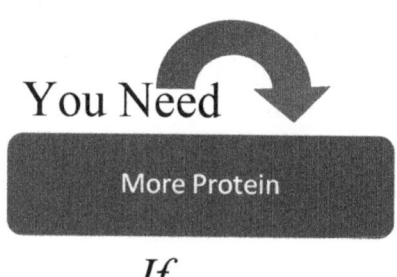

You Need

More Protein

If . . .

If your wet hair feels weak, gummy and limp. Hair stretches and stretches before breaking

form of breakage is the hair's increased porosity and shoddy protein infrastructure, which encourages moisture to flow into the fiber, but allows moisture to exit the fiber unopposed.

A secondary cause of this form of low protein breakage is simply over-conditioning the hair with moisturizing products or keeping the hair in a damp or wet state for long periods of time. In these situations, shoddy cuticle structure is again the instigator of hair breakage. Without solid protein backing and infrastructure, the hair's natural elasticity can kick into overdrive. Healthy hair will stretch because it has natural elastic properties, but stretching can damage textured hair, particularly in regions of the fiber where there is little natural protein support. Re-

search has shown that the naturally protein-free areas of the cuticle—the endocuticle and CMC portions of the cortex—are most damaged by stretching. (1) There is a point where a stretch becomes too much for the hair to withstand, and recognizing this threshold is very important for protecting against breakage.

Hair typically breaks when stretched beyond roughly 25 percent of its natural length. The closer to the scalp the stretching occurs, the longer the hair will stretch before it breaks. The resistance to stretching higher up the shaft is because hair is generally healthiest when it first emerges from the scalp. Toward the ends of the hair, there is more damage and so less leeway for stretching before breakage will occur. This further underscores the point that ends should be handled gently and with expert care. At the critical stretching point, the cuticle scales loosen from the cortex and the hair is irreparably damaged. Before protein-deficiency breakage occurs, however, your hair will give off several warning signs. Hair will seem to go limp first and will stretch considerably in this weakened state prior to breaking. This is an indication that structural protein components of the hair are deficient and can't properly balance the elasticity level of the hair.

Determine Your Level of Breakage: "Breakage Zoning"

After determining the source of your breakage, you may find it useful to categorize your level of breakage to help with product selection and correction. There are three main breakage levels or zones—minimal (Zone 1), moderate (Zone 2) and heavy (Zone 3)—for each major cause of breakage. Classifying your approximate level of breakage will help you select the proper product and strength to correct your imbalance without tipping the balance too far in the opposite direction. You will find product recommendations for hair correction in each breakage zone in the Regimen Builder to follow.

Products and weather conditions can cause your hair to change breakage zones quickly. Stronger processes such as chemical relaxers and colors can take minimal Zone 1 breakage to severe Zone 3 breakage almost instantaneously. Be proactive about hair breakage and follow the cues and signs your hair gives. Remember, you do not have to wait for breakage to act!

As you work to correct your protein/moisture balance, always remain flexible and cognizant of your hair and how it is feeling. You may find that as you complete the steps in the regimen appropriate for each breakage zone, your hair will self correct before you are able to complete all of the steps. You may also find that you have to repeat a zone regimen for a week or two before the balance returns. The possibilities are endless! Always pay close attention to what your hair is telling you. This will help you know when to stay the course and when to redirect your efforts. Learning to "read" your hair takes practice, and you will make a few mistakes along the way. The mistakes and successes are all important parts of the learning process, and will help you avoid problems in the future!

Finally, the suggested breakage correction regimens that follow are just that: suggestions.

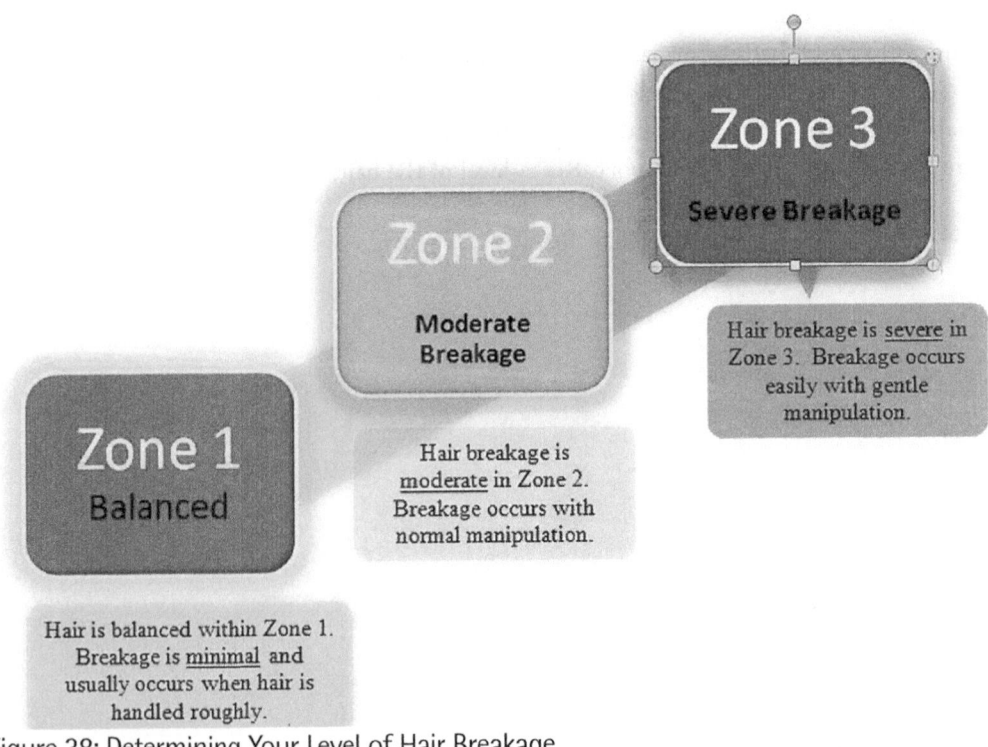

Figure 38: Determining Your Level of Hair Breakage

You should feel free to alter and adjust the regimens to suit your hair's needs, your tastes and your lifestyle. There is a wealth of beauty and clarity in experimentation. No two heads of hair are the same, and what works for one cannot possibly be expected to translate—product for product and step by step—to 100 percent success for others.

As you follow the steps in each corrective regimen, you must pay attention to and evaluate your hair at each step. It is possible that your condition may correct itself in the first one or two steps of each regimen, so it may be unnecessary for you to follow the regimen from beginning to end. You also may need to adjust the conditioning times to reap the best benefits and to suit your own hair and lifestyle. Conditioning needs depend on your personal level of breakage, prior treatments, specific product use and level of hair porosity. You must learn to read your hair's cues! Some regimens, particularly the moisture-deficiency (low moisture) breakage corrections, will require weeks of use before results appear. You must be diligent and patient and use these regimens as flexible guidelines.

Zone 1 Breakage (Balanced Hair)

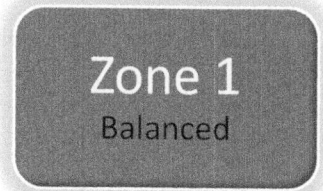

Zone 1 is the healthy "green zone" in which hair is balanced and daily breakage is minimal to nonexistent. Because our textured strands are such delicate fibers, despite even our very best efforts, we cannot expect to have no breakage whatsoever. Therefore, occasional breakage here and there is still considered balanced.

When breakage does occur in Zone 1, it is typically after an intense styling episode.

The rule of thumb for breakage counts in Zone 1 is fewer than five broken strands on non-wash days and less than ten broken hairs on wash days. Essentially, Zone 1 breakage is so minimal that you can count broken hairs on one hand. No large clumps of hair should be lost to breakage during detangling in this zone. Shed hairs will give the illusion that more breakage is taking place than is truly the case, but shed hairs should not be factored into your breakage assessment. In Zone 1, slight fluctuations in the protein/moisture balance may occur but do not result in noticeable amounts of breakage.

Zone 2 Breakage

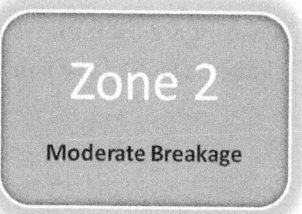

Zone 2, the "yellow zone," is where much of our breakage occurs. This is the intermediate stage between healthy, unbroken hair and severe damage and breakage. Zone 2 breakage is usually the result of minimal Zone 1 breakage either being neglected or misdiagnosed and given improper protein or moisture treatment. For instance, this may occur if more protein conditioning is given to hair that needs moisture or if porous hair with an inadequate protein backbone receives too much moisturizing treatment.

Daily breakage in this zone is slightly higher than in Zone 1 and occurs more easily, even with normal manipulation. The rule of thumb for breakage counts in Zone 2 is no more than ten to fifteen hairs lost on non-wash days and no more than fifteen to twenty hairs on wash days. In Zone 2, hair covers your sink and floor after styling. Medium to large clumps of hair may be lost after detangling and comb-out. Hair should be properly treated at this point to avoid further damage.

Zone 3 Breakage

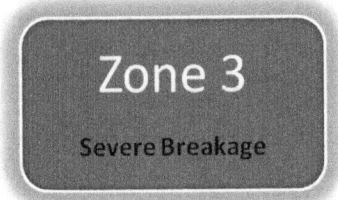

Zone 3, the "red zone," is the hair breakage zone encountered when hair breakage and damage issues have gone unresolved in the previous zones. Hair breakage in this zone is chronic and heavy. Zone 3 breakage is most often the result of Zone 2 breakage allowed to continue untreated for extended periods of time. Signs of thinning, short pieces, patchy hair loss in areas and sparsely filled areas are common. A see-through "hemline" along the ends of the hair is the greatest indicator and telltale sign of Zone 3 breakage run amuck.

Daily breakage is extremely common in Zone 3, even with low-manipulation styling. Large clumps of hair are lost routinely during comb-outs and on wash days. Hair covers your sink, floor and back after styling. The rule of thumb for breakage counts in Zone 3 is more than ten to fifteen hairs lost on non-wash days and more than fifteen to twenty hairs lost on wash days. Chemical treatments such as relaxing and permanent coloring can transform minimal Zone 1 breakage into severe Zone 3 breakage almost overnight. The proper corrective treatments must be followed diligently over a period of time to return hair experiencing Zone 3 breakage to a healthy balance. Ultimately, some cutting may be required to usher in the balanced, healthy hair.

Breakage Correction for Moisture Deficiencies
Zone 1 Low Moisture Breakage Corrective Regimen

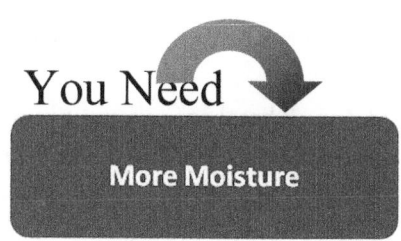

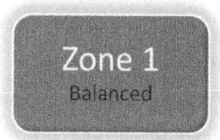

Since Zone 1 hair is considered balanced, any low-moisture breakage typically is corrected in one moisturizing deep-conditioning session. The mildest forms of Zone 1 breakage can be corrected by simply treating the hair once or twice a day with a water-based moisturizer. For Zone 1 low moisture breakage, follow these steps:

1. Choose a sulfate-free shampoo from the Regimen Builder.
2. Detangle your hair. Then, thoroughly saturate the hair with warm water for one or two minutes to remove any topical debris on the strands and scalp.
3. Apply your shampoo. Gently massage your scalp with the pads of your fingers.
4. Rinse out your shampoo thoroughly.
5. Apply a moisturizing conditioner from the regimen builder for ten to fifteen minutes, with or without heat.
6. Rinse out the conditioner in cool water. Allow the hair to cool first if heat was used.
7. Apply your leave-in conditioner if desired. At

this point, you should be able to determine, using the wet assessment method and touch testing, whether or not your next step needs to include a product with more moisture or more protein.
8. Apply a moisturizer.
9. Finish with an oil to seal the hair.

Zones 2 and 3 Low Moisture Breakage Corrective Regimens

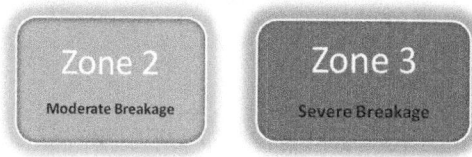

Correcting Zone 2 and Zone 3 low moisture breakage will require much more intensive conditioning with moisturizing deep conditioners. These levels of breakage can take several weeks to repair, and the suggested regimen may need to be followed for several consecutive washes. For Zones 2 and 3 low moisture breakage, follow these steps:

1. Select a sulfate-free shampoo from the Regimen Builder
2. Detangle your hair. Then, thoroughly saturate your hair with warm water for one or two minutes to remove any topical debris on the strands and scalp.
3. Apply your shampoo. Gently massage your scalp with the pads of your fingers.
4. Rinse out the shampoo thoroughly. Apply a moisturizing conditioner from the Regimen Builder for fifteen to twenty minutes, with heat.
5. After allowing the hair to cool, rinse out the conditioner with cool water, blot hair dry with a microfiber towel and apply your leave-in conditioner. For Zone 2 and 3 hair, you will need a moisturizing leave-in conditioner (see Regimen Builder).
6. Apply a moisturizer.
7. Finish with an oil to seal the hair.

Breakage Correction for Protein Deficiencies

Zone 1 Low Protein Breakage Corrective Regimen

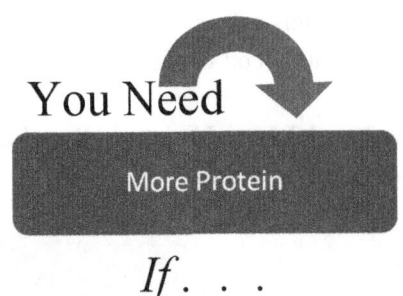

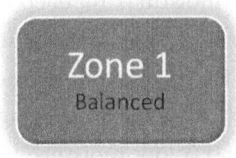

Zone 1 low protein breakage is typically corrected in one protein deep-conditioning session. The mildest forms can be corrected by simply moisturizing the hair twice a day with a water-based moisturizer that contains protein. The best protein products for Zone 1 breakage are light instant conditioners, leave-in conditioners and protein-based moisturizers. Follow the same shampoo and conditioning steps required for the Zone 1 Moisture Deficiency Corrective Regimen above, substituting in protein-rich conditioners, leave-ins and moisturizers from the Regimen Builder where moisture products are referenced.

Zones 2 and 3 Low Protein Breakage Corrective Regimen

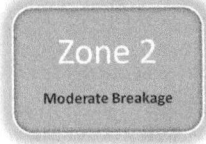
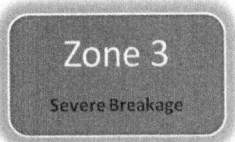

Mild Zone 2 breakage may require only the use of a moderate protein-based conditioner or protein-based moisturizer once or twice each week. For some, one treatment will restore the hair's balance because protein-deficiency breakage is generally easier to correct than moisture-deficiency breakage.

If your breakage is on the border of Zone 2, heading into Zone 3, a mild reconstructive treatment may be in order. Zone 3 low-protein breakage will require a heavier protein-reconstructor treatment.

1. Detangle your hair. Then, thoroughly saturate your hair with warm running water for one or two minutes to remove any topical debris on the strands and scalp.

2. To support the deepest penetration of protein, you may first wish to use a low-level sulfate shampoo or mild clarifying formula to lift debris and products from the hair. Apply your shampoo, and gently massage your scalp with the pads of your fingers.

3. Rinse out the shampoo thoroughly.

4. Apply a protein-rich conditioning product or treatment that corresponds to the level of protein deficiency. Cover the hair with a plastic cap, and apply heat for 10-15 minutes or for the time indicated in the directions on the product package. Heat use is optional but recommended to support maximum product penetration.

5. Rinse out the conditioning treatment with cool water. If heat has been used, allow the hair to cool for several minutes before rinsing thoroughly.

6. Apply a creamy moisturizing conditioner for another ten to fifteen minutes. Additional heat use is optional.
7. Thoroughly rinse the conditioner from the hair, blot dry and proceed to detangle. (If heat has been used, allow the hair to cool for several minutes before you rinse.)
8. Apply a protein-rich leave-in conditioner if desired.
9. Apply a protein-rich moisturizer.
10. Finish with an oil to seal the hair.

NOTE: Since protein-deficiency breakage is relatively easy to correct, using protein-based products from beginning to end of this regimen may flip your balance in the opposite direction. In fact, you may find that your balance is restored at the shampoo or protein conditioner stage. Monitor your hair as you complete this regimen. As you feel your hair begin to strengthen, you may switch over to more moisturizing products.

Ambiguous Hair

You've tried the moisture, you've tried the protein—or you are not sure where to begin tackling your hair issues. Occasionally, over the course of a new regimen, you may notice times when your hair is simply unreadable and does not respond to your attempts to treat it. Many times, hair that does not respond to treatment is burdened with product buildup. Even the lightest products can accumulate and build up on the hair shaft, rendering our moisturizing and protein-replacement efforts futile. At other times, unresponsiveness to treatments may be due to an underlying problem with the hair that is unrecognized or has been misdiagnosed. In other words, you may have been applying the wrong treatments.

The following regimen is a remedy for hair that is not responding to your attempts to treat it. This treatment also can be done as a once-monthly maintenance step in your regular schedule. Since this is a stripping wash (essentially removing all products and natural oils from your hair and getting it back to the bare essentials), this treatment should always be done sparingly—never more than once or twice per month—and must be followed by deep conditioning. Subsequent cleansings should be done according to your hair's needs and always with a gentle, sulfate-free shampoo whenever possible.

NOTE: If you are recovering from protein overload, this sample regimen does not apply to you. Protein-induced breakage takes a few weeks or several washes to clear up. Although your hair may not appear to be responding to treatment, each shampoo and conditioning treatment is restoring your moisture balance and lessening the protein's hold on your hair. Remember, since protein-rich products bind to the cuticle, depending on the strength of the protein or period of time during which these products were used, they may take a longer time to remove.

Corrective Regimen for Ambiguous Hair

1. Choose a clarifying shampoo or a strong sodium lauryl and/or ammonium lauryl sulfate regular shampoo. Any shampoo with clarifying ability will be fine.
2. Thoroughly saturate your hair with warm water for one or two minutes to remove any topical debris on the strands and scalp.
3. Apply your shampoo, and gently massage your scalp with the pads of your fingers.
4. Rinse out the shampoo thoroughly with warm water.
5. Apply a mild protein conditioner and leave on for about ten minutes, with or without heat.
6. Rinse out conditioner with cool water. (If heat has been used, allow the hair to cool for several minutes before you rinse.)

7. Apply a moisturizing deep conditioner. Cover with a plastic cap and apply heat for ten to fifteen minutes.

8. Alternatively, to speed the process, combine steps 5 and 7 and apply the two conditioners together. Then cover hair with a plastic cap. Apply heat for ten to fifteen minutes.

9. Rinse under cool water. Remember to cool down the hair first if heat was used.

10. Blot the hair dry with a microfiber towel.

11. Apply a leave-in conditioner if desired.

12. Detangle, and apply a moisturizer.

13. Finish with an oil to seal the hair.

This treatment should effectively free up the hair shaft and allow you to better determine the cause of your hair breakage problems.

Chapter 7: Getting Started with a Healthy Hair Care Product Regimen

The main reason that many of us have failed to reach our hair goals is because we follow regimens that lack the proper protein and moisture conditioning components. We should always begin with a more moisture-friendly product regimen in the early days of regimen building. Why do we start with moisture?

The reason for emphasizing moisture over protein is that many of us (before our hair-care awakening) have naturally moisture-deficient hair care routines. Rarely do hair problems arise as a result of over-conditioning and excess moisture. About 99 percent of the time, poor moisturizing and conditioning are the issues that spawn our hair care interventions. Hair care beginners should get in the habit of hydrating and conditioning their hair twice a week for the first four to six weeks of their regimens. Once a healthy hair baseline has been established, reducing the number of cleansings/deep conditionings to once per week works rather well for most.

Getting the Most Out of Frequent Hydration

In order to garner maximum benefit from regular hair hydration, three important things must be in order.

First and foremost, hydration success is in the products we use. Our hair can be safely shampooed and conditioned several times a week or even daily, as long as proper moisturizing and conditioning products are used. Many of us simply use the wrong shampoos and conditioning products! Harsh shampoo detergents and shaft-coating conditioner agents work against the hair's moisture balance and dry out textured tresses.

Cleansing the hair with a moisturizing shampoo that does not contain sodium lauryl sulfate (SLS) or ammonium lauryl sulfate (ALS) cleansing agents is the first step toward successful, frequent cleansing.

Likewise, the hair should be deep conditioned with a quality conditioner that contains few heavy oils (especially mineral oil or petrolatum). Silicone ingredients are okay as long as they do not directly follow water in the ingredients list. The conditioner you choose should address a particular protein or moisture need and should be rotated continuously at the next wash with a different conditioner designed to meet the opposite protein or moisture need in order to maintain the hair's protein/moisture balance from week to week.

On Frequent Hair Hydration

Over the years, I've e-coached many women on the value and importance of increasing the frequency of their "hair washing" in the first few weeks and months of their new healthy hair care regimen. Many of them found that their hair was much fuller and softer to the touch after adding in an additional wash each week.

In most healthy hair regimens, the first change one sees is a change in the hair's thickness. Changes in thickness often always precede visual changes in length. This increase in thickness is primarily due to a restoration of the hair's preferred moisture balance and the inability of shaft-coating hair products to negatively affect the hair's natural volume and body.

Next, improvements in your hair's moisture level must be balanced with a proper protein structure in order to prevent hair breakage. Hair that is frequently conditioned will eventually require protein supplementation to ruggedize the hair fiber. Many of us have not benefited from regular hydration because we do not know how to pick up on the cues our hair gives when it needs additional protein, or moisture. The wet-assessment method described in the Protein and Moisture Balancing chapter will help you learn how to address your hair's protein and moisture conditioning needs accurately.

The third key to frequent hair hydration is putting protective measures in place to reduce hygral fatigue (see Oil and Butter Basics section). Hygral fatigue is simply the damage that occurs to the hair fiber from the repeated process of expansion (when wet) to contraction (when dried). Beating hygral fatigue is all about maintaining the innate protein architecture of the hair shaft. If the protein structure is intact, the hair fiber will resist excessive expansion when wet. Ensuring a proper protein structure through timely protein conditioning is essential. A polar oil, such as coconut oil, may be used as a pre-shampoo treatment to strengthen hair fibers and reinforce the hair's protein structure prior to cleansing. Polar oils bind to the proteins in the hair shaft and reduce the amount of expansion in wet hair fibers so that they can better endure frequent hydrating. (26)

The Regimen Builder will walk you through the types of products you will need to put together your healthy hair care regimen strategy.

The Regimen Builder

We've now seen how the ingredients in our hair products and the basic care techniques we employ can affect our hair—for better or for worse. Now it's time to start narrowing down product choices to develop a hair care product regimen that works. What makes a hair product or brand great ultimately depends on the user and her hair goals. Some individuals prefer to make and use their own natural products using things from the earth, while others much prefer the convenience of a commercially-packaged, off-the-shelf product. Still others prefer the quality of high-end salon products to everyday bargain brands. No matter your personal product preference, healthy hair can be achieved through all of these product-selection routes.

Natural Products vs. Commercial Products

Some natural-living enthusiasts argue that almost all commercially available products contain chemical compounds that should be avoided in favor of all-natural products. Though this position requires a grand shift in our way of thinking about products, and may be a lofty call to action for some, it is a significantly valid position that should not be dismissed lightly. Preliminary research has uncovered possible links between some commercially available product ingredients and increased incidence of cancer and other health problems in the black community. (25) Research into the health risks of chemicals has focused primarily on commercially available products containing hormones (i.e., estrogens/placenta), phthalates (found in plastics) and popular preservatives known as parabens. While no firm link has been found to exist between hair products and cancer incidence to date, reducing exposure to even a few chemicals in hair products, cosmetics or everyday foods is a step toward better overall health, hair and peace of mind.

In the end, product selection is a matter of personal choice. Ideally, we want products that are as natural as possible. The fewer difficult-to-pronounce names a product formula contains, the better for our hair and our health. Many times, however, we simply do not have easy access to all-natural products, either because they are cost prohibitive or just aren't as easy to pick up at a local store. Ultimately, the product-selection process depends on the user's goals and involves quite a bit of trial and error. With the exception of products that are specifically designed to change the shape and composition of the hair fiber—traditional, commercial shampoos, conditioners and moisturizer products that are not 100 percent natural or organic still have much to offer in the way of improved cosmetic hair appearance. Remember, although products are important, techniques always trump products and brands when it comes to healthy hair care.

Finally, there are simply no universal hair products that work well for everyone. In addition, there is no guarantee that any hair product will meet the expectations and claims presented on its bottle. Because the U.S. Food and Drug Administration (FDA) regards hair products as cosmetics, they are not regulated with the same intensity as products classified as drugs, nor must they undergo stringent safety and effectiveness testing. In fact, there is no guarantee that the ingredients advertised on a cosmetics or hair-product label are complete or that those listed are even in the product! Always exercise caution when trying new hair products for the first time, especially those from unknown manufacturers.

Science of Black Hair Street Interview

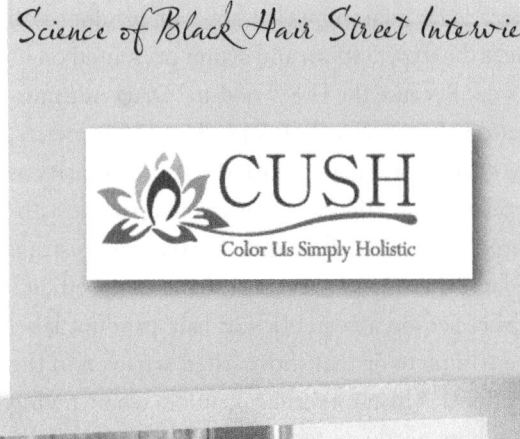

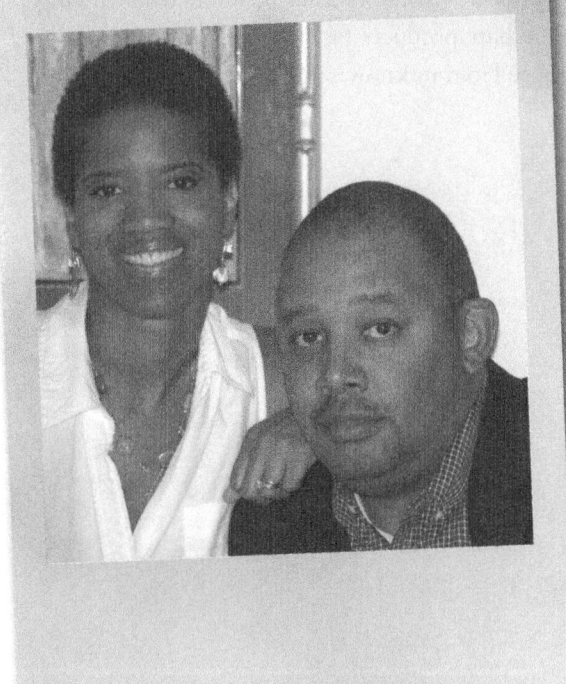

Name: Joe and Toni Parker
Occupation: Husband and wife team who co-founded Color Us Simply Holistic, LLC (CUSH) Cosmetics. CUSH is a hair product company that specializes in developing chemical-free product alternatives for the hair and cosmetics industries. **The Science of Black Hair** spoke with Toni Parker:

Q: **Tell us more about CUSH Cosmetics. What was your inspiration for taking the natural product challenge?**

A: *I was diagnosed with high blood pressure about seven years ago and wanted to look for ways to lower it naturally. My daughter was three years old at that time and she had asthma. The doctors wanted to put her on steroids. I thought to myself: There is no way we can give her steroids and have that become a way of life for her at three. So I started looking into natural alternatives to help me lower my blood pressure and to help her control her asthma. What I discovered in my research absolutely shocked me. For the first time, I understood that the foods we were eating and the products we were putting on our bodies and in our hair, absolutely impacted our health. I knew in that moment that I wanted to be a change agent in the black community to help get us back on track in terms of our overall health.*

My husband has a background in the personal care/cosmetics industry, and I had been asking him to create a natural cosmetics line for me. However during that time, he was in charge of engineering for a major cosmetics company and was too busy to hear me! So, I just kept doing research and eventually went on to become a Certified Holistic Health Coach. I did a major overhaul of our personal diets and our skin care products. I also continued to press my husband to create something that we could market. Six years and many months of research later, he came to me and said that he was ready to launch a product line. CUSH Cosmetics was born!

Q: **The term "natural" has different meanings for different people. What does natural mean to you? What is the CUSH cosmetics philosophy on product ingredients?**

A: *To us, natural has only one meaning: the product does not contain harsh chemicals, preservatives or synthetic fragrances. The CUSH philosophy is simply to use the best and safest botanicals, essential oils and other natural ingredients to formulate high-performing, salon quality skin and hair care products at affordable prices.*

Q: **In your opinion, which product ingredients are the worst offenders for black hair and black health?**

A: *On my list of the top 5 ingredients that consumers should absolutely avoid are 1.) sulfates, 2.) betaines, 3.) parabens, 4.) phthalates, and 5.) synthetic fra-*

grances. *Preliminary research has found that many of these ingredients not only strip our skin and hair of its natural oils, but some have even been linked to kidney damage, skin rashes, asthma, reproductive problems, birth defects, and even cancer risk.*

Q. What do you think of the trend toward "natural, chemical-free" products in mainstream hair care lines? Are manufacturers falling short?

A. *Unfortunately, mainstream hair care lines still have a long way to go in terms of creating truly, authentically green cosmetics. They continue to fall short, especially where African Americans are concerned because they simply do not see demand for safer cosmetics coming from us. We are not telling manufacturers that we do not want parabens or synthetic fragrances in products that are marketed to us. Think like a manufacturer. It is much cheaper for companies to use parabens as a preservative, for example, than greener alternative preservatives. This affects overall price to the end user: the cheaper the ingredients, the lower the retail price. Yet, having said that, many high-end products continue to be manufactured using these cheaper, harmful ingredients, but are sold at very expensive prices.*

Q. What challenges does CUSH Cosmetics face as a small, organic product retailer?

A. *Our biggest challenges of course are marketing and advertising. It really does work. The more we are on social media sites and working with bloggers and sites like The Science of Black Hair, the more we generate business. It would be great if we had the budget and/or the connections to broaden our base and start to do more magazine advertisement, or QVC/Home Shopping Network advertisement, and attend more trade shows.*

Q. What is your favorite CUSH and non-CUSH hair product and why?

A. *I have my favorite regimen. I absolutely love the Hydratation Supreme Shampoo, the Hydrate Me Leave-In Conditioner, the Moisturize Me Leave-In Conditioner, and the Mango Pomade by CUSH. The combination of those products leaves my hair feeling moisturized and my curls and coils nicely defined. My favorite non-CUSH product is Kinky Curly's Curling Custard. First of all, it meets my safety standards and secondly, it gives my coils a nice light hold.*

Q. What can we expect from CUSH Cosmetics in the next 5 years? Plans for expansion?

A. *In the next 5 years, I see CUSH as a regular player in the hair and skin care market. I really want to continue to grow our salon business as well so that women of color can have options when they are getting their hair done professionally. When a woman is conscious about what she is putting on her hair and skin, she can request products from her stylist that she is confident won't harm her or her baby. I would also like to have a few "brick and mortar" store fronts in place... and possibly a spa. That's my big dream.*

About the Regimen Builder

The hair care market changes at a lightning-fast pace. New products regularly enter the market as others exit, and formulas are always being tweaked as science or ingenuity dictate. Given the dynamic nature of the market, it is impossible to create an exhaustive product list. This Regimen Builder contains a few representative products as a guide. To build your regimen, simply choose one (or two when indicated) product from each category.

> Remember, when you are working to achieve a protein/moisture balance in your hair-care regimen this balance can be achieved in many, many ways. For example, you could decrease application of your leave-in conditioner to every other week to reduce the moisture or protein load that product might create—or you could simply substitute another product from the opposite end of the protein/moisture balance to counterbalance the leave-in's effect if you would like to continue a weekly leave-in conditioner strategy.

NOTE: Products suggested in the regimen-building lists that follow can be found online and in traditional retail outlets. These products have been assigned a protein or moisture profile that is based on user testing, product claims and the ingredients list. Inclusion in the Regimen Builder is not a specific endorsement of the product's claims; rather, the products included have been found to have widespread appeal in the healthy black hair community. Products included here also contain ingredients that have met a certain standard as far as promoting better hair moisturization and supporting the protein integrity of black hair fibers. For an updated list of products, visit the Science of Black Hair on the web at www.blackhairscience.com.

Shampoo

If you have decided to include shampoo in your hair care regimen, it is recommended that you select the gentlest formula for your textured tresses. Natural and sulfate-free formulas are typically easier on black hair. Two types of shampoo are recommended for your regimen: one gentle cleansing weekly shampoo and one clarifying shampoo for monthly use. If you require a chelating shampoo for no-lye relaxer buildup or regular cleansing in a hard-water environment (see Chapter on Hair Product Selection Basics: Shampoo Basics), please select one of these as well.

Sulfate-Free Gentle Cleansing Shampoos
USE: Once or twice weekly.
Abba Pure Gentle Shampoo
Abba Pure Moisture Shampoo
Abba Pure Basic Shampoo
Abba Pure Color Protect Shampoo
Abba Pure Curl Shampoo
AG Hair Cosmetics Colour Savour Sulfate-free Shampoo
AG Hair Cosmetics Recoil Curl Activating Shampoo
Alba Botanica Cocoa Butter Dry Repair Hair Wash
Alba Botanica Coconut Milk Extra Enrich Hair Wash
Alba Botanica Gardenia Hydrating Hair Wash
Alba Botanica Honeydew Nourishing Hair Wash
Alba Botanica Mango Moisturizing Hair Wash
Alba Botanica Plumeria Replenishing Hair Wash
Alba Botanica Daily Shampoo
Alterna Color Hold Repair Shampoo
Alterna Color Hold Shine Shampoo
Alterna Color Hold Straight Shampoo
Alterna Scalp Therapy Shampoo
Alterna Clarifying Shampoo
Alterna Color Hold Repair Shampoo
Alterna Volume Restore Shampoo
Anita Grant Babassu Lavender Rose Shampoo and Shower Bar

Anita Grant Peppermint Babassu Shampoo Bar

Anita Grant Organic Kelp + Ylangylang Babassu Shampoo Bar

Aubrey Organics BGA Protein + Strengthening Shampoo

Aubrey Organics Egyptian Henna Shine-Enhancing Shampoo

Aubrey Organics GPB Glycogen Protein Balancing Shampoo

Aubrey Organics Green Tea Clarifying Shampoo

Aubrey Organics Honeysuckle Rose Moisturizing Shampoo

Aubrey Organics Island Naturals Replenishing Shampoo

Aubrey Organics J.A.Y. Desert Herb Revitalizing Shampoo

Aubrey Organics Rosa Mosqueta Nourishing Shampoo

Aubrey Organics White Camelia Ultra Smoothing Shampoo

Auromere Ayurvedic Sulfate-Free Aloe Vera-Neem Shampoo

Avalon Organics Awapuhi Mango Moisturizing Shampoo

Avalon Organics Biotin B-Complex Thickening Shampoo

Avalon Organics Extra Moisturizing Olive and Grapeseed Shampoo

Avalon Organics Nourishing Lavender Shampoo

Avalon Organics Clarifying Lemon Shampoo

Avalon Organics Shine Ylang Ylang Shampoo

Avalon Organics Smoothing Grapefruit & Geranium Shampoo

Avalon Organics Strengthening Peppermint Shampoo

Avalon Organics Tea Tree Mint Treatment Shampoo

Avalon Organics Tea Tree Scalp Treatment Shampoo

Avalon Organics Tear-Free Baby Shampoo

Avalon Organics Volumizing Rosemary Shampoo

Aveda Scalp Benefits Balancing Shampoo

Aveda Damage Remedy Restructuring Shampoo

Aveda Dry Remedy Moisturizing Shampoo

Aveda Men's Pureformance Shampoo

Bed Head Foxy Curls Frizz-Fighting Sulfate-Free Shampoo

Bed Head Superstar Sulfate-Free Shampoo for Thick Massive Hair

Bee Mine Peppermint & Tea Tree Nourishing Shampoo

Blended Beauty Soy Cream Shampoo

Body and Bath Omega-3 Hemp Moisturizing Shampoo

Burt's Bees Baby Bee Shampoo

Burt's Bees Color Keeper Green Tea & Fennel Seed Shampoo

Burt's Bees More Moisture Raspberry & Brazil Nut Shampoo

Burt's Bees Rosemary Mint Shampoo Bar

Burt's Bees Super Shiny Grapefruit & Sugar Beet Shampoo

Burt's Bees Very Volumizing Pomegranate & Soy Shampoo

CHI Ionic Color Protection System Sulfate Free Shampoo

Curl Junkie Curl Assurance Gentle Cleansing Shampoo

CURLS Pure Curls Organic Clarifying Shampoo

CURLS Curlicious Curls Cleansing Cream Organic Shampoo

CURLS Curlie Cutie Cleansing Cream Organic Shampoo

CUSH Hydration Supreme Conditioning Shampoo

DermOrganic Conditioning Shampoo

Design Essentials Natural Curl Cleanser Shampoo

DevaCurl No-Poo Cleanser

DevaCurl Low-Poo Cleanser

Dr. Bronner's Almond Liquid Soap

Dr. Bronner's Citrus Orange Liquid Soap

Dr. Bronner's Eucalyptus Liquid Soap

Dr. Bronner's Lavender Liquid Soap

Dr. Bronner's Peppermint Liquid Soap

Dr. Bronner's Rose Liquid Soap

Dr. Bronner's Tea Tree Oil Liquid Soap

Elasta QP Creme Conditioning Shampoo

Elucence Moisture Benefits Shampoo

Giovanni Smooth as Silk Shampoo

Giovanni Tea Tree Triple Treat Shampoo

Giovanni 50:50 Balanced Shampoo

Giovanni Golden Wheat Shampoo

Giovanni Root 66 Max Volume

Giovanni Wellness Shampoo with Chinese Botanicals

Hair Rules Aloe Grapefruit Purifying Shampoo

Hair Rules Daily Cleansing Cream

Jane Carter Solution Hydrating Invigorating Shampoo

Jason Natural Tea Tree Scalp Normalizing Shampoo

Jason Natural Biotin & Peppermint Strengthening Shampoo

Jason Natural Grapefruit and Aloe Smoothing Shampoo

Jason Natural Lavender & Rosemary Curl Defining Shampoo

Jason Natural Tall Grass Shampoo

Jason Natural Rosewater & Chamomile Normalizing Shampoo

Jason Natural Plumeria & Sea Kelp Moisturizing Shampoo

Jessicurl Hair Cleansing Cream Shampoo

Jonathan Product Infinite Volume Shampoo

Jonathan Product Weightless No Frizz Shampoo

Jonathan Product Hydrating Shampoo

Jonathan Product Green Routine Nourishing Shampoo

Herbal Choice Natural Tea Tree Shampoo

Karen's Body Beautiful Bodacious Beauty Bar (Shampoo Bar)

Karen's Body Beautiful Cool Clarifying Shampoo

Karen's Body Beautiful Ultimate Conditioning Shampoo

Kenra Platinum Shampoo

KeraCare 1st Lather Shampoo

KeraCare Hydrating Detangling Shampoo

KeraCare Naturals Cleansing Cream

Kinky-Curly Come Clean Moisturizing Shampoo

Kiss My Face SaHaira Shampoo for Dry Hair

L'OrealEverstrong Hydrating Shampoo

L'Oreal Everpure Smooth Shampoo

L'Oreal Everpure Volumizing Shampoo

L'Oreal Everstrong Reconstructing Shampoo

L'Oreal Hair Expertise Everstrong Sulfate-Free Fortify System Bodify Shampoo

MOP C-System Clean Shampoo

MOP C-System Hydrating Shampoo

MOP C-Curl Enhancing Shampoo

Neutragena Triple Moisture Cream Lather Shampoo

Organix Awakening Mocho Expresso Shampoo

Organix Energizing Passion Fruit Guava

Organix Enriching Cucumber Yogurt

Organix Fortifying Lavender Soymilk Shampoo

Organix Healing Mandarin Olive Oil

Organix Hydrating Tea Tree Mint Shampoo

Organix Instant Repair Cocoa Butter Shampoo

Organix Moisturizing Grapefruit Mango Butter

Organix Nourishing Coconut Milk Shampoo

Organix Rejuvenating Cherry Blossom Ginseng Shampoo

Organix Revitalizing Pomengranate Green Tea

Organix Smoothing Shea Butter Shampoo

Organix Soft and Silky Vanilla Silk Shampoo

Organix White Tea Grapeseed Shampoo

Oyin Grand Poo Bar

Phyto Phytojoba Gentle Regulating Milk Shampoo (Dry Hair Formula)

Pureology Essential Repair Shampoo

Pureology Hydrate Shampoo

Pureology Nanoworks Shampoo

Pureology Pure Volume Shampoo

Pureology Super Smooth Shampoo

Qhemet Biologics Egyptian Wheatgrass Cleansing Tea Shampoo

Queen Helene Mint Julep Shampoo

Scruples White Tea Sulfate Free Restorative Shampoo

SheaMoisture Raw Shea Butter Moisture Retention Shampoo

SheaMoisture African Black Soap Deep Cleansing Shampoo

Silk Elements ColorCare Sulfate-free Shampoo

Softsheen Breakthru Fortifying Moisturizing Shampoo

TIGI S-Factor Health Factor Sulfate-Free Daily Dose Shampoo

Trader Joe's Nourish Spa Shampoo

Trader Joe's Tea Tree Tingle Shampoo.

I've selected _____ _____ as my weekly gentle cleansing shampoo.

Clarifying Shampoos

USE: Once monthly or as needed every one to two weeks to remove product buildup.

Alba Botanica Daily Shampoo

Alterna Clarifying Shampoo

Artec Texturline Daily Clarifying Shampoo

Carol's Daughter Rosemary Mint Purifying Shampoo

CURLS Pure Curls Clarifying Shampoo

Elucence Volume Clarifying Shampoo

Hair Rules Aloe Grapefruit Purifying Shampoo

Jessicurl Gentle Lather Shampoo

Kenra Clarifying Shampoo

Kiss My Face Aromatherapeutic Shampoo

Ouidad Clear & Gentle Essential Daily Shampoo

NOTE: For gentle clarifying, most sulfate shampoos fall under this category.

I've selected _____ _____ as my monthly clarifying shampoo to back up my weekly gentle shampoo.

Chelating Shampoos

USE: After swimming or monthly for basic anti-hard water maintenance. For extreme hard water

cases, use a gentle chelating shampoo every one to two weeks to control mineral buildup.

Alba Botanica Daily Shampoo

Artec Texturline Daily Clarifying Shampoo

Bumble and Bumble Sunday Shampoo

Curl Junkie Daily Fix Cleanser

Elucence Moisture Acidifying Shampoo

Joico Resolve Chelating Shampoo

Kenra Clarifying Shampoo

KeraCare DeMineralizing Treatment

Nexxus Aloe Rid Gentle Clarifying Shampoo

Nexxus Phyto Organics Kelate Purifying Shampoo

Ouidad Water Works Shampoo

Paul Mitchell Shampoo Three

Redken Hair Cleansing Cream Shampoo

I've selected _____ _____ as my chelating shampoo to combat pool chlorine residue and/or mineral deposits from hard water or relaxer treatments.

Conditioner
Moisture-Based Conditioners

Conditioning products take care of the bulk of protein and moisture balancing in a healthy hair care regimen. The moisturizing conditioner you choose is the heart of your healthy hair care regimen. It is the product that makes up for lower quality products in other areas of the hair care regimen. Select one moisture-based conditioner for weekly use. Note that some of the moisturizing deep conditioners listed below contain various types of lightweight proteins that may respond differently to different types of textured hair. Individual results may vary with products. A little trial and error will be required to determine the conditioning products that best suit your hair's needs.

Battling Hair Breakage with Moisture Conditioning

Correcting hair dryness and breakage with moisture conditioning is often necessary to keep the hair in great condition. Used at the correct frequency, the moisturizing conditioners listed below will relieve "low moisture" hair breakage in all three zones of the breakage zone system described in the Protein and Moisture Balancing chapter of this book. Because moisture/water infusion is the primary objective of moisturizing conditioning, and the act of cleansing provides considerable moisture by default, the conditioning products used can vary wildly in their actual moisturizing ability and still be quite effective. In Zone 1 balanced hair, moisturizing conditioning may take place once per week without heat for ten to fifteen minutes or less. For Zone 2, low moisture breakage, moisturizing conditioners should be used to deep condition once or twice per week, with or without heat, for fifteen minutes. For Zone 3 low moisture breakage, these conditioners should be used at least twice per week, with heat, for at least thirty minutes.

Moisturizing Deep-Conditioning Products

USE: At least once a week.

AtOne Botanicals Reconstructor w/ Moisture Recovery

Aubrey Organics Honeysuckle Rose Conditioner

Aubrey Organics Rosa Mosqueta Conditioner

Aubrey Organics White Camellia Conditioner

Aussie Aussome Volume Conditioner

Aussie Moist Conditioner

Avalon Organics Awapuhi Mango Moisturizing Conditioner

Avalon Organics Lavender Nourishing Conditioner

Avalon Organics Ylang ylang Glistening Conditioner

Aveda Color Conserve Conditioner

Aveda Dry Remedy Moisturizing Conditioner

Back to Basics Bamboo Straightening Conditioner

Back to Basics Rich Moisture Coconut Mango

Back to Basics Vanilla Plum Conditioner

Bee Mine Bee-U-Ti-Ful Deep Conditioner

Biolage Hydratherapie Conditioning Balm

Blended Beauty Herbal Reconditioner

Bumble and Bumble Alojoba Conditioner

Bumble and Bumble Seaweed Conditioner

Burt's Bees Super Shiny Grapefruit & Sugar Beet Conditioner

Carol's Daughter Tui Hair Smoothie

Crème of Nature Professional Nourishing & Strengthening Treatment

Curl Junkie Healthy Condition Daily Conditioner

Curl Junkie Hibiscus & Banana Deep Fix Moisturizing Conditioner

Curl Junkie Curl Rehab Moisturizing Hair Treatment

Dove Advanced Care Sheer Moisture Conditioner

Dove Beautiful Care Conditioner

Dove Moisture Rich Color Conditioner

Dove Damage Therapy Daily Moisture Treatment

Elasta QP DPR-11 Deep Penetrating Remoisturizer

Elucence Moisture Balancing Conditioner

Frederic Fekkai Technician Color Care Conditioner

Frederic Fekkai Glossing Conditioner

Frederic Fekkai Luscious Curls Conditioner

Frederic Fekkai Shea Butter Moisturizing Conditioner

Giovanni Smooth as Silk Deeper Moisture Conditioner

Herbal Essences Hello Hydration Moisturizing Conditioner

Herbal Essences BodyEnvy Volumizing Conditioner

Herbal Essences Color Me Happy Conditioner

Herbal Essences None of Your Frizzness Smoothing Conditioner

Herbal Essences Totally Twisted Curls and Waves Conditioner

Jane Carter Nutrient Replenishing Conditioner

JASON Plumeria & Sea Kelp Moisturizing Conditioner

Jessicurl Aloeba Daily Conditioner

Jessicurl Too Shea! Extra Moisturizing Conditioner

Jessicurl Weekly Deep Conditioning Treatment

Joico Moisture Recovery Conditioner

Joico Moisture Intensive Treatment Extra Conditioning Conditioner

Kenra Moisturizing Conditioner

Kenra Nourishing Masque Deep Conditioning Treatment

Keracare Humecto Crème Conditioner

Keracare Moisturizing Conditioner for Color-Treated Hair

Kerastase Nutritive Masquintense Nourishing Treatment

Kinky Curly Knot Today Conditioner/Detangler

L'Anza Healing ColorCare Color-Preserving Conditioner

Mizani Moisturefuse Moisturizing Conditioner

MOP C-System Moisture Complex Conditioner

MYHoneyChild Organic Shea Butter Hair Paste

MYHoneyChild SO DEEP Conditioner

MYHoneyChild Olive You Deep Conditioner

Neutragena Triple Moisture Daily Conditioner

Neutragena Triple Moisture Deep Recovery Mask

Nexxus Humectress Ultimate Moisturizing Conditioner

Organix Nourishing Coconut Milk Conditioner

Organix Hydrating Tea Tree Mint Conditioner

Oyin Honey-Hemp Conditioner

Pantene Pro-V Color Preserve Smooth Conditioner

Redken Real Control Conditioner

Tigi Bed Head Moisture Maniac Conditioner

Trader Joe's Refresh Conditioner

I've selected _____
_____ as my weekly moisturizing conditioner.

Protein-Based Conditioners and Treatments

Protein-based conditioners help keep black hair strong. Select one protein conditioning treatment from the light or moderate protein lists for use every two weeks. Also select one protein treatment from the moderate or heavy/intense lists for more intensive protein conditioning every four to six weeks. Many of these treatments will yield strengthening results in one or two conditioning sessions.

Battling Hair Breakage with Protein Conditioning

Correcting hair breakage with protein conditioning is often necessary to keep the hair in great condition. Unlike moisturizing conditioning, in which frequency of application plays a primary role in breakage correction, the correction achieved using protein conditioning is more directly affected by the strength of the individual protein product. For Zone 1 low protein breakage, light protein-based products are best. For Zone 2 low protein breakage, moderate protein conditioning is required. For Zone 3 low protein breakage, intense protein conditioning is necessary.

Protein-Based Conditioners and Treatment Products

USE: Every two to six weeks, or as needed..

Light Protein Products

Aubrey Organics Glycogen Protein Balancing (GPB) Conditioner

Aveda Damage Remedy Conditioner

Garnier Fructis Length & Strength Fortifying Cream Conditioner

Got2B Soft One Minute Emergency Repair Creme

Herbal Essences Long Term Relationship Conditioner

Joico Moisture Recovery Treatment Balm

Joico K-Pak Reconstruct Conditioner

Mane and Tail Original Conditioner

Motions Moisture Silk Protein Conditioner

MYHoneyChild Banana Creme Conditioner

Neutrogena Triple Moisture Deep Recovery Mask

Organic Root Stimulator Replenishing Pak

Ovation Cell Therapy Crème Rinse Moisturizer

Paul Mitchell Super Strong Daily Conditioner

Phytospecific Intense Nutrition Mask

Redken Extreme Conditioner

Rusk Sensories Calm 60 Second Hair Revive

Trader Joes Nourish Spa Balance Moisturizing Conditioner

Vitale Pro Super Conditioner

NOTE: The protein conditioning treatments in this category are suitable for correcting Zone 1 breakage.

Moderate Protein Products

Aphogee Keratin 2 Minute Reconstructor

Elasta QP Breakage Control Serum

Elucence Extended Moisture Repair Treatment

Frederic Fekkai Protein Rx Reparative Conditioner

Giovanni Smooth As Silk Extreme Protein Treatment

LeKair Cholesterol Plus Strengthening Conditioning Cream

Motions Critical Protection and Repair (CPR) Treatment Conditioner

Nexxus Keraphix Restorative Strengthening Conditioner

Ovation Cell Therapy Conditioner Hair Treatment

Queen Helene Cholesterol Hair Conditioning Cream

NOTE: The protein conditioning treatments in this category are suitable for correcting Zone 2 breakage.

Heavy/Intense Protein Products

Affirm 5 n 1 Reconstructor

Aphogee Two–Step Protein Treatment

Dudley's DRC 28 Hair Treatment and Fortifier

Elasta QP Breakage Control Serum

Elucence Extended Moisture Repair Treatment

Joico K-Pac Deep Penetrating Reconstructor

Mizani Kerafuse Intensive Strengthening Treatment

Motions Critical Protection and Repair (CPR) Treatment Conditioner

Nexxus Emergencee Strengthening Polymeric Reconstructor

Nexxus Keraphix Restorative Strengthening Conditioner

Organic Root Stimulator Hair Mayonnaise Treatment for Damaged Hair

NOTE: The protein-conditioning treatments in this category are suitable for correcting Zone 3 breakage.

I've selected _____
_____ as my light weekly protein-based conditioner.

I've selected _____
_____ as my intensive protein conditioning treatment.

Water-Based Moisturizers and Leave-In Conditioners

Moisturizers are a must-have in every healthy hair-care regimen. Select one water -based moisturizer and one protein-based moisturizer. The best water-based moisturizers do not contain heavy, hair shaft-coating oils such as mineral oil and petrolatum; rather, they contain a mixture of water, humectants and natural oils or butters. Leave-in conditioners can also double as water-based moisturizers in most hair care regimens so that fewer products are used overall.

Moisturizing Leave-In and Water-Based Moisture Products

USE: After hair is shampooed and conditioned, or every one to three days as needed to for hydration.

Bumble and Bumble Leave-In Conditioner

Curl Junkie Hibiscus & Banana Honey Butta Leave-In Conditioner

CURLS Curl Soufflé Organic Curl Cream

Hollywood Beauty Carrot Oil Moisturizer

Hollywood Beauty Olive Oil Moisturizer

Jane Carter Solution Hair Nourishing Cream

Kinky Curly Knot Today Leave-In Conditioner

Kenra Platinum Color Care Botanical Detangler

Kenra Daily Provision Leave-In Conditioner

Luster's S-Curl No Drip Activator Moisturizer

Neutrogena Triple Moisture Silk Touch Leave-In Conditioner

Organic Root Stimulator (Olive Oil) Moisturizer

Organic Root Stimulator (Carrot Oil) Moisturizer

Oyin's Frank Juice Nourishing Herbal Leave-In Conditioner

Oyin's Greg Juice Nourishing Herbal Leave-In Conditioner

Paul Mitchell The Detangler

Profectiv Damage Free Anti-Tangle Leave-In

Proline Lite Comb Thru Creme Moisturizer

Silk Elements MegaSilk Leave-In Hair Moisturizing Crème

Silk Elements Megasilk Olive Moisturizing Treatment

Soft Sheen Carson StaSoFro Hair and Scalp Spray

Soft Sheen Carson Wave Nouveau Coiffure Daily Humectant Moisturizing Lotion

NOTE: Most braid sprays also work well as water-based moisturizers.

I've selected _____ _____ as my leave-in and/or water-based moisturizer.

Protein-Based Leave-Ins and Water-Based Moisture Products

USE: After hair is shampooed and conditioned, or every one to three days as needed for protein support.

Cantu Shea Butter Break Cure Treatment

Cantu Shea Butter Grow Strong Treatment

Cantu Shea Butter Leave-In

Chi Keratin Mist

Elasta QP Mango Butter

Infusium 23

Mane N Tail Conditioner

Profectiv Break Free Leave-In

Profectiv Break Thru Treatment

Profectiv Mega Growth Treatment

Profectiv Healthy Ends Treatment

Salerm 21

I've selected _____ _____ as my protein-based leave-in conditioner/water-based moisturizer.

Oils and Butters

Select one or more oils from the list.

Natural Oils

USE: After moisturizer to provide a seal. These oils may also be used alone in pre-shampoo and hot-oil treatments, added to relaxer creams, or as carriers for essential oils.

Almond

Argan

Castor

Coconut

Flaxseed

Jojoba

Hemp

Olive
Palm
Palm Kernel
Peanut
Safflower
Sesame
Soybean
Sunflower
Sweet Almond
Wheat Germ
Ximenia

Natural Butters

USE: After moisturizer to provide a seal.

Avocado
Cocoa
Coffee
Mango
Shea

Commercial Oil and Butter Products

USE: After moisturizer to provide a seal.

Carol's Daughter Healthy Hair Butter
CUSH Mango Pomade
Nutiva Coconut Oil
Dabur Vatika Oil
Dabur Amla Oil
Oyin Burnt Sugar Pomade
Oyin's Whipped Pudding

I've selected _____
_____ as my oil/butter sealant.

Essential Oils (optional)

Several drops of the following essential oils can be added to shampoos, conditioners and moisturizers to boost their potency and achieve particular scalp and hair benefits. Pregnant women, those who are nursing and those with sensitive skin conditions should check with a medical practitioner prior to using essential oils for hair or skin.

Essential Oils

Cedarwood: Astringent/cleanser and dandruff-fighter.
Jasmine: Scalp stimulant. Controls sebum production.
Lavender: Soothes dry, itchy scalps.
Peppermint: Scalp stimulant. Great for soothing itchy, inflamed scalps.
Rosemary: Scalp stimulant.
Tea Tree: Scalp stimulant and dandruff-fighter. Controls sebum production.
Thyme: Scalp stimulant.
Ylang ylang: Scalp stimulant. Controls sebum production.

Carrier Oils

Almond
Grapeseed
Jojoba
Olive
Sesame
Shea butter (melted)
Soybean
Sweet Almond

Ancillary Hair Products (Stylers and Curl Definers)

Ancillary hair products are the products responsible for sculpting, smoothing, slicking, curl defining, and adding an extra bit of polish and control to textured tresses.

Hair-Friendly Gels, Jellies, Whipped Creams and Puddings

100% Aloe Vera Gel
Afroveda PUR Whipped Hair Gelly
Aveda Light Elements Defining Whip
Aubrey Organics Mandarin Magic Ginkgo Leaf and Ginseng Root Hair Jelly
Blended Beauty Curly Frizz Pudding
Blended Beauty Happy Nappy
Curl Junkie Aloe Fix Lite Hair Styling Gel
CURLS Curl Souffle Organic Curl Cream

CURLS Goddess Glaze Organic Gel
CURLS Whipped Cream
DevaCurl Set it Free
Ecostyler Gel
Fantasia IC Polisher with Sparklelites
Garnier Fructis Cream Gel
Jane Carter Solution Curl Defining Cream
Kinky Curly Curling Custard

Heat Protectants
BioSilk Silk Therapy
CHI Silk Infusion
FHI Heat Hot Sauce
got2b Guardian Angel Heat Protect N' Blow Out Lotion and Gloss Finish
John Frieda Frizz-Ease Thermal Protection Hair Serum
Kenra Straightening Serum

Nexxus Heat Protexx
Redken Smooth Down Heat Glide Smoother
Sedu Anti-Frizz Polishing Treatment with Argan Oil
Tigi S-Factor Heat Defender Flat Iron Shine Spray

Setting Lotions/Design Foams
Design Essentials Compositions Foaming Wrap Lotion
Dudley's Fantastic Body Texturizing Setting Lotion
Giovanni Sculpting/Setting Lotion
Lottabody Texturizing Hair Setting Lotion
Jane Carter SolutionWrap and Roll
KeraCare Foam Wrap
Mizani Setting Lotion

Chapter 8: Low-Manipulation Hair-Maintenance Strategies

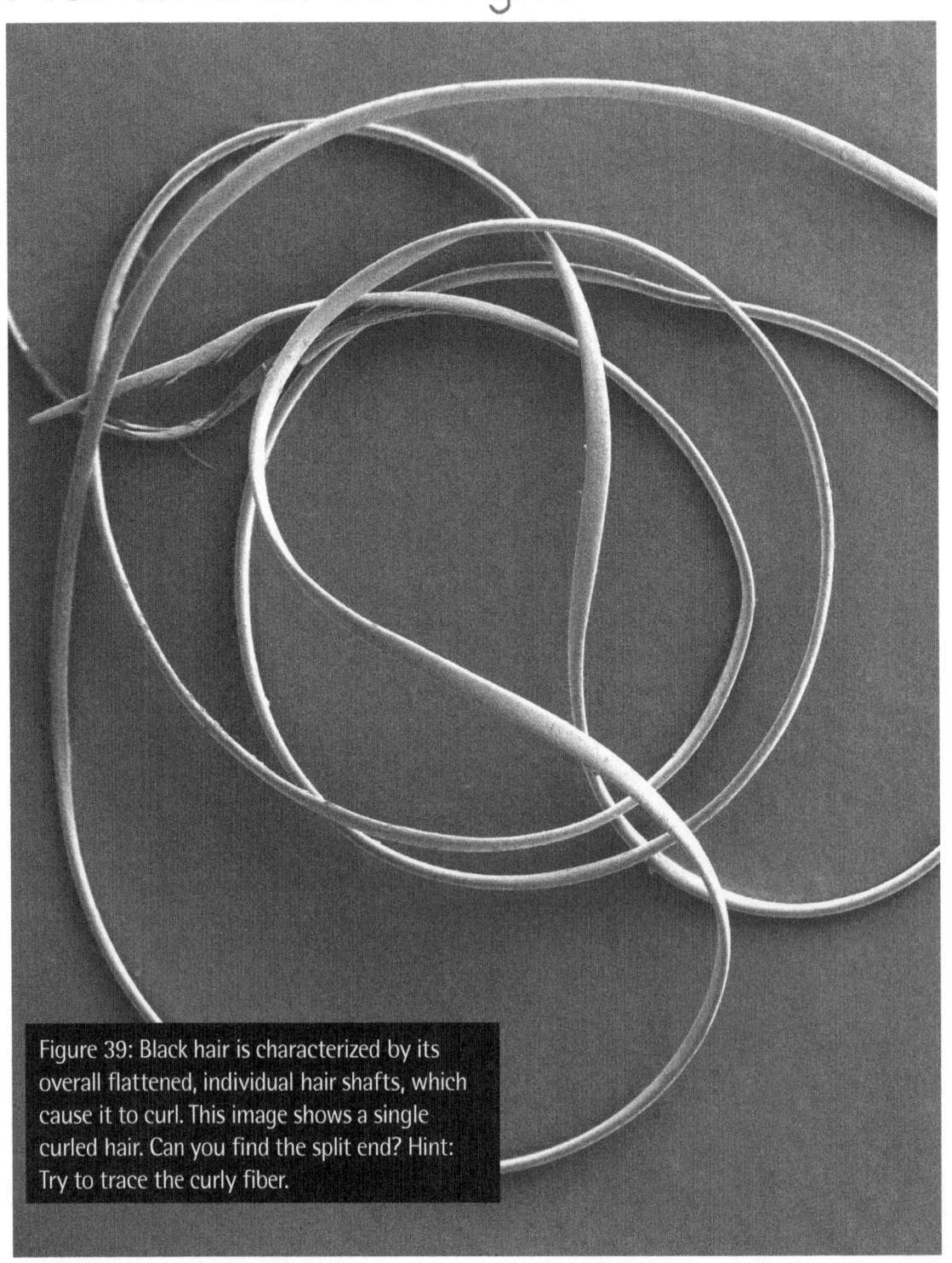

Figure 39: Black hair is characterized by its overall flattened, individual hair shafts, which cause it to curl. This image shows a single curled hair. Can you find the split end? Hint: Try to trace the curly fiber.

We've learned the basic formulations of hair care products, their general placement within a hair regimen, and have made some preliminary product choices to build a new regimen. Now it is important to fold the product choices into an overall low-manipulation hair care strategy. Low-manipulation care and styling are a must for textured hair. Our hair strands' flattened, cross-sectional profiles, and each strand's natural tendency to curl and coil around its neighbors, together make regular handling and styling manipulation detrimental to our hair over time.

In its natural, unprocessed state, our hair's cuticles are slightly lifted at the points along the hair fiber where the strand either coils or bends. This lifted cuticle structure means that the cuticles simply do not hug the cortex tightly along the entire length of the strand. In addition to exposing the cortex to the possibility of direct damage, this inherent tendency toward lifted cuticles in our hair increases the friction factor between individual hair fibers. With chemical relaxing or color-treatment, the cuticle lifting normally present at bend points becomes more pronounced and the cuticle scales lift along the entire processed length of the hair fiber. Wherever the hair's cuticles are lifted, the potential for friction and tangling between individual fibers increases. The roughened surfaces of each strand brush past and catch on one another leading to tangling and breakage. This tangling occurs wherever cuticle lift is present, especially near the ends in both natural and relaxed hair.

Friction and tangling, unfortunately, are precursors to hair breakage. If reductions in hair friction and tangling can be achieved, then overall breakage will decrease. To reduce breakage and reach greater lengths, black hair should be handled minimally. The less our textured hair is handled, styled and combed into submission, the less stress, breakage and tension our hair fibers will endure. Whether you are bombarding your hair with heat,

weaves and hair colors or are simply switching hair products in rapid succession in search of that surefire fix, doing too many things to your hair at once will prevent it from thriving.

> We often see the great success of low-manipulation hair care regimens best among our children. Children's hair care tends to be very simple. Their hair is not typically styled elaborately or with heat. In addition, children tend to wear their hair in its natural, unprocessed state and in long-term styles such as braids or plaits that can stay in place for several days at a time. All of these factors make the growth environment for children's hair ideal and reduces their potential for hair breakage.

As we age and move into adulthood, we often grow more creative with our styling techniques and methods. Wigs, weaves, relaxers, colors and heat become a regular part of daily hair care for many of us—and over time, our hair may begin to suffer from stress. It's not too late, to get back some of the simplicity of childhood. The following chapters encourage you to explore the many ways that you can apply a hands-off (or hands-on!) approach to your healthy hair care regimen. Let's begin with hair tools.

Protective Styling Tools

Just as proper product selection is important in a healthy hair care regimen, the selection of proper hair styling tools is another important aspect of regimen building and protective styling. These tools help us secure our hair, move our hair out of the way, straighten it, smooth it, curl it and style it to perfection. Styling tools may be as simple as our fingers, or as specialized as a pair of hundred-dollar thinning shears or a standing, hooded-dryer unit. We often use our hair combs, brushes, hair clips, hair rollers and pins without giving them much thought, but for textured hair types in particular, selecting suitable hair tools is extremely important. Poorly-made, or improperly used, hair tools can ravage textured tresses, stripping precious cuticle layers and moisture from our delicate strands. The effects of using poorly-made hair tools on the hair each day often proves costly for textured hair in the long run. Are your hair tools working for or against you in your quest for healthier, longer hair?

To jumpstart your healthy hair regimen and proper protective styling, you will need to do a quick inventory and evaluation of your current hair tool arsenal. So gather your combs, brushes, clips, clamps and scissors, and take a minute to determine if your tools make the final cut.

Hands

Our hands are probably the most overlooked styling tools we have at our disposal. In fact, we came into this world with these tools in our arsenal! Because of their superior, built-in flexibility, hands are able to work the magic that combs and brushes simply cannot. Styling with hands is a more controlled process than styling with conventional tools. Snags and tangles can be loosened with minimal hair fiber breakage because finger-combing and smoothing puts very little stress on delicate hair fibers. Expert finger-combing and smoothing takes practice, and tends to work best on natural hair, transitioning hair, and curly set styles that can be maintained by simply fluffing. Like other styling tools, hands must be kept in good condition. Your fingernails should be smooth and snag-free, and your hands should be soft, moisturized and callous-free to prevent hair damage.

Combs

You'd be hard pressed to find a home that does not have one of these tools, but combs and textured tresses—natural or relaxed—have a love-hate relationship. Our hair's unpredictable bends and tendency to tangle and mesh with oth-

er hairs, even when chemically straightened, presents an interesting challenge to hair combs. The finer the comb's teeth, the greater the challenge combing presents. In a low-manipulation styling regimen, detangling perfection is not a goal. Major tangles should always be removed with the fingers and large-tooth combs first to the greatest extent possible. Combs with excessively small teeth should be avoided as much as possible for most daily styling. Too many teeth equal too many opportunities for breakage. These tiny combs are not necessary for most textured styles.

> **Remember:** Before combing textured hair, textured tresses should always be moisturized with water and/or lubricated with a moisturizer or oil to reduce frictional forces between individual textured fibers. This lubricating (or plasticizing) enhances the hair's pliability and reduces hair breakage. After lubrication, the hair should be slowly finger-combed to navigate and negotiate the hair's larger natural bends, tangles and coils. Finally, slowly comb the hair in a graduated, step-down manner—using a large-tooth comb first to detangle, and then successively smaller-toothed combs as desired until the hair has been successfully detangled.

Beware of Sharp Seams

The first thing to check for when you consider using a particular comb is whether or not the teeth are intact, and whether or not they have serrated edges or seams running along their centers. Combs with broken or chipped teeth are snag hazards that can shred textured hair and lead to breakage. When a comb has seams running along the teeth, it becomes a hair-torture device. Seams and serrations scratch the cuticles and cause tearing and splits. Seams indicate that your styling tool was mass produced and made from a mold with thousands of others like it.

Using these types of combs, or any tool with seams, is like going through your textured hair with a shredder!

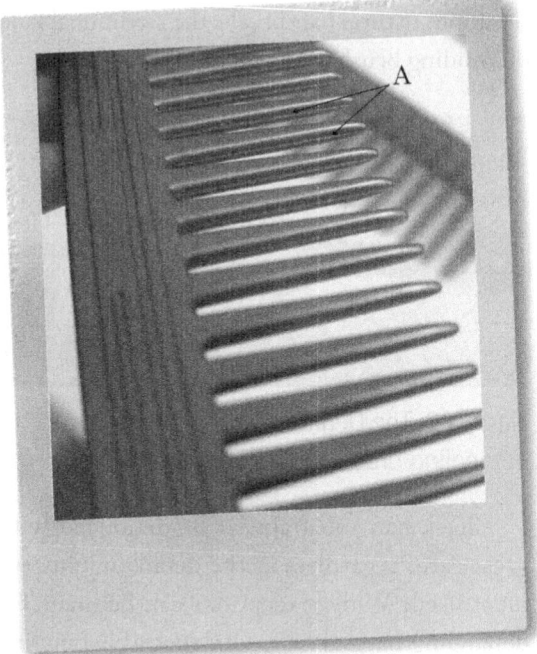

Figure 40: Comb seams can be difficult to spot, but always take note of any tiny plastic ridges lining the teeth of your combs and clips. These seams can snag and shred delicate strands with every passing and use.

Seamless combs are the combs of choice for healthy, textured hair. These combs are available in a variety of sizes and styles to meet nearly every styling need. The most popular seamless combs are made from wood, bone (now resin), high-quality, polished plastics, hardened organic materials, and faux shell and horn materials. Seamless combs are made and polished entirely by hand to eliminate the harsh seams that can snag the hair and damage cuticles. Many of these combs are heat-resistant, and will last a lifetime. Seamless combs can be purchased from many beauty supply stores and verified online vendors such as www.tenderheaded.com or www.hairsense.com.

If your hair is long or thick, opt for combs with longer teeth. Shorter comb teeth tend to pull and snag the top layers of hair and do not really penetrate well through the hair's thickness for most textured hair types. Longer teeth are more hair friendly and require less manipulation and effort to work through the hair.

Detangling/Shower Combs

Detangling combs are another good healthy hair care option for textured hair types. Traditionally, shower combs have rounded tips and longer teeth for handling longer or thicker hair types. These large-tooth combs come in a variety of teeth designs and orientations, and often have hooked ends for hanging the comb in the shower.

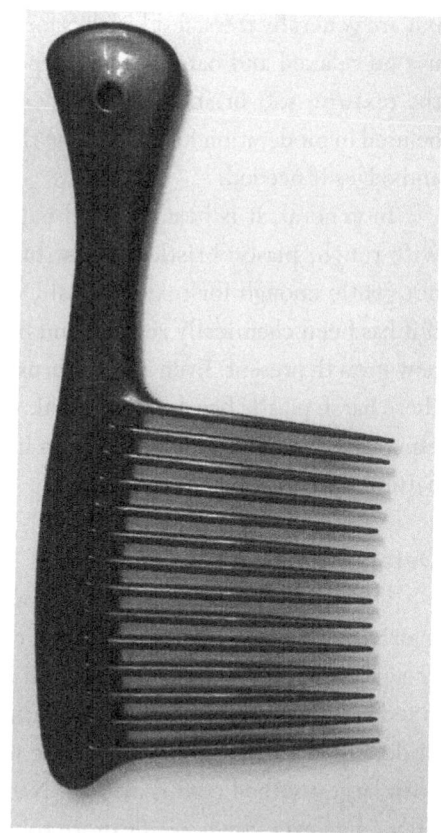

Figure 41: This detangling comb has longer teeth for easier detangling. It is great for removing shed hair.

Brushes

Brushing textured hair, relaxed or natural, is risky business. Many healthy hair care advocates advise against any and all brushing, while others are firmly pro-brushing. One thing is for sure, the "hundred-strokes-a-day" advice from your grandmother's great-grandmother was not meant for textured hair! Textured hair always thrives best when manipulation of any kind is kept to a minimum. You will be surprised how well a small- or medium-tooth comb, a little water, your hands and a scarf can perform the duties of a brush!

While brushing is tough on the hair cuticle, some brushes are safer than others for textured hair types. Natural boar-bristle brushes are pricey but are generally the safest brushes for moderate use on relaxed and natural hair. Depending on the texture, soft-bristle baby brushes may also be used in moderation for smoothing the hairline and edges if needed.

In general, it is best to avoid hair brushes with rough, plastic bristles. These brushes are not gentle enough for textured hair, especially if it has been chemically relaxed and has a bit of new growth present. Even a gentle brushing with these harsh plastic brushes will break your hair, especially at the fragile demarcation line where natural texture meets relaxed hair.

Detangling Brushes

Detangling brushes, like the popular Denman®, may be used to detangle damp, conditioner-soaked hair, in particular, natural hair. Relaxed hair does not often fare well with this sort of detangling strategy and should be detangled with large-toothed combs instead. Natural hair fibers, however, are *generally* more robust fibers than chemically relaxed strands and respond well to gentle, sectioned detangling with brushes that have flexible, comb-like teeth. These brushes also tend to distribute product through thick, massive coils better than combs. Because kinky, coily natural hair fibers are generally not structured or equipped to withstand thorough dry detangling, strands should always be moistened or dampened prior to removing tangles with hair tools. In this situation, natural hair breaks the traditional rule of avoiding brushes on wet hair.

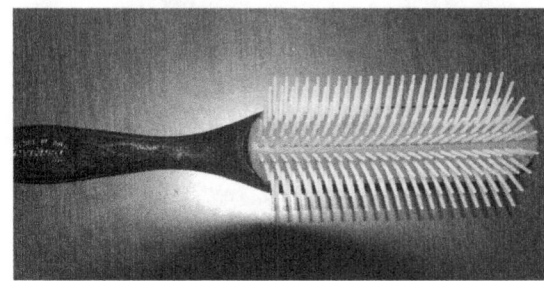

Figure 42: The Denman® is a popular detangling brush with comb-like teeth.

Black hair must always be detangled with great care, regardless of the detangling instrument used. While exceptions can be made for detangling natural hair with special detangling brushes, it is still advisable to avoid brushing wet hair with other types of brushes. Brushing textured hair in its weakest state will cause it to overstretch, weaken and break under the pressure. In addition, it is important to avoid brushing through completely dry hair with any type of brush. Semi-dry, moisturized and oiled hair is best able to cope with brushing because the extra elasticity and pliability in this hair reduces the breakage burden.

Clips, Clamps and Claws

Clips, clamps, and claws suffer from some of the same pitfalls as combs: namely, serrated or seamed teeth and edges. Always ensure that your hair clamps and clips are well-made. Serrated teeth and rough seams can cut and tear through delicate textured tresses as you pin your hair up. Always clip up loosely twisted hair gently, and avoid placing the clips so tightly that they scrape or rub your scalp. Only use clamps, clips and claws that have hinge pieces that are in great working condition. Poorly made hinges can snag your hair as you are placing or removing the clamp. To remove a clip, gently hold and support your hair as you slowly take it out. Never pull or release the clip from your hair without bracing the hair first.

Hairpins

Hairpins are useful for keeping textured hair styles in place. When evaluating hairpins, always be sure that they have soft, rounded tips and that those rounded tips are intact. If a bobby pin has a sharp edge or a rounded tip that is beginning to lift, discard it immediately.

When worn frequently and in the same position in the hair, hairpins can repeatedly crease and bend the cuticles, causing damage. When wearing clips, clamps or pins of any kind, be sure that you change their positions regularly so as not to stress the hair in a particular area. Do not abruptly slide hairpins into the hair or quickly pull them out of the hair. Separate the prongs of bobby pins slightly before guiding them into the hair. Follow the same procedure for removing bobby pins to protect your hair against damage.

Good Hair Days® hairpins are an alternative to traditional hairpins. Good Hair Days® pins are designed with open prongs at the bottom and a loop at the top for easy insertion or extraction from the hair. These snagless hairpins are the ultimate in pin-up style protection. Find these hairpins at www.goodhairdays.com.

Scrunchies, Hair Ties and Bands

Securing the hair with hair ties, scrunchies (decorative fabric-covered elastic rings) and hair bands is a great way to organize and style the hair. Textured hair should be thoroughly moisturized before applying any type of holder, and moisturizing attention should be focused in the area where your holder will rest on your hair. Ideally, scrunchies and bands should be made

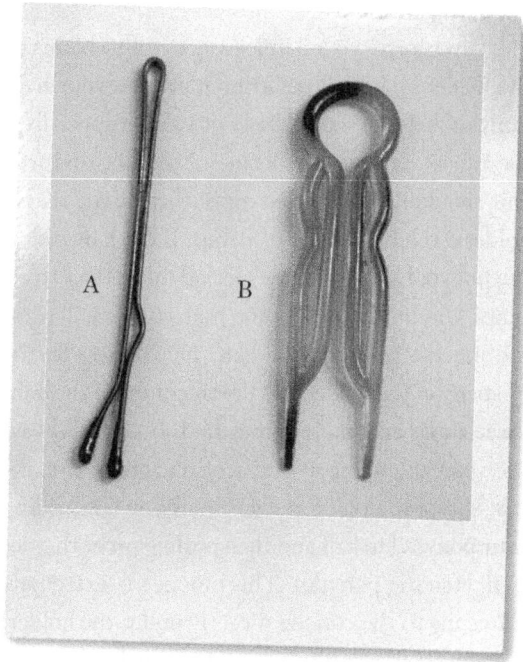

Figure 43: The open prong hair pin configuration to the right (B) is ideal for textured hair types.

of silk or satin fabrics to guard against rubbing and moisture loss from the hair into the fabric. Cotton fabrics can steal moisture from your hair throughout the day. To add a protective benefit to hair bands, ties and holders, dip these tools in your favorite oil before securing them around the hair. Avoid metal crimps or hard glue pieces on holders as these can snag the hair. Rubber bands should be avoided altogether due to their high potential for causing hair fiber stress and breakage.

TIP: Need a quick, hair-safe ponytail holder? Simply remove the feet of a pair of new pantyhose or stockings by making a horizontal cut across the leg with a pair of scissors. Next, make another horizontal cut across the legs 1.5 to 2 inches above the first cut. Increase the distance between the horizontal cuts to make a holder with firmer hold.

Safe and Secure

Always give your hair leeway to shift a bit inside the holder by loosely securing it around your hair. Ponytail holders should be kept loose, especially if the hair is very wet. As a rule of thumb, textured hair should not be circled more than twice with a holder if the hair is wet or damp. If the hair is dry, the ponytail should not be circled more than three times. Circling the holder too many times will place too much tension on the hair. Depending on the elasticity of the holder and the thickness of the hair, three times around still may be too tight. Always use your judgment. If you are struggling to make that last loop, don't force it. Finally, avoid dividing your ponytail in half and then pulling on both sides to tighten the ponytail. This practice is extremely damaging to the cuticles directly under the holder, since the holder is being forced upward against the natural alignment of the cuticles.

Short or Layered-Hair Ponytails

If your hair is slightly layered, or if your hair is shorter than shoulder length, you may run into issues placing and using ponytail holders in a protective way. At these lengths, the ends of shorter hair layers tend to get clamped down tightly by ponytail holders. If you cannot successfully ponytail your hair without clamping down on your ends, opt for a clipped-up style instead.

Scissors

For self trimmers, scissors are an important tool for carrying out your "ends-maintenance" regimen. A great pair of scissors can mean the difference between clean-cut ends and badly cut, chronically re-splitting ends. Dull blades do not cut hair cleanly, and simply push hair around inside the blades before executing the cut. Such blades can easily damage your otherwise healthy ends, leaving them vulnerable to breakage. Remember, shears for hair-cutting should be used only for this purpose. Using your shears for anything else will dull them over time. For most do-it-yourself trimmers, a standard scissor brand such as Goody® will suffice.

Caring for Your Styling Tools

All combs and brushes (and clips and clamps, on occasion) should be cleaned regularly, according to frequency of use. Combs and clips can be soaked in a simple solution of warm water and soap or clarifying shampoo. After soaking for ten minutes, rinse under warm running water, and wipe dry with a clean towel or cloth.

Pre-soak brushes in soapy water (clarifying shampoo plus water), and then use a comb to loosen, lift and remove any hair that may be stuck in the bristles. Allow the combed-out brush to soak for a few more minutes. Rinse and air dry.

Protective Shampooing and Conditioning Strategies

The best products in the world are of little benefit to our hair if we don't put them to use with effective styling and handling techniques.

Low manipulation is perhaps most critical during shampooing and conditioning sessions. Because natural, unprocessed hair often has a stronger protein infrastructure, it can tolerate frequent wetting, shampooing and conditioning better than chemically weakened relaxed hair fibers. But chemically relaxed hair fibers desperately need the moisture available to them from weekly hydration and conditioning sessions. In addition, regular protein conditioning becomes absolutely essential for those with chemically relaxed or color-treated hair because chemical treatment induces protein damage.

Black Hair Logistics

We've all seen those commercials and movies in which actresses furiously scrunch shampoo lather through their hair and pile it high in huge, soapy balls atop their heads. Many of us probably are guilty of the same haphazard shampooing technique. Unfortunately, this cleansing method is used mainly for dramatic effect on television and works poorly in real life.

Textured hair cleansing requires organization. Black hair should never be lathered and piled in a frothy mass upon the head. Roughing up the hair in this manner increases the frictional forces between the cuticle scales of individual hair fibers. Friction between hair fibers, as previously discussed, leads to excessive tangling, matting and damage to the hair fiber when it comes time to rinse, making the comb-out process nearly impossible. Instead of going for a good scrub, manipulation of textured hair should be in one direction only—DOWNWARD—during shampooing and conditioning sessions. The force of water, with the support of our fingers (exclusive of our nails), should direct shampoo and conditioner DOWN the hair fiber, smoothing the cuticle layers DOWNWARD as it flows.

There are two basic hair-cleansing techniques that once incorporated in a healthy hair care regimen, will help further minimize hair breakage and reduce tangles on wash day. Both methods begin with strategic disentangling of the hair fibers prior to the start of the cleansing process.

Low-Manipulation Detangling for Textured Hair

Our hair must be thoroughly prepared and disentangled prior to shampooing and conditioning, or any other form of styling. Detangling the hair before cleansing eliminates tangles that will become harder to remove once the hair has become saturated with water. Generally speaking, matted, tangly, dry hair translates to even more matted, tangled wet hair. However, moving fingers or combs through textured hair can be a feat whether the hair is natural, has considerable new growth or has been recently relaxed. Special care must be taken to reduce and manage hair breakage as we prepare the hair for cleansing.

Remember, black hair should always be handled with gentle care, and detangling must always

be a slow, deliberate process. Textured hair is quite elastic and can handle considerable styling manipulation before breakage occurs. But even healthy hair fibers will break if they are subjected to rapid stress and force. Quick, short combing bursts cause the most damage because our hair's internal bonds do not have enough time to take advantage of their natural elasticity to maneuver against the force of the comb. The cross-linked bonds in our hair fibers need time to stretch and accommodate styling stressors, whether that stress comes from a comb or our fingers. If black hair is manipulated too quickly, the hair will simply snap under pressure. Techniques differ from person to person, but a few basic steps should be followed to insure that combing manipulation does not interfere with your growth plans.

Detangling Breakdown: Pre-cleansing Technique

1. Plasticize To Decrease Friction

Most textured tresses do not take well to dry detangling and combing without succumbing to breakage. Before you begin detangling or combing through your hair, a plasticizer (either a moisturizer or a lubricant) should be applied to the hair beforehand. A plasticizer is a product that improves manageability by softening the hair from within or by coating and surrounding the hair fiber. The plasticizing product may be water, moisturizer, leave-in conditioner, oil or regular conditioner. The amount of plasticizer added to the hair depends on whether your hair is being detangled for cleansing (in which case, a generous amount of product can be used) or whether you are detangling to style for the day (in which case, less product will likely be used). Personal preference also plays a role in the type of product used.

Pre-shampoo treatments (see Special Conditioning Treatments), discussed in the coming sections, are another way to plasticize the hair prior to shampooing. These treatments work well

Reminder

Wet hair's extra elasticity makes it more fragile and weaker than dried hair. You should always exercise great care when detangling or styling the hair at this vulnerable time. Always make sure that your hair is properly balanced with protein to resist the extra stretching, weakening, and breaking.

for removing stubborn tangles in most textured hair types, relaxed or natural. Plasticizing with conditioner or oil works well for coarser or tightly coiled hair types that need additional time to soften prior to detangling and shampooing.

2. Separate Hair into Manageable Sections

Taking on a full head of tangled hair with the wrong technique, tools and no game plan is a recipe for disaster and unnecessary breakage. If your textured hair is thick, or lengthy, the divide-and-conquer approach is a beneficial detangling tactic for organizing and styling your textured hair without breakage. To begin the detangling process, divide moistened hair into several sections, using your fingers to create the parts. If your hair is relaxed, you will need four or five sections. If your hair is natural, more sections may be needed. The more sections you create, the easier and more thorough the detangling result will be. Loosely braid, twist or clip up each section of water-misted, conditioned or oil-saturated hair. If your hair is too short to braid, then the hair may be fastened with ponytail holders to organize the cleansing if desired. Closely cropped hair may be cleansed without sectioning.

3. Fingers: The Ultimate Detangler

Detangling textured hair is an art. Textured hair, unlike straight hair, is not designed to greet combs with ease. When we deal with textured hair, it is important to make use of our hands as

much as possible to reduce the stress of detangling and styling manipulation. The hands are the most effective detangling tool we have at our disposal. Our hair is organic. It likes to be gently touched, guided and fluffed. Our fingers are wonderfully equipped to accomplish these tasks. Fingers can feel for tangles that plastic combs cannot perceive. Fingers are also able to apply and remove pressure from the hair as kinks and curls are detected, and can navigate those tangles most easily to complete a style.

Hair that is finger-combed often tends to be thicker and longer than hair that is detangled with combs exclusively. In addition, removing naturally shed hair is easiest when the hair is finger-combed. As shed hair fibers begin their descent from the scalp, fingers can gently work this shed hair out and defend the rest of the hair against additional tangling, damage and breakage.

Finger-combing is not simply a matter of smoothing or running the fingers through textured hair. It involves the careful separation of enmeshed strands. In finger-combing, sectioning is encouraged so that small groups of strands and then, eventually, single strands may be isolated. This is why sectioning is recommended following plasticizing.

To begin, select a section of hair to be finger-combed. Starting with the last few inches of the section, begin detangling the hair gently with your fingers. When you meet a tangle, do not force it. Immediately release the tangled section and start from the bottom again. Any time you meet resistance, immediately stop and redirect your detangling efforts.

4. Comb Through

Follow your finger detangling with a thorough detangling with a large-toothed, seamless comb with eight to fourteen teeth. Detangling brushes also work well for gently detangling natural hair. Ideally, combing strokes should be limited to the fewest needed to get the job done.

Start with your comb at the very end of a section. Lightly stroke the surface of the hair with the comb while working your way deeper and deeper into the section. Add more and more hair to the detangling stroke as the hairs on top become untangled.

Work your comb back up toward the scalp slowly as you detangle and move through each section. When a comb's tooth approaches an unconformity, or textured bend, the moving force of the comb may stress and then eventually break the hair if the combing force is not redirected. You may find that bracing the hair by holding it mid-shaft just above where you are detangling

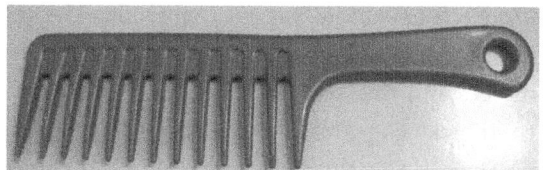

Figure 44: The wide spacing between this comb's teeth makes it ideal for negotiating tangles in both relaxed and natural heads of hair.

decreases the combing tension and allows for better handling and detangling. Tearing or ripping through tangles always leads to thinning and breakage over time. Do not force it!

> **TIP:** Never attempt to comb completely through a tangle. If you encounter a tangle, redirect your comb. Use your fingers to carefully free single strands from the larger tangle. Then, start again from the ends with your comb and work your way back upward along the section of hair.

Comb each section of your hair once through from the root down through the ends, bracing your hair along the way. Use the same technique with a progressively smaller comb if desired. Once you have detangled a section to your sat-

isfaction, pin it up or rebraid it out of your way. After thorough detangling, you are ready to proceed with regular styling or move on to the low-manipulation hair-cleansing techniques.

Hair-Cleansing Techniques
Water Temperature

Water temperature plays an important role in black hair care. For something that is dead, our hair responds quite well to different types of stimuli. Just as the hair's cuticle layers respond to pH by lifting and constricting, they also respond to hot and cold water temperatures. Warm water expands and lifts the hair cuticles, while cold water contracts and tightens them.

It is best to cleanse black hair in water that is warm, not hot. If the water used to cleanse your hair is too hot, it may damage the cuticles and leave the hair feeling dry and parched in the process. Hot water causes the cuticles to lift dramatically, and repeated hot cleansings can cause them to peel and crack. If your textured hair is color treated, using hot water to shampoo and condition your hair may cause your color to fade rapidly and lose its vibrancy. Warm water is easiest on black hair and protects hair colors so that they last longer.

The final rinsing of conditioner should be done with water that is cooler than the water used to shampoo the hair. Cold-water rinsing is a mechanical or physical way of tightening and constricting the cuticle layers. It should be done as the final step of any hair-cleansing session. The cool water rinse will make the cuticles lie flatter and tighter, enhancing the hair's shine as light bounces off of it. The water does not have to be bitterly cold, but it should be cool enough for your scalp to feel invigorated by the rinsing. Water as cool as you can stand is the rule of thumb.

Make sure that you thoroughly rinse the conditioner product from your scalp and hair. Leftover conditioner residues can dull the hair and leave a film-like coating on the scalp. This film may flake off when dry and create a dandruff-like appearance.

Water Pressure

Using the shower to shampoo and cleanse the hair is very convenient for a number of reasons. Body and hair can be taken care of in one session, and the force of the water from the showerhead helps lift and remove stubborn dirt and debris from the hair. High water pressure, however, can be a source of unexpected damage for black hair. Black hair is extremely fragile when it is wet, and great care must be taken to ensure that it is not damaged by rough handling. Some showerheads eject streams of water in a concentrated fashion that can be too much for delicate textured hair fibers.

If your shower releases high-pressure water, decrease the water pressure by turning down the water, adjusting the showerhead's settings, or using a cup to pour water over your head. If you are not opposed to it, you may also wash your hair separately in the tub and then switch to a shower for your body cleansing.

Over-the-Sink Washing

Shampooing and conditioning the hair over the sink can be tricky, and it is best to have someone to help you with this if at all possible. The best way to wash hair over the sink is face up, just as it is done in a salon setting. As you may realize, trying this technique at home is sure to be an uncomfortable, backbreaking task! It is much easier to wash the hair face down in the sink at home. However, this method presents a possible tangling challenge when you begin the comb-out.

When we lean forward over the sink or tub to shampoo our tresses, the hair and cuticles are oriented in the opposite direction of the recommended DOWNWARD comb-out. When we rise from the sink to detangle the hair, we are forced to flip the hair backward before starting to comb it downward. The manipulation and potential for

tangling in this situation can be high. Washing the hair face down over the sink at home is advisable only if you are using the Braided Cleansing method described below.

Breakage-Free Hair-Washing Strategy 1: Braided Cleansing

Shampooing and conditioning black hair is best done on four to five loosely braided sections. These braided sections keep the hair organized and reduce normal friction and breakage between the hair strands. When the hair is bound during a wash, the tendency toward tangling is reduced because the hair does not have an opportunity to wander far from its original position.

Each hair braid has a strength that the individual hairs it is made of do not possess. To understand this concept, try breaking a single toothpick. Easy, right? Now bundle five or six toothpicks together and try to break them. It seems to take superhuman strength to break the bundle of toothpicks! There is certainly strength in numbers, and this is as true of your hair as it is of the toothpicks. As your hair grows longer, you will truly understand the utility of this divide-and-conquer method of hair organization for cleansing. You will find that using the braided sections method for cleansing makes your hair very soft and pliable. It is the preferred low manipulation method for cleansing the hair at home.

Braided cleansing can be done in two basic ways. One option is to keep the braids intact throughout the entire shampoo and conditioning process. This method reduces overall breakage, but shampoo and conditioner can linger if the hair is not rinsed very well. The second option is to unbraid and address each section of hair separately as you shampoo and condition. This method is best for those who simply wish to keep their hair organized during a session and allows the user to focus product and effort on individual areas of the hair while ensuring thorough rinsing.

After detangling your hair, take advantage of your detangling sections and braid the hair into four (or more) sections. The braids should be looser at the top near the scalp and should tighten toward the ends. Keeping the braid looser at the top will give you room to massage the scalp underneath. Tightening the braid at the end will help it stay together once the water hits it. Do not braid the end too tightly because if this part of the braid is really thin, it can be difficult to unbraid once it is wet. For extra protection, or on shorter hair, you may choose to secure the braids on the end with a hair tie or loose band.

For braided cleansing, follow these steps:

1.) Thoroughly wet and rinse braided hair in warm water for one to two minutes to free it of product buildup and residue. Use the pads of your fingers to gently lift the hair, squeezing and smoothing it to loosen buildup.

2.) Squeeze shampoo about the size of a quarter into your hand and then distribute the shampoo throughout the braided hair sections, concentrating on the root and scalp areas. The initial application of shampoo should be used to lift oils, sweat and product from the scalp area. The length of the hair will receive the shampoo runoff.

3.) Allow the shampoo to sit on the hair undisturbed for about a minute. This gives the ingredients in the shampoo formula an opportunity to bind to dirt, debris and products to lift them in the first rinsing.

4.) Next, work the lather downward along the braid in a squeezing, milking fashion. The shampoo and water mixture will penetrate the braid and loosen dirt and product buildup without removing the hair's natural oils.

5.) Thoroughly rinse the hair in warm water.

6.) If your lather is weak and the hair is quite soiled, repeat steps 2 through 5.

7.) Apply a small amount of conditioner, about the size of a quarter, to each section, focusing on the ends. Allow the conditioner to remain on the hair for at least ten minutes, with or without heat.

8.) Thoroughly rinse out conditioner with cool water. If heat is used, allow the hair to cool down before rinsing.

Breakage-Free Hair-Washing Strategy 2: Freeform Cleansing

If you elect to forego the plaited sections, you may simply shampoo your hair in the usual way, making sure that you keep the hair strands hanging downward throughout the session. The strategy and technique are quite similar to the first method, except that greater care must be exercised when dealing with free-ranging textured hair. These fibers are more delicate because they don't benefit from the strength-in-numbers protection that braids afford.

After detangling the hair as described above, follow these simple steps for freeform hair cleansing:

1.) Thoroughly wet and rinse loose hair in warm water for one to two minutes to free it of product buildup and residue. Use the pads of your fingers to gently lift the hair, squeezing and smoothing to loosen buildup.

2.) Squeeze shampoo about the size of a quarter into your hand and then distribute the shampoo throughout the hair, concentrating on the root and scalp areas and avoiding any bunching and scrunching. The initial application of shampoo should be used primarily to lift oils, sweat and product from the scalp area. The length of the hair will receive the shampoo runoff.

3.) Allow the shampoo to sit on the hair undisturbed for two to three minutes. This gives the ingredients in the shampoo formula an opportunity to bind to dirt, debris and products to lift them in the first rinsing.

4.) Next, work the lather downward along the hair shafts in a squeezing, milking fashion.

5.) Thoroughly rinse the hair in warm water.

6.) If your lather is weak and the hair quite soiled, repeat steps 2 through 5.

7.) Apply small amounts of conditioner (about the size of a quarter) to the hair, focusing on the ends, until the hair is saturated with conditioner. Allow the conditioner to remain on the hair for at least ten minutes, with or without heat.

8.) Thoroughly rinse out conditioner with cool water. If heat is used, allow the hair to cool down before rinsing.

Low-Manipulation Deep Conditioning

Textured hair should always be conditioned after a shampoo product is used. Deep conditioning, however, is an intervention designed primarily for damaged, porous hair. Despite this, all hair can benefit from deep conditioning. For the purposes of this conditioning discussion, the term *damaged hair* refers to black hair that has been compromised by relaxers, permanent hair colors or any styling processes (excessive heat styling, for example) that affect its protein structure and cuticle. While healthy hair can benefit from deep conditioning, damaged hair requires it.

Regular conditioners are primarily surface-acting products. Their task is to seal the outer cuticle and shield it from external trauma. Healthy hair with a strong, intact cuticle resists the entry of conditioner and limits its activity to the outer cuticle layers. Regular deep conditioning keeps healthy hair on the up-and-up. When hair is damaged, the outer cuticle layers are not uniform, and there are often gaps in cortical protection. Under these circumstances, conditioners are able to get in and do more repair work on damaged or compromised hair, in addition to supporting better barrier function against moisture loss. Because the protective action of conditioners lasts for only a few days, more dedicated and regular deep conditioning efforts must be in place. To obtain optimal hair condition for damaged hair,

deep conditioning must become a part of your total healthy hair care regimen.

When warm water is introduced to our hair, the hair fiber swells and the cuticles lift to accommodate the swelling. Conditioners correct the disrupted cuticle orientation by smoothing the scales and reorienting them downward. Conditioners also help to normalize the pH of the hair and provide a layer of protection against trauma from detangling and styling until the next conditioning.

To get the most out of deep conditioning, follow these steps:

1. After shampooing, gently squeeze excess water from the hair. Displacing the water from the hair fiber makes room for needed conditioning compounds to bind and integrate with the hair fiber.

2. Thoroughly saturate your hair with conditioner, concentrating the conditioner product on the ends of your hair. (It is good to get into the practice of applying hair products from the ends up, especially conditioners and moisturizers.) If you have decided to cleanse your hair using the Braided Cleansing method, you may either choose to unbraid the sections to apply deep conditioner or simply slather the conditioner over the braids.

3. Once the conditioner has been applied, cover the hair with a plastic cap for deep conditioning. Heated deep conditioning is most effective, but the natural warmth from your scalp, held in by the plastic conditioning cap, is also a good deep-conditioning environment.

4. Rinse out the conditioning treatment with cool water. If heat is used, allow the hair to cool for several minutes before you rinse out the treatment.

How Long Should I Deep Condition?

The length of conditioning time required for thorough conditioning depends on several factors including the hair's porosity, the type of conditioner used, and whether or not heat will

The CCC Method

Often times, the middle and crown areas of the hair do not receive adequate conditioning, especially when the hair is conditioned at home. Many times, this is simply a result of the limitations of our anatomy, which make reaching certain areas along the back of the scalp difficult. To ensure full coverage of the conditioner, a helpful conditioning method is one I call the Comprehensive Conditioner Coverage (CCC) method. This method is a highly detailed conditioner-application method that ensures maximum conditioner coverage throughout the hair. In the CCC conditioning method, conditioner is applied to the hair as though it were a relaxer. The hair is divided into four sections and then finger parted at 1-inch intervals. Conditioner is placed on the hair fiber along each section in a thick layer that—unlike relaxers!—extends from the roots down to the ends of the hair fiber for maximum coverage.

be used. A good rule of thumb is that deep conditioners should be left on the hair until the hair softens. With heat applied, this timing can be anywhere from five to fifteen minutes and will ensure maximum penetration and conditioning of the fiber. Without heat, you should allocate at least ten minutes for regular conditioning after washes and at least ten to fifteen minutes for deep conditioning the hair. Damaged or porous hair will take in the conditioner and soften at a faster rate, with or without heat. Positively charged conditioners are strongly attracted to the negatively-charged, damaged areas along the fiber, so the more damage, the more conditioner binding and uptake you will get. Some conditioners—for instance, instant conditioners—contain ingredients that are much too large to penetrate deep into the fiber. No matter how much heat is used to encourage fiber penetration, these types of conditioners are not deep conditioners and can only coat the hair to protect it.

Low-Manipulation Towel Drying

You will want to have a microfiber towel ready to dry your hair. Microfiber towels, although typically not as fluffy as regular cotton towels, are preferable because they quickly absorb water from the hair with minimal contact with the fiber. They do not contribute or create substantial frictional force upon the hair fiber, making them much easier on textured hair. Hair wrapped in a microfiber towel also dries faster than hair wrapped in standard drying towel. If you do not have microfiber towel on hand, a standard cotton T-shirt has a similar drying effect and is easy on textured strands.

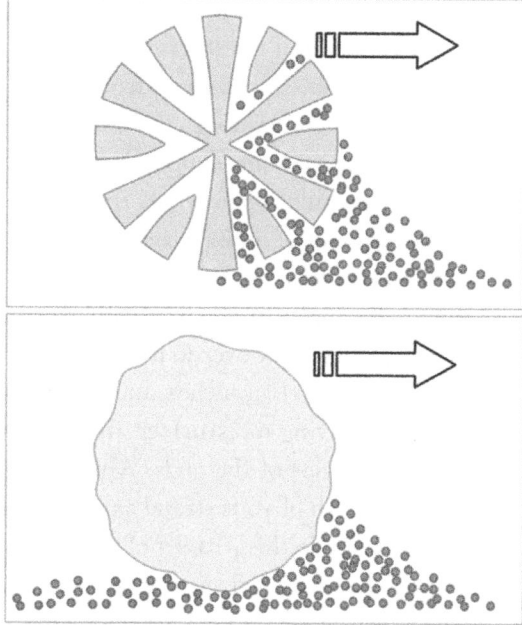

Figure 45: Cross Section of microfiber absorbency (top) compared to cotton absorbency shown below. No residue remains after contact with microfiber fabric .

Once you have conditioned and rinsed your hair, use your hands to carefully press excess water from the hair. Next, use the microfiber towel to gently blot the hair. Avoid scrunching, rubbing and sliding the towel down your wet tresses with tension. Simply pat and squeeze the excess water out of the hair. For naturals with coily, curly and kinky hair types, microfiber towels will help preserve curl definition as you dry your hair.

Low-Manipulation Moisturizing

The divide-and-conquer technique used for detangling also works well for moisturizing the hair with water-based cream moisturizers. This method is perfect for focusing on the precious ends of your hair. After establishing your hair sections, simply use a finger coated in a bit of cream moisturizer to make ½- to 1-inch partitions throughout the hair.

Follow the steps below to apply cream moisturizers:

1.) Once you have partitioned a section, take a pea-size amount of moisturizer and apply it to your hair three inches away from the tips of the ends. Gently smooth the moisturizer down from this point, supporting the sectioned hair strand as you do so. You may adjust the amount of moisturizer used to suit your tastes and to account for product consistency. Be sure that you have fully treated your ends, but don't overdo it!

2.) Move up three to four inches, and repeat the process, applying moisturizer all the way down to the tips of the ends. Always support the length of your strand as you move down. Continue this pattern of application until you have reached your scalp.

3.) Repeat on each section until you have moisturized your entire head of hair.

With this technique, you will go over the hair ends in each section with two to four passes, depending upon the length of your hair. This is vital. The lower parts of the hair shaft are naturally more porous and dry because they are older. The higher up on the hair strand you move, the newer the hair and the less moisture it needs to remain in tip-top shape. This technique takes that fact into account, gifting the lower parts of your hair with more moisture than the base.

For those who are truly on the run, those with fine hair and those who are wearing styles such as weaves, braids and twists that do not lend themselves to the use of cream moisturizers, hair misting is a better moisturizing option. Invest in a misting bottle and fill it with your favorite liquid water-based moisturizer or diluted conditioner. Sprays are an inexpensive way to keep your hair moisturized without a lot of fuss.

Keep in mind that a little goes a long way in the application of moisturizers. Too much, and your hair may have a limp, greasy feel. Your hair should feel moist, not wet, after applying your moisturizer (unless that is the feel you are going for). You may need to experiment with different amounts of different moisturizers to find the consistency and amount that works best for your hair and lifestyle. Some individuals prefer spray or mist-type moisturizers, others prefer light creams, while still others prefer thick, heavy, butter-type products. Your preference may vary depending on the style you are wearing and your hair type. If you have just straightened your hair, using a spray or mist type moisturizer may not work as well for you as it would with someone who has chosen a wash-and-go or bun style.

Special Conditioning Treatments and Methods

Pre-shampoo treatments are hair treatments applied before the shampoo stage. These treatments are optional moisture or softness boosters (depending on the medium used) and help dry hair regain its suppleness and elasticity. For those who use harsher shampoos, pre-shampoo treatments help the hair preserve some of its natural oils and emerge from the shampooing stage less stripped and fragile.

These treatments can be done with either warmed conditioner or oil, or with a combination of both. Water-based conditioner products work best for penetration into the hair fiber, while oils are better cuticle-nourishing elements. Pre-shampoo treatments are usually done twenty to thirty minutes prior to washing or as an overnight treatment before the wash. Pre-shampoo treatments can be performed on dry or damp hair. Some people find that doing pre-shampoo treatments on dampened hair allows the fiber to absorb moisture-boosting products with greater ease. Others find that their dry hair receives the treatments better. You will need to experiment to discover what works best for you.

Hot-oil vs. Pre-shampoo Treatments

Hot-oil treatments are very similar to pre-shampoo treatments. They differ mainly in the stage of the washing cycle in which they are applied. Unlike pre-shampoo treatments, hot-oil treatments tend to follow the shampoo stage rather than precede it. Increasingly, however, many people are finding utility in applying hot-oil treatments at the pre-shampoo stage as well. Hot-oil treatments also tend to include oils exclusively, whereas pre-shampoo treatments are quite varied.

You should experiment with these treatments in order to determine where they best fall in your new healthy hair-growing regimen. You may decide to forgo them altogether as they are not an absolute requirement for improving the condition of the hair. These are simply icing-on-the-cake treatments. Pre-shampoos are highly personal; experiment with timing and different ingredients to find the technique that works best for you.

Perfecting Pre-shampoo/Hot-Oil Treatment Techniques

First, determine if you would like to conduct your treatment with a warmed conditioner, an oil mix or both. The following oils are most commonly used for hot-oil treatments:

- Almond
- Amla
- Argan
- Avocado butter (melted)
- Castor
- Coconut
- Jojoba
- Olive
- Shea butter (melted)
- Dabur Vatika

Other oils may be added or substituted for these staples. For those who choose to use conditioners, the easiest to use are really inexpensive instant conditioners such as Suave and VO5 brands. They are light and moisturizing, and you can use a little or a lot without feeling guilty! (The amount you use will vary depending upon hair thickness and length and the thickness of the warmed oils/conditioners.)

Treatment Checklist
- applicator bottle
- ½ cup or more oil or conditioner
- ¼ cup honey
- small bowl
- comb, hair clips, plastic cap, and towel/dryer

Get Your Hair Together

This treatment is best done on hair that is detangled and parted into sections. You may do as many large sections as you desire, but three or four will be easiest to work with.

Get Your Mix Together

Warm the oils, conditioner and honey in a small microwavable bowl at ten-second intervals. Check the mixture for warmth, and remove it when it becomes too warm for your fingers. Stir the mixture, and allow it to sit briefly. When the mixture has cooled just enough not to scald, transfer the warmed liquid or cream to your applicator bottle. (Alternatively, you may simply use your hands to apply the pre-shampoo concoction.)

Application: One Step at a Time

Work with one section of hair at a time. Use clips to tie back the other sections of hair while you concentrate on one. If you have chosen to use an applicator bottle, simply finger part your hair within each section and apply the warmed concoction to your scalp and hair. Do not attempt to part through your hair perfectly with a comb, especially if you are several weeks post-relaxer. Finger parting will work just as well. You want to part, lift, apply, part, lift, apply. Be sure that you coat both sides of the hair strand with your mixture. Use your hands to distribute the remaining concoction throughout the length. If you do not want oily hands, gloves will work here as well.

Time to Bake

When your hair is covered with the mixture from root to ends, it is now time to trap in some warmth with the plastic conditioning cap. Once your cap is secure, you may wrap your head with a warmed towel from your dryer. Alternatively, you may forgo the towel and simply sit under a hooded dryer wearing your plastic cap. Keep your hair covered for twenty to thirty minutes. (Another option is to use no heat at all, but this method will require that you keep the mixture on your hair much longer (until the hair begins to soften) to achieve the same conditioning level the heat creates.)

Rinse and Shampoo

Remove the towel and/or plastic cap from your hair and rinse with warm water. The length is the part of the hair that truly benefits from pre-shampoo/hot-oil treatments, so keeping a bit of the oil there while you shampoo is helpful.

Finally, shampoo and condition your hair as normal. Remember, the final hair rinse should be done with water as cool as you can stand. This will help to seal the cuticle mechanically. Your hair should feel full, soft and strong from the pre-shampoo or hot-oil treatment. Any oiliness, greasiness or stickiness following your treatment is the result of inadequate rinsing.

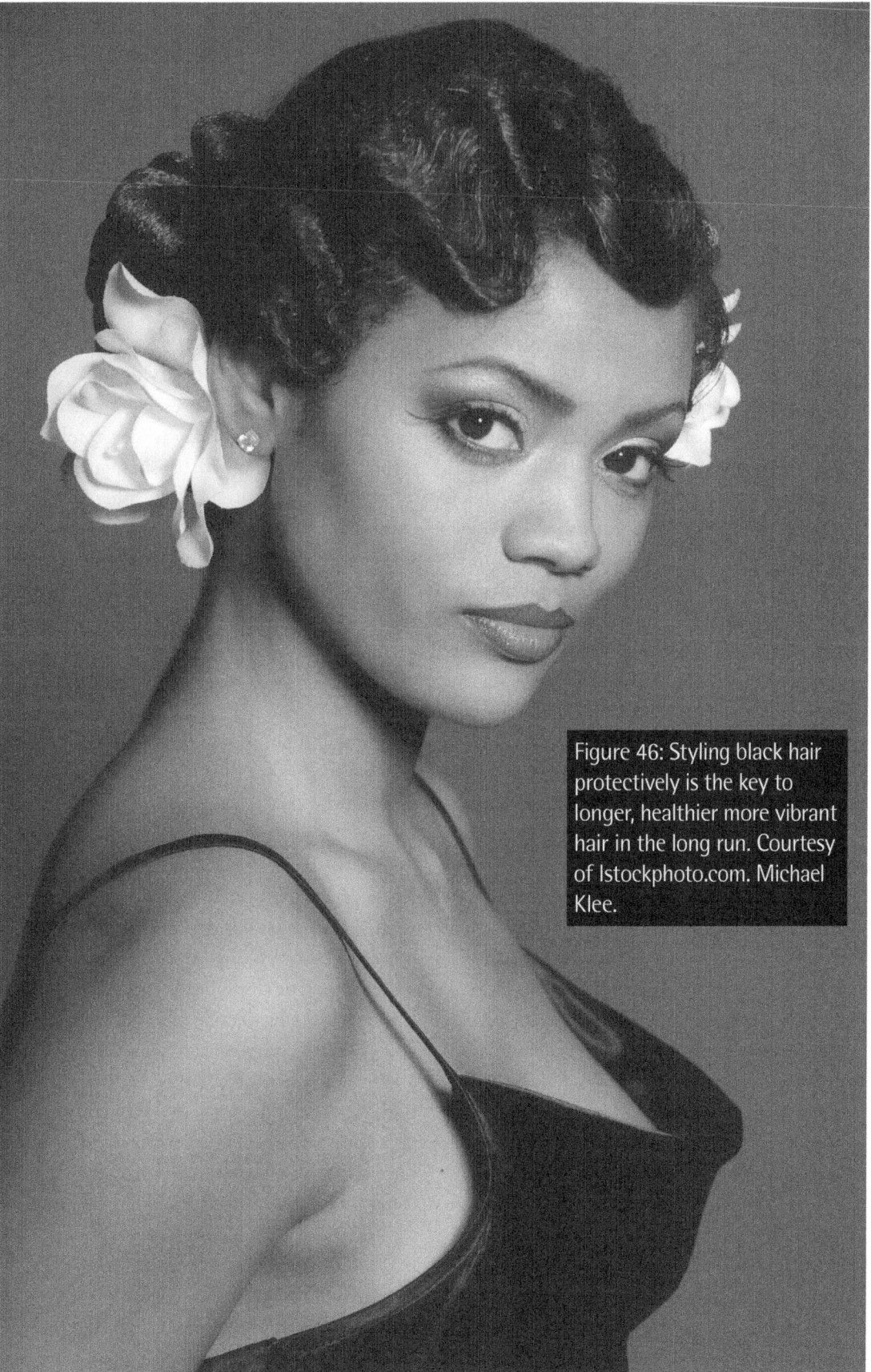

Figure 46: Styling black hair protectively is the key to longer, healthier more vibrant hair in the long run. Courtesy of lstockphoto.com. Michael Klee.

Protective Hair Styling

Black hair is very fragile. It must be treated like fine silk to reach its greatest length potential. For those of us who are all too familiar with the shoulder-length plateau, protective hair styling is the ultimate key to hair ends preservation.

In addition to the fact that we are dealing with older, more fragile hair at shoulder length, the shoulders themselves are very much an anatomical obstacle to increased hair length. When our hair is worn straight, our already delicate older hair ends repeatedly brush the shoulders in the open air, creating an overall tendency toward dryness. When our hair rubs back and forth against the shoulders, the hair's natural flat cuticle orientation is disrupted, the cortex loses precious internal moisture, and the hair grows ever more prone to splitting and breakage. Our shirt and blouse fabrics create harmful friction forces with our hair ends that can lead to splitting and cracking of the cuticle. Unless a shirt's fabric provides great slip for the hair (for example, silk or satiny materials), it is able to draw precious moisture from your hair and become an additional source of friction against the cuticles. Simply stated, wearing textured hair down and loose, regularly, encourages breakage at the very ends.

Remember, the ends of the hair are characterized by a natural decrease in cuticle thickness and protection as normal wear and tear has worn the bottom scales. A cycle develops in which the ends become dry, rough and finally split. The hair may be trimmed again and again to compensate for this roughening of the cuticle and damage to the ends. Without comprehensive protective styling, the ends of the hair will continue to fray as they rub and slide back and forth across cotton shirts and blouses. If this continues over the course of several months or years, the hair will never grow past this point and may even retreat.

Hard-to-grow-long textured hair should be worn up and off the shoulders to protect it from common environmental hair stressors that lead to hair breakage. Our textured hair is diverse, and a variety of protective styling options are ours for the choosing. Common protective hairstyles include carefully styled hair buns, chignons, braids, head wraps, roller sets, spiral sets and other curly hairstyles. Short hair and most natural hairstyles are already protective in that they keep our hair up and off the shoulders.

Types of Protective Hairstyles

Protective hairstyles preserve our hair in several ways. Some reduce day-to-day combing and styling manipulation with brushes, curling irons, blow dryers and flatirons, while others reduce the hair's primary exposure to environmental stressors like the air, sun, wind, rain and humidity. The two most common protective-styling categories are complete protective styles and low-manipulation protective styles.

Complete protective styles keep the ends of the hair entirely out of sight. They can be achieved without heat and are 100 percent protective of the ends of the hair. Low-manipulation protective styles may expose the ends of the hair to some degree, but they drastically cut down on day-to-day hair manipulation. Low-manipulation protective styles are typically long-term-wear styles such as twists and spiral sets that do not need to be combed daily. These styles can be smoothed or fluffed back into place with the fingers. Some protective hairstyles can be classified as both complete and low manipulation. A good regimen will contain a healthy mixture of both types of styles for variety. Taken together, these protective styling measures greatly reduce our hair's breakage burden so that greater length can be achieved over time.

Is Protective Styling Necessary?

Remember, protective styling is a comprehensive method of hair care that extends far beyond simple hairstyling. While protective hairstyling is a highly effective hair preservation tool and proven hair growing method, it is not an absolute requirement for growing the hair. Our hair can be grown with regimens that keep the hair loose and free. In fact, there are many, many women with textured hair who wear their hair in loose, free-form or hanging styles twenty-four hours a day, seven days a week and grow their hair to great lengths without incident. But hair care trade-offs of one kind or another are quite common. Those who wear their hair loose or free tend to follow regimens that are protective in other ways. For example, their regimens may not include regular hair coloring, they may not relax their hair, or they may follow other types of low-manipulation or low-heat styling regimens. While protective hair styling is not a hard-and-fast rule for hair growth, this form of hair care fits neatly into the overall, healthy hair care low-manipulation strategy of shampooing, conditioning and detangling to support healthy black hair growth and retention.

If you have had problems in the past with growing out your hair, protective hairstyling may be a viable option for you. Hair care regimens that emphasize protective hairstyling stand a greater chance of producing healthier, longer hair faster than regimens in which the hair is regularly worn out and manipulated. If daily protective hairstyling does not appeal to you, then similar results can be achieved by incorporating protective styles on a more flexible schedule. Simply incorporating a few protective styles into your regimen each week will make a difference in the quality of your hair and its ability to retain length.

Protective Styling for Shorter Hair

Hair shorter than shoulder length is a protective style all on its own. Short hair does not produce frayed and splitting ends after rubbing against clothing, shoulders and chair backs throughout the day. With hair at this inherently protective length, the hair can be worn loose

fairly often. The only styling concern for short hair is ensuring its protection from the elements: air, wind, rain, heat and cold—which can quickly dry out the hair. Luckily, this concern can easily be mitigated by simply moisturizing and sealing the ends of the hair each day.

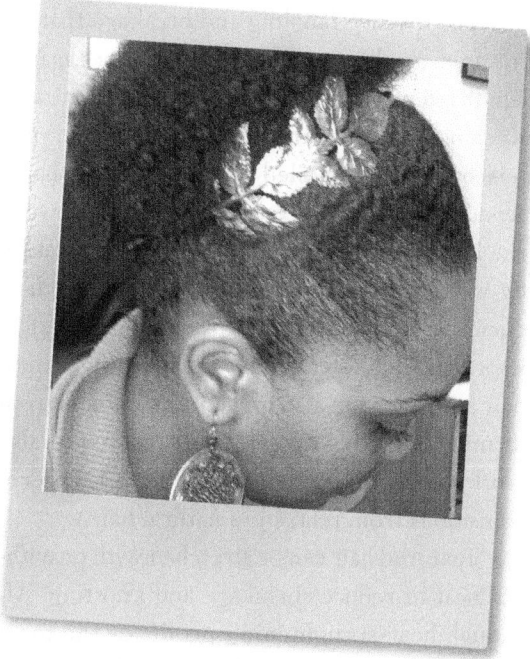

Figure 47: Short hair is both stylish and protective.

The best styles for hair that is shorter than shoulder length are curly styles including braid-outs, twist-outs, Bantu knots, straw sets, roller sets and anything pinned up. Some women like to wear braids to help them grow past this awkward length/styling stage. Once your hair reaches shoulder length, bunning your hair as a protective measure becomes an option.

Protective-Styling for Natural Hair
Working with Knots

A common problem that many kinky and tightly coiled naturals face is single-strand knotting. Single-strand knots occur when individual kinky, coiled strands wrap around themselves or connect and entwine with other strands. Such knotting often increases when textured hair is allowed to shrink back tightly to the scalp after cleansing, and is worn in this shrunken state. Wash-and-gos, braid-outs, twist-outs and other free-flowing natural styles are common triggers for single-strand knotting, especially on longer natural hair.

The massive tangling and breakage that result from single-strand knotting can work against length retention in natural hair quite dramatically. Keeping natural strands well moisturized, protein-balanced, and oiled cuts down on the hair's tendency to tangle by reducing friction between the hair fibers. Reducing styling manipulation by wearing the hair in confined styles such as cornrows and buns also helps to protect against knotting. Finally, stretching or elongating natural hair as it dries can also prevent these knots from forming along the strand. (These techniques also work well for those who are planning long-term transitions from relaxed to natural hair.)

Textured hair can be stretched with or without heat to reduce shrinkage and knotting. Although heat-straightening produces the most dramatic results, this technique is detrimental to a healthy hair care regimen when used for extended periods of time. Coarser, textured hair types can often handle regular heat manipulation, but finer, textured types may falter under such a regimen. Trial and error will help you determine where you fall.

Heat-Free Natural Hair-Stretching Techniques

Hair stretching is an effective styling tool for shrinkage-prone natural hair. Stretching may be used to keep single-strand knots and other tangles in check or simply to show off more length with natural hair. Although natural hair can be stretched while it is dry, it is best stretched while wet or dampened.

Natural-Hair Banding

Banding is a stretching technique that involves stretching the hair by placing small cloth ponytail holders or bands along the length to keep it stretched. Banding can be done on wet or dry hair; however, wet or damp hair will lengthen more easily and "remember" the banding set longer than dried hair. Simply separate the hair

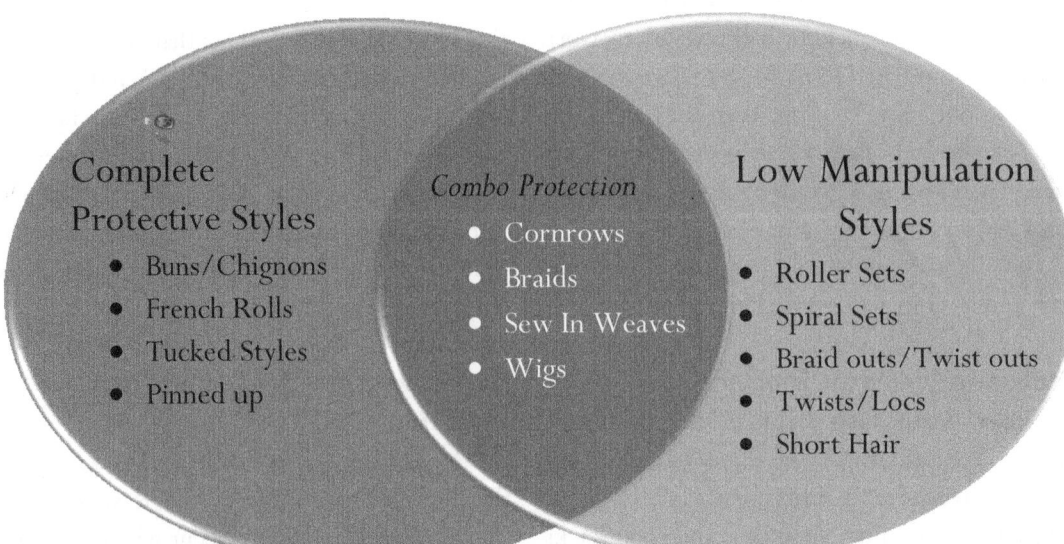

Figure 48: Types of Protective Hair Styles. The ideal protective style is one that requires little daily manipulation, hides the ends, and has been achieved without heat.

into eight to ten sections. Dampen and detangle one section of hair at a time and place a band at the base of the hair to create a standard ponytail. Continue to place bands along the length of the hair for each section at ½- to 1-inch intervals until you reach the ends. Band the entire head of hair in this manner, and allow the hair to air dry. Alternatively, a hooded dryer unit may be used. The result will be stretched-out, lengthier natural tresses that can be styled in a variety of longer styles. Band the hair to add length to two-strand twists, puffs and other natural styles.

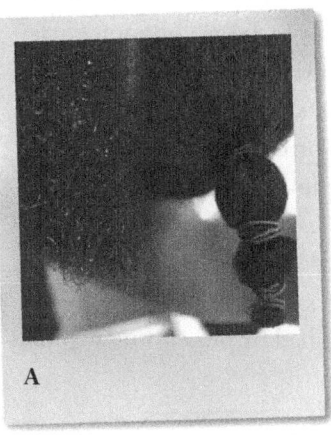 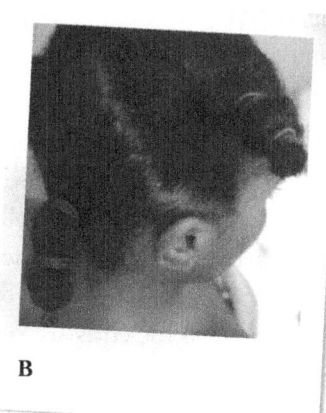

A   **B**

Figure 49: Banding works well for all hair types and lengths. This method can give additional length to even the shortest, shrinkage-prone natural hair. Notice how the back hair section in photo A is already beginning to contract and shrink back to the scalp as it dries. This section retains much more of its length when it is banded (B).

Braids and Twists

Twisting and braiding the hair in 1- to 1 ½-inch-square sections while damp also loosens kinky textured hair. Better lengthening results can be achieved with the twists, however, due to the sharp Z-shaped bends and angles that braids create in the hair. A similar effect can be observed on regular braid-out styles which tend to appear shorter than twist-out styles because of this angling/crinkling. Small braids and twists tend to work best for stretching the hair. If larger twists and braids are done to save time, these should be made tighter at the base of the hair to ensure that the part of the strand closest to the scalp is lengthened.

Roller setting and/or lightly blow drying natural hair (on a cool setting) are additional ways to stretch out textured locks so that they resist knotting.

Reducing Unwanted Frizz on Natural Curls

Frizz is the greatest enemy of those who desire natural, defined curls and coils. The best way to achieve crisp, bold curls and coils on textured hair is to apply a leave-in conditioner product to the hair while it is sopping wet. You can pat the hair with a T-shirt or microfiber towel to absorb the excess water. (Using a regular terry cloth towel will ruin your curl definition and cause the cuticles to ruffle—which leads to frizz.) Mix a bit of light styling gel with a serum in your hands. Scrunch this mixture through your hair by gently cupping the hair in the palm of your hands and squeezing upward in a slow, deliberate motion. (Some people find that bending forward while scrunching improves curl definition and volume.) The gel will help to set the style, while the serum will smooth your hair and block external moisture in the environment—another contributor to unwanted frizz!—from entering the hair. In addition, tighter coils and curls can be encouraged by adding a little light moisturizing gel to a small section of hair, smoothing with the fingers or brushing through with a hair-safe detangling brush for even distribution, and finally twisting the section with the fingers in the direction of the desired curl. Keep in mind that some frizziness is natural for some hair types. If curls cannot

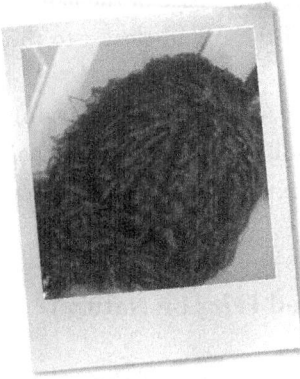
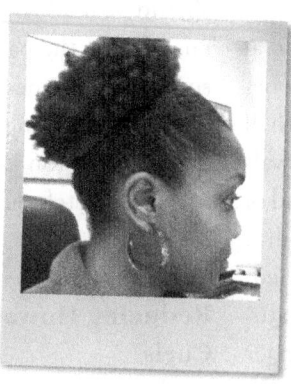

Figures 50, 51: Twist out style on relaxed hair. Hair was flat twisted to scalp after washing and conditioning. The twists were dried under a dryer, then released and fluffed. Moisturizer and oil were scrunched through for shine. Figure 51 shows a twistout style pulled into a puff on shorter natural hair.

be defined despite your best product efforts and techniques, it may be time to embrace and learn to work with some natural frizziness.

Common Protective Styles
Braid-Outs and Twist-Outs

Braid-outs can be accomplished by either plaiting the hair in four to five large sections or by corn rowing. The hair is simply braided and then released after a set time, which can be as short as thirty minutes to as long as a day or two, to produce the style. Braid-outs can be set on wet or dry hair. As with any style, wet setting produces the sleekest, longest-lasting results. Braid-out waves are Z-shaped and slightly angular. The ends of the hair may be curled with soft rollers or left to hang free.

Twist-outs are similar to braid-outs and can be accomplished by flat twisting the hair down toward the scalp, or simply twisting two sections of hair from the roots to the ends. The

twists are then released and unraveled to get twist-out waves. Like braid-outs, twist-outs can be set wet or dry (see Figures 50 and 51). Wet set twist-outs last longer than twist-outs set on dry hair, and the wet set waves are much more defined and polished. Twist-out waves are usually softer and have more of an S-shape than braid-out waves. Like braid-outs, the ends of twist-out styles can be curled using rollers or left free.

Roller Sets

Roller sets can range from small, straw-like sets to large, bouncy curls, depending on the size of the rolling tool used. These sets are great long-term-wear styles (see Figures 52 and 53) that need very little day-to-day care. The smaller the rod or roller used to set these curls, the longer-lasting the style. A typical roller set done on 1- to 2-inch rollers can last three to five days if the curls are refreshed by pin curling nightly.

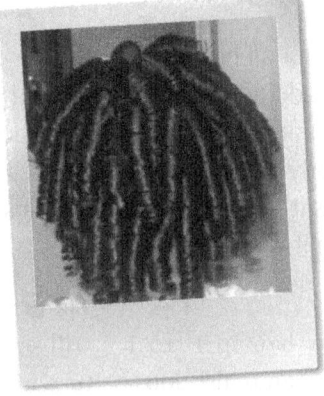
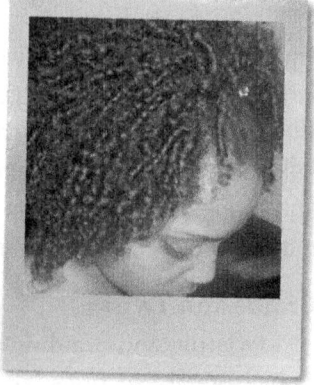

Figure 52 (above left): Spiral Set. Hair was set on basic hair rollers (approximately nickel-width diameter). Style can be worn "as is" or picked apart for beautiful volume.

Figure 53 (above right): Straw set after a week of wear. Hair was shampooed and conditioned then set using drinking straws as rods. Small perm rods will create a similar effect and style. Hair can be moisturized and fluffed to maintain throughout the week.

Smaller, tighter roller sets including straw sets can last as long as two weeks with very little maintenance.

Roller setting is a protective style that typically requires heat. Although sets may be air-dried, these sets generally do not have the sleekness of heat-supported sets. Fortunately, the heat required for rollersetting (hooded dryer heat) is a safer source of heat than traditional blow dryer heat. Quality hooded dryers warm hair gradually over the course of thirty to forty-five minutes, avoiding the damage that often comes with rapid heating. When we take this relatively safer heat, and consider the longer term nature of the styles achieved and the low manipulation required to maintain these styles, we find that these styles have protective effects. Finished sets can be worn curly or picked apart for volume and style changes throughout the week.

Ponytails and Puffs

Ponytails and puffs are also effective protective styles. These simple, low-manipulation styles can help keep the hair up and off the shoulders. Ponytails with relaxed hair are best done on almost dry, moisturized hair as relaxed hair is very prone to damage from stretching and breakage when wet. Relaxed hair can be smoothed, moisturized and sealed daily to maintain the style. Natural puffs, however, are best created on very moist hair (not wet!). To maintain the puff style, natural hair can be re-moistened, stretched and shaped gently to create more length and volume.

Keep in mind that the tightness of the bands and holders (see Figure 54) used to secure these styles determines how protective the style is. If pulled too tightly, ponytails and puffs can put stress on the delicate hairline and lead to thinning and breakage. Bands are too tight if wearers can feel tension along the hairline when the head is turned, or if simple facial expressions like smiling result in tugging. Stress around the

ponytail holder also can cause hair breakage and mid-shaft splitting. Oiling ponytail holders can reduce some of the natural friction against hair in confined, ponytail or puff styles.

Avoid placing holders or ties on hair that is dripping wet. Pulling our hair taut and into a fixed holder while it is sopping wet can be terribly damaging to our tresses over time. Hair is stretched and is most elastic when wet. As our hair dries, it naturally begins to contract. While the stretched hair is trying to return to its normal state, it is still being held taut in its stretched position by the ponytail holder. Over time, the area near the holder grows weaker from the stretching and the hair's inability to properly contract during drying. The end result is breakage. It is always best to create any ponytail, puff or bun style on hair that is moisturized

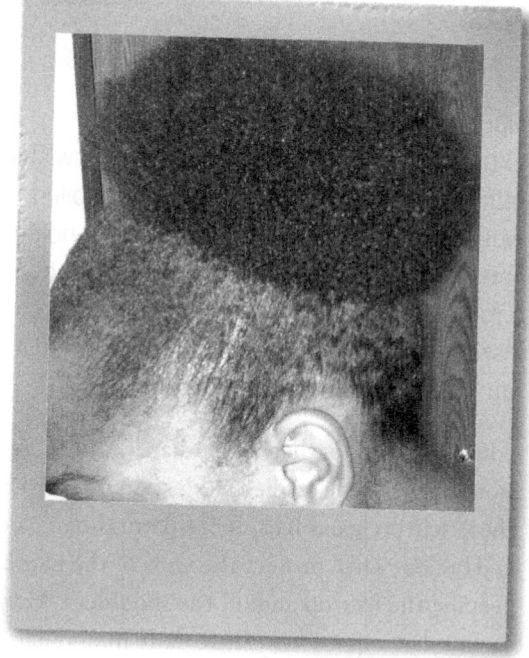

Figure 54: Simple afro puff protective style. Puff was styled on damp hair. Light hair butter and Ecostyler® gel products were distributed to sides and edges to prepare for drawing of the puff. Puff was drawn using a tie fashioned from a cut leg of hosiery. Damp hair was tied down around puff with a satin scarf for ten minutes to increase sleekness.

and almost completely dry to avoid "wet holder stress." Once hair is completely dry, loosening holders that were styled on damp hair is strongly advised. Alternating the positions of ponytails and puffs is also encouraged to fight breakage.

Buns, Chignons and Updos

Buns, chignons and updos are classic protective hairstyles that take the ponytail/puff

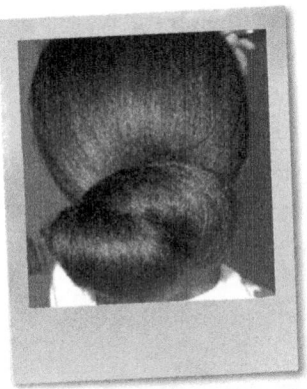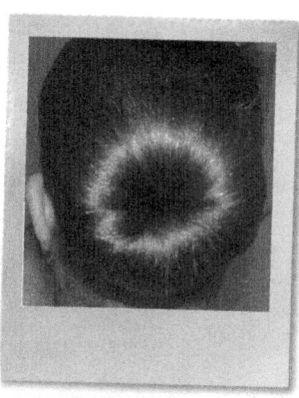

Figure 55: Simple bun styles. Buns are extremely versatile protective styles. In twisted bun configurations, hair is simply ponytailed, wound, and pinned around the ponytail holder. The "donut" or sock bun is created by using a form that resembles a donut. Ponytails are inserted into the donut's interior and are then fanned and secured around the circle.

concept a step further and enhance the protection of those styles. These styles can be worn by those with relaxed hair, loose natural hair, locs and braids. They protect the ends of the hair by keeping the hair up and off the shoulders. Many such styles require very little daily maintenance over the course of a week and can be refreshed by simply moisturizing, oiling and fluffing with the fingers.

The bun is one of the easiest protective styles to achieve, but it is more protective at certain lengths. If, for instance, the hair is so short (usually between neck and shoulder) that the holder sits on the hair ends when the bun is created,

then the style is less protective. Waiting until the hair is fully shoulder length or just below to begin bunning is a better option.

Buns can be styled either wet or dry, but caution should be exercised when wet bunning textured hair.

Two-Strand Twists

Two-strand or double-strand twists are popular hairstyles among women with natural hair. Twists are a very convenient hairstyle that can be worn on hair in its early natural stages and beyond (see Figure 56). Once set, they can be worn for days at a time, making them a great low-manipulation protective style. One set of twists has the ability to evolve into a variety of other styles over the course of a week with simple unraveling and fluffing. Twists can also be used as a styling tool to simply stretch natural hair for lengthier styles,

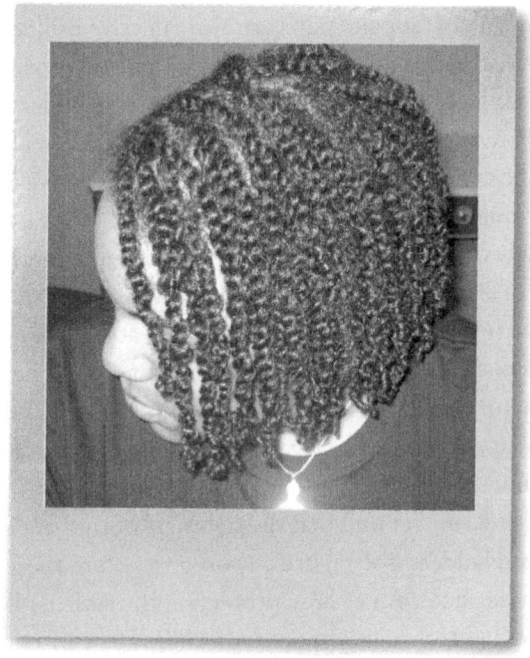

Figure 56: Simple two strand twists. These twists can be worn as a style, or as preparation for twistouts and other styles. Courtesy of Georgette Whaley of Soul Sister Hair Care, Houston TX.

or as a precursor styling step for styles such as chunky afros or chunky puffs.

While two-strand twists can be done on dry hair, like most sets, the best definition is achieved when the twists are wet set. Any additional styling looks you may get out of a set of twists will also be less defined if the twists are set on dry hair. Light gels and hair butters are great product tools to use at the initial twisting stage to improving twist definition, style longevity and shine.

Twist maintenance generally involves daily misting with a spray moisturizer to keep the twists fresh and moisturized throughout the day. Sealing the twists with an oil or butter product will give them additional polish and will help lock in important moisture.

Hair can be shampooed and conditioned easily in two-strand twists. This is a great option if you want to avoid the handling associated with parting and re-parting a new set of twists after a wash.

Locs

Locs are simply organized (or unorganized!) bundles of natural hair. Contrary to popular belief, this bundled hair still requires cleansing, protein/moisture conditioning and protective oils to remain pliable. As with textured hair in general, heavy, shaft-coating, grease-like products that include beeswax and/or petrolatum ingredients should be avoided when possible. These ingredients can accumulate in the core of the loc. Because locs can unravel with heavy conditioning, deep conditioning locs should be reserved for once-monthly maintenance. Weekly moisture mists and oil sealing are preferable methods for infusing locs with needed moisture.

Locs are already somewhat protective in that daily combing and brushing maintenance are no longer causes of cuticle abrasion. Coloring and regular twisting and handling, however, can easily damage delicate locs. Loc wearers can get more

protection out of their locs by simply styling longer locs in updo styles, ponytails and curly styles. Ideally, new growth should be twisted into locs once it reaches ½ inch in length. This translates into retwisting no more than once a month to keep manipulation low.

Coils and Comb Twists

Comb coils are a good low-maintenance style for those with natural hair. These coils are great for new naturals with very short hair. With proper care, these twists (see Figure 57) can last three to four weeks, depending on the wearer's hair-growth rate. If comb coils are worn for any longer than this three-to-four-week period, coils may begin to form early locs. For this reason, comb coils are often used as a loc-starting method.

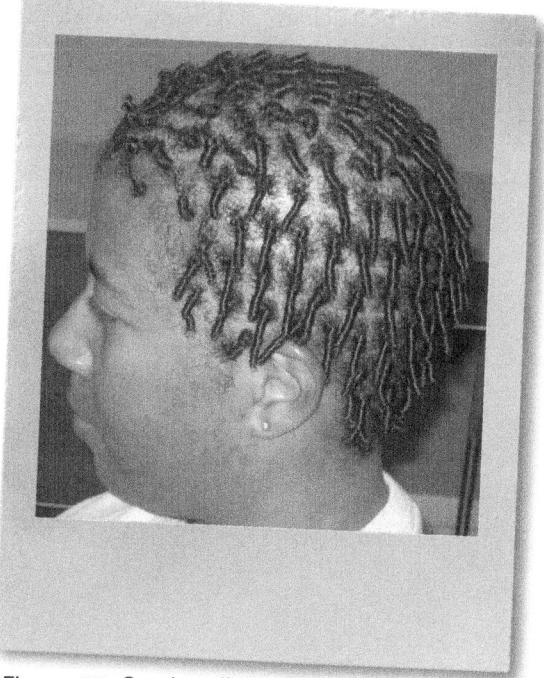

Figure 57: Comb coils are a great short hair style for natural hair. Courtesy of Robyn Allen (pictured) & Georgette Whaley (stylist) of Soul Sister Hair Care, Houston TX.

For styles like comb coils and early-stage locs, introducing water to the hair will spoil the style. In this case, it may be better to directly cleanse the scalp with a cotton ball dabbed in a diluted astringent like Seabreeze®. Essential oils like witch hazel and lemongrass are natural astringents that are great to use for controlling excessive oiliness and keeping the scalp clean. Astringent-type products can be harsh, so do use them sparingly on the scalp to remove stubborn buildup. Dry shampoos are also popular with frequent braid and weave wearers but may not work well for those with styles such as comb coils that unravel easily.

Step-By-Step

No matter how well written a book may be, all books face considerable disadvantages when it comes to conveying styling steps in an effective manner. From hair styles, to makeup looks, to baking a cake or roasting a holiday hen—some topics simply lend themselves better to the visual realm. Hair styling is one of those topics.

I like to think of writing a hair styling chapter like singing a song. I can write the lyrics to the most beautiful song in the world and even show you the score on paper, but that song does not come alive for you until you hear it sung by someone with talent. This chapter of the book presents a variety of protective styles and highlights the benefits of each style. Care instructions are discussed in detail throughout the section, but for step-by-step styling guidance *(to hear the song sung well)*, I encourage you to seek out the many, many free online styling tutorials available on popular video sharing sites like *YouTube*®. Simply put, nothing beats visual media for describing how to best achieve styles and looks.

Science of Black Hair Street Interview

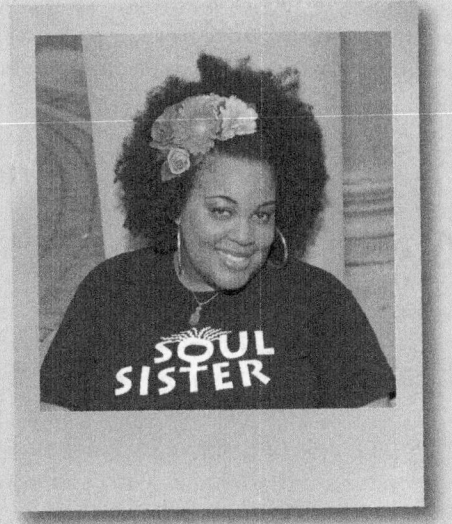

Name: Georgette
Occupation: Natural Hair Stylist/Loctician (Soul Sister Natural Hair Care Salon- Houston, TX)

Q: How long have you been natural? What was your inspiration?

A: My hair has been 100 percent natural since May of 1994. One day I went to the barber shop and did what is now referred to as the Big Chop, and I've been all-natural ever since! I decided to go natural during my second year of college. I was going through a period of self discovery, and I realized that I had no clue what my real hair texture looked like. My hair had been chemically relaxed since I was about five years of age. I was inspired by some of the other students on campus who wore their hair in locs, Afros and braids. I wanted this "freedom hair"! I was also a big fan of Cree Summer from the television show "A Different World." I was mesmerized by her springy, gravity-defying tresses! On top of all that, my hair was overprocessed and damaged and was falling out! I realized if I didn't stop abusing my hair it might all fall out and never return!

Q: What is your hair regimen/routine?

A: I try to leave my hair alone. I shampoo and condition it about once a month. During the warmer months, I keep it in two-strand twists to help keep my scalp cool. During the colder months, I still wear my two-strand twists a lot, but I am more apt to wear a twist-out style and my Afro. As a hairstylist working on my clients' hair all day, my hair is the last thing I want to have to deal with! I do keep my hair healthy. I try not to pull and tug on it too much. I often sport what has now become my trademark: a flower (or two or three) in my hair.

Q: Tell us about your nighttime hair regimen.

A: I sleep on a satin pillowcase every night! Even when I travel, I slip my pillowcase over the hotel pillow! Cotton pillowcases make my hair very dry! Cotton sucks the moisture out of your hair as you sleep. I also sleep in a satin cap.

Q: How do you keep your hair moisturized?

A: To be totally honest, what works best for me is nothing at all. Whatever oil or products I use on my hair, I put them on after the shampoo and conditioning process. Everyone's scalp secretes its own natural oils. I rely on that to keep my scalp and hair moisturized. Sometimes I add a little pure shea butter to my hair if it needs a little extra. There are billions of products out there, all claiming to do this or that. Some are very inexpensive, and some are very pricey. Unfortunately, people of African descent are constantly looking for that miracle in a jar or bottle, when in actuality they may not need anything! Your hair and scalp work together naturally. If you take care of both, you will have everything that you need.

Q: What is your signature hairstyle?

A: Two-strand twists! That is the best style ever! You can unfurl them and do a twist-out. You can roll them and wear them curly. You can plait them and wear them crinkly. You can do updos with them. Bantu knots. The options are endless! The best thing about them is that they allow you to not have to comb or brush your hair every day.

Q: What was your biggest hair mistake?

A: My biggest hair mistake with my natural hair was to let someone press and flat iron it straight several years ago! It took me a few years after I got it straightened to get it healthy. I will never do that again!

Q: What do you like best about your hair? Least?

A: I love the freedom that it allows me! No longer do I have to worry about being caught in the rain—I can ride with all the windows down! Being natural is the best choice I have ever made for my hair! I know that we are all made in God's image. That image is no longer altered! There is nothing I like least about my hair! I love it!

Q: How long have you been styling natural hair? Did your cosmetology training prepare you for addressing the needs of natural hair?

A: I have been a natural hairstylist/loctician since 1997. I got my first job in a salon in 1998. Cosmetology school did nothing in regard to natural hair! There was only one chapter in my textbook that discussed "ethnic hair," and it was referred to as "overly curly," as if there can ever be too much curl! I managed to start and finish cosmetology school with a head full of virgin hair! I knew when I started school that I wanted to do natural hair care. I was told that I wouldn't be successful because "nobody wants to wear no nappy hair!" Boy, were they wrong! I have maintained a large and faithful clientele all these years!

Q: Tell us about Soul Sister Natural Hair Care. What was your inspiration for starting your own salon?

A: What I do at Soul Sister Natural Hair Care is not a job to me. It's more like a ministry! I may never become a millionaire, and I may never get the accolades or exposure that some of my fellow hairstylists do. All of that doesn't matter! Whenever the Lord calls me home, I will be thankful that I was able to have a positive impact on the lives (and hair) of others.

I was inspired to start my own salon because I wanted a place of nurturing for my clients. If they never receive love, patience, care and understanding anywhere else, they will receive that in my chair!

Q: What products do you use in your salon? What's your favorite style or specialty style?

A: I use Organic Root Stimulator products in my salon. I use their entire natural hair-care line and their shampoos and conditioners. It is one of the few product lines that actually does what it claims to do! I also appreciate the fact that they are a black-owned business—just like me!

I won't say I have a favorite or specialty style. I will say that I love transforming people! They come in one way and leave a totally different person! There is just something awesome about getting your hair freshly coiffed! It seems like it puts an extra gleam in your smile and pep in your step!

Q: What is the biggest hair problem you see coming into the salon?

A: I haven't seen any major hair problems in my salon. The only problems I have seen is when people first transition from relaxed to natural and there is a lot of breakage and thinning. I enjoy watching my clients' hair flourish as it blossoms in its natural state.

Q: As a stylist, what advice would you share with others who are contemplating a Big Chop, newly natural or more advanced in their natural journey?

A: If you are contemplating the Big Chop, just do it! Waiting gives the devil time to try and change your mind! Before you know it, you will have a head full of natural hair!

If you are newly natural, hang in there! You will have closets, drawers and cabinets full of different products! It may all seem so overwhelming. Just be patient and educate yourself, and you'll be just fine!

If you are a long time natural head, you are set on your path. As your hair grows... so will you!

Q: What are your long-term business plans for Soul Sister Natural Hair Care?

A: My long-term business plan is to continue to keep my clients happy! That has always been my goal! I want to continue to spread my "nappy gospel" to the masses through my podcast, The Soul Sister Show. I want my words of encouragement to reach the corners of the earth!

For those who want to check it out, tune in to www.thesoulsister.com and www.thesoul-sistershow.podomatic.com.

Wigs, Braids and Weaved Styles

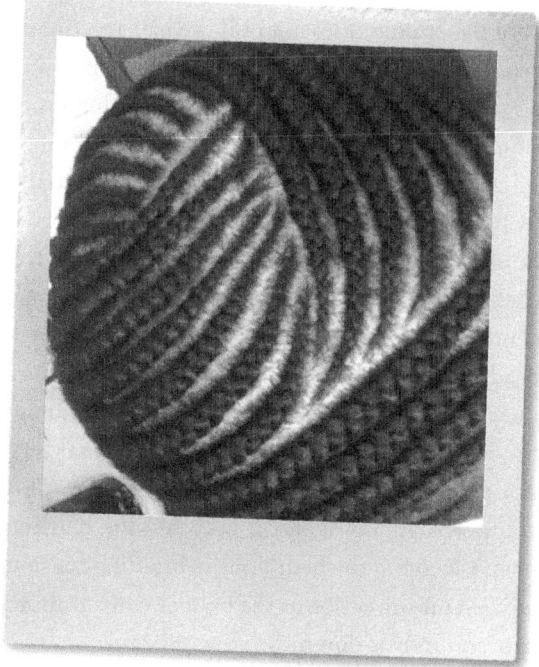

Figure 58: Cornrows are a protective style that must be carefully styled in order to maintain its protective effectiveness.

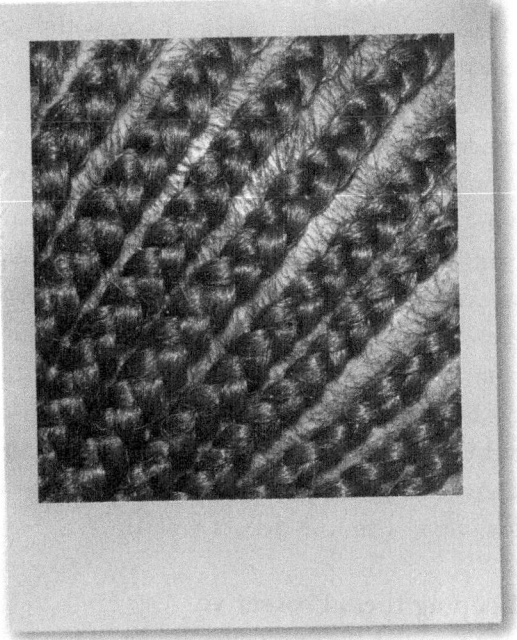

Figure 59: Always evaluate the condition of your hair prior to braiding or weaving. Notice the slight gapping and irregular spacing between the rows as we progress to the right of the picture. Long term braiding and weaving can lead to hair follicle damage and hair loss.

Another major category of low-maintenance protective styles includes weaves and braided styles. Weaves and braids are an excellent way to add spice and variety to your hair care regimen. They allow you to go from color to color, from curly to straight, or from long to short in the blink of an eye, with very little damage to your own beautiful tresses. They also cover and protect our hair from regular manipulation that can lead to breakage. Braids or twists are particularly versatile and can be worn up, down, long, short, pulled back—you name it! These styles are some of the best protective styles because they are extremely low maintenance, require no heat and can be worn for weeks at a time. Many also hide the hair ends completely, another protective plus for our hair.

While weaves and braids are great styling options that give our own hair lengthy breaks from manipulation and styling, the misuse of these styles in a hair care regimen can result in hair loss, breakage and thinning in affected areas. In many cases, the hair-growth benefits that should accrue from wearing these styles are often forfeited due to negligent hair care. Many of us acquire a set of braids, a weave or a wig thinking that we are eternally free and absolved from any further dealing with our very real hair hidden underneath. Weeks pass without the hair ever receiving an ounce of fresh water or moisture. This is a recipe for hair breakage if ever there were one.

Preparing for a Weave or Braids
Evaluate Your Hair

Before you put in the first braid or lay the first track, you must evaluate the condition of your hair. Black hair must be in tip-top shape prior to the addition of extensions or weaves of any kind.

Breakage, thinning or shedding issues with your hair must be resolved before jumping into braids or a weave because once your hair is woven or braided, it will be much harder for you to access your hair and treat any underlying problems. Do not start your braids or sew in your weave if your hair is breaking for any reason. The subsequent weeks of confinement will only aggravate breakage problems with your hair. When you finally remove your extensions or weave, the problem will still be there waiting for you—only amplified by your lack of attention to it. Thoroughly shampooing and deep conditioning your hair prior to starting all long-term-wear hair styles is a must!

Keeping them Protective

To get the most protection out of the hair braiding process for sew-ins, cornrows and braided extensions, follow these steps *before* arriving at your braider's shop:

1.) Thoroughly shampoo and deep condition your hair.
2.) Detangle hair with a large-tooth comb.
3.) Moisturize the hair with a water-based moisturizer and seal the hair with oil.
4.) If you have new growth or if your hair is natural, blow out the roots with a blow dryer on the COOL setting. (This will cut down on breakage since some braiders are hard on the hair and will rake through delicate tresses from root to tip with a rattail comb.)
5.) Be sure that all tangles have been removed by gently going through your hair with a comb. Carefully moisturize and oil the hair again for protection during the braiding process (and afterward, when your hair will be obscured by the braid extensions).
6.) Braiders should be working with clean, conditioned, moisturized and sealed hair only.

Once seated in the braider's chair, you should remain involved in the process to avoid leaving the shop with a damaging style that is too tight and works against your healthy hair goals. Make sure the braider does not pull the hair too tightly around the edges. The hair on the hairline and edges is very delicate and cannot take high tension loads for extended periods of time.

Support the beginning of each braid initially by placing an index finger at the start of the row or braid while the braider is advancing down the line. As you anchor the braid with your finger, gently introduce a counter force toward your forehead, or in the opposite direction of the braider's motion. This will reduce braiding tension along the hairline by introducing an oppositional tension to counter the braider's tugging motion. This counterbalancing method prevents the hairline from receiving the brunt of the braiding tension force in one direction as the braider collects more hair and moves down the row or braid.

Once your braids are installed, take note of your hair's condition. If you notice any of the following symptoms, your braids are too tight:

- small red or white bumps forming along partings, and at the hairline and edges
- an extra-shiny look to partings and exposed areas of your scalp
- white-tipped hairs sticking up from your braid where it starts at the hair line
- excessively dry, flaking skin along parts, particularly at the frontal hairline

Braided and twisted styles may loosen over time as the hair begins to grow out, but the danger here is that tension on delicate follicles can cause irreparable damage. Ultimately, damage to the hair follicles affects the quality of hair you can produce in the future.

For individual braided extensions, make sure the parted sections are in proportion to the size of the braid. If the parted section is small, do not allow the braider to overload your hair by creating a braid larger than the section. Placing a large braid on top of a small section of hair will increase your hair's breakage potential as it struggles to support the weight of the braid.

For cornrows, a similar principle applies. The best types of cornrows for growing black hair are "advanced" cornrows (also known as Ghana cornrows, banana cornrows or step-up cornrows). Advanced cornrows generally start small and incorporate additional pieces of weave hair as the cornrow advances along its line. Because they grow larger only as the line advances, this type of cornrow is less likely to put stress on growing hairlines. The same "too-tight" warning signs apply for all cornrows, braids and weaves.

Maintaining Braids and Weaves

Shampooing and conditioning hair that has been braided or protected with a weave hairstyle is very important for maintaining the health of the hair. Like hair worn in other protective styles, hair worn in braids and weaves still needs to be rinsed and or washed on a weekly basis. Diluted shampoo and conditioner are most effective for cleansing braids and weaves to prevent build up. Shampoos and conditioners can be transferred to squeeze bottles or applicators for precise placement between tracks, along cornrow lines and along the length of braid extensions. Textured hair in these confined styles also needs to be treated with moisturizing and protein sprays throughout the week to remain strong. Because of their mist and drip action, sprays can reach hair that creams and oils cannot. You will need to follow the same moisture and protein-balancing principles and rules with these sprays as you would with any other product if your hair is to remain in good condition. Finally, sealing braids, twists and other styles when possible with oils or butters also helps textured hair retain precious moisture.

Cornrows

Cornrows should be cleansed every seven to ten days or as your hair and style dictate. A stocking cap placed over the cornrowed style can help prevent frizzing and extend the life of your braided style. Begin by rinsing the rows in warm water to remove buildup. Then, carefully squirt or pour the diluted shampoo mixture onto your scalp and hair to saturate. Carefully smooth the cornrow lines with your fingers, and gently work the shampoo lather down the braids in a squeezing, milking fashion. Always move your fingers downward along the braids and lines. Avoid scrunching or roughing the hair as much as possible. Rinse out the shampoo thoroughly with warm water, and repeat the process with diluted conditioner. Rinse. Gently pat the hair dry with a microfiber towel. Do not rub the rows. Allow the hair to air dry. Spray-based moisturizers are preferable for cornrowed protective styles. Moisturizers may be sealed with an oil or butter by smoothing the oil product into the palms of your hands to create a thin film. Then, gently press your hands down onto the cornrows, allowing the fingers to carefully smooth over and press the oil along the lines. Again, rubbing the rows should be avoided as much as possible. A hooded dryer set on low may be used to speed the drying process.

Individual Braids and Twists

Individual braids call for the same cleansing routine as cornrowed braids. In addition, you may find that braiding single or individual braids into larger braids facilitates the cleansing process. Braids may be cleansed every seven to ten days or less often as your hair and style dictate. A cup may be used to gently pour warm water onto the scalp and down the braids for cleansing light dirt and debris. Repeat the process with your diluted shampoo mixture. Gently work the shampoo lather down the braids in a squeezing, milking fashion. Again, take care to avoid scrunching or roughing the hair as much as possible. Rinse out the shampoo thoroughly with warm water, and repeat the process with diluted conditioner.

Rinse. Gently pat the braids dry with a microfiber towel. Allow the hair to air dry. Finally, apply a moisture or protein-based spray for conditioning. Add a bit of oil or butter to each braid to seal. A hooded dryer set on low may be used to speed the drying process.

Weaves

Weaves can be shampooed and conditioned while you shower. It is important to keep your hair oriented DOWNWARD just as you would when shampooing your own free-form hair to prevent excess tangling and frizzing. Fill a squeeze or applicator bottle with diluted shampoo and work the watery shampoo between your tracks. Thorough rinsing of shampoo with warm water is a must! Conditioner may be diluted and applied to weaves in the same manner as braids. Remember to rinse out conditioner completely with cool water. Always make sure that you fully dry your hair under wigs, weaves and braids once you have rinsed or washed it. Damp hair lurking in a dark, warm environment is a recipe for odors, mildew and bacterial growth.

NOTE: For all braided or weave styles, conditioner may create buildup on braids that can lead to an excessively itchy scalp if it is not diluted properly and rinsed well.

Create a Protective Balance

It is important to strike a balance with weave techniques. While weaves are the perfect protective style for decreasing manipulation and helping textured hair to grow out, they can also stand in the way of your ability to effectively maintain and treat your scalp and hair.

Remember, our hair needs regular rest periods between braid and weave applications. These rest periods allow us the opportunity to thoroughly examine the condition of our hair and apply the correct moisture and protein treatments to keep it growing without breakage. Rest periods between weaves or braided styles should be two to four weeks in duration, and wear periods should be no longer than eight to twelve weeks at a stretch. Today's weave hair often looks good and holds up much longer than twelve weeks; nevertheless, our hair requires attention and basic maintenance to prevent excessive tangling and matting.

Keep in mind that our hair sheds around the clock as a natural response to living. When your hair is confined by a braid or weave, the shed hair falls from the scalp but is trapped in the braid and is unable to fall completely. It must wait until style "take down," when the hair is freed. This is one obstacle we face with woven and braided styles. Hair that has not been properly maintained under a weave may begin to suffer from extreme breakage and matting when braids or weaves are removed because the natural shedding compounds tangling.

Finally, weaves and braids should not be a permanent solution to your hair's care. We shouldn't allow ourselves to become so dependent on hair weaves that we begin to despise and neglect our own hair underneath.

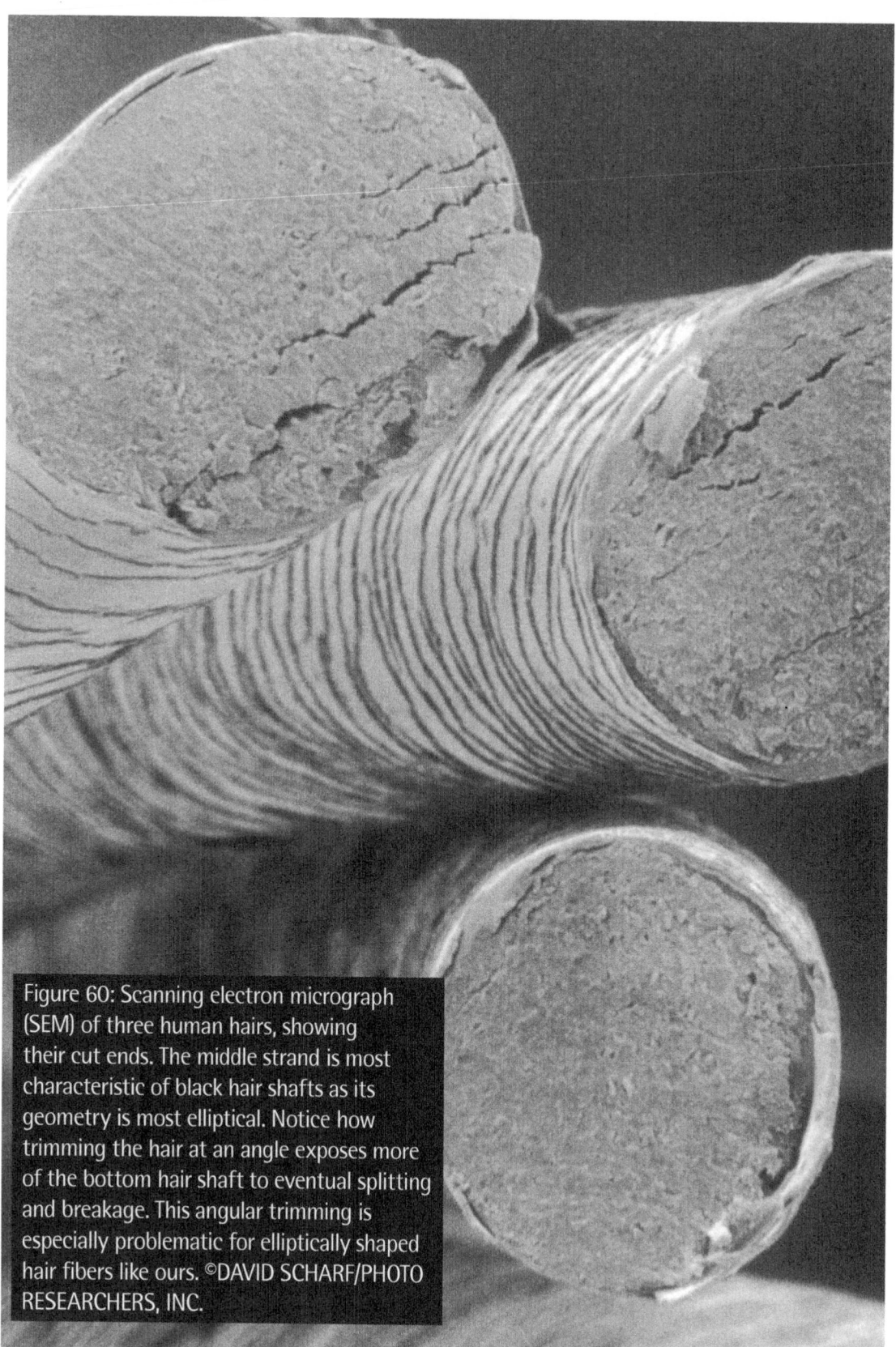

Figure 60: Scanning electron micrograph (SEM) of three human hairs, showing their cut ends. The middle strand is most characteristic of black hair shafts as its geometry is most elliptical. Notice how trimming the hair at an angle exposes more of the bottom hair shaft to eventual splitting and breakage. This angular trimming is especially problematic for elliptically shaped hair fibers like ours. ©DAVID SCHARF/PHOTO RESEARCHERS, INC.

Hair Trimming: Manicuring the Ends

You've seen her: The lady with lengthy hair that grows thinner and stringier as your eyes reach the ends of it. The length is respectable, but she's holding on to thin, unkempt ends. Why?

Or maybe this person is you: You've finally grown your hair some, and then a friend, a stylist or family member abruptly informs you that you need a trim. You relent, and your hair turns out shorter than you imagined. From this day forward, you fear all scissors. In fact, it will take an act of Congress or Parliament to get another pair of shears near your head again! Why?

Trim fear.

We've all had a bout or two (or three) with trim fear. Maybe you've had a few bad experiences with trims (that ended up turning into cuts) or are just trying to reach your hair goals as soon as possible. Either way, trims are just not your cup of tea. There is nothing wrong with wanting to keep your hair securely on your head, but a problem occurs when we start holding on to thinning ends for the sake of length, regardless of their condition. If done correctly and executed strategically, however, trims can be a beneficial part of your hair growing regimen. Think of trimming as manicuring the ends of your hair. Well-manicured ends are aesthetically pleasing, stronger hair ends that resist breakage. When combined with a proper protective hairstyling routine, the need for ends maintenance (trimming) naturally decreases as the ends are preserved in their manicured state.

Whether we like it or not, trimming is the only permanent solution to hair damage. Products formulated to "repair" damage and mend split ends can temporarily improve the look and condition of the hair by gluing or sealing split hair shafts together. Protein treatments can bond to the weak points along the strands to strengthen them, and moisture treatments can increase the elasticity and water content of the strand—but the reparative and reconstructive effects of these treatments only last for several washes, days or weeks at the most. Because all hair damage is cumulative, and our hair is no longer living tissue once it leaves the comfort of the follicle, hair must be treated continuously. Hair cannot repair itself. Once damaged, hair can never be repaired to predamaged condition, no matter how well you take care of it from the point of damage onward. You cannot add more cuticle layers to damaged hair. At some point, such hair must be removed, or it will break and fall off of its own accord.

Trimming Like Clock-work

One trimming myth in particular has proliferated in the hair care world with a fervor unmatched by any other. This myth holds that trimming textured hair on a set schedule actually grows the hair. This is simply not the case. Trimming on a strict six-, eight-, or ten- week schedule, sadly, has relegated many black women to membership in the shoulder-length-for-life-brigade. When such a strict trim schedule is instituted, often, individual growth factors are not considered. The hair trimmed usually equals or surpasses the hair grown in, and of course, the hair never seems to gain much length over time.

On the other end of the spectrum, some healthy hair advocates are completely anti-trim. And, understandably so. When black hair is cut, it loses length—a matter of simple mathematics. The no-trim approach works best, however, for those with healthier hair to start with. For those just setting out on a healthy hair care path, trimming may be necessary to get the hair ready to achieve greater length. Initial trims may delay your hair goals, but need not stop you from reaching them altogether. Unfortunately, avoiding trims entirely can lead to massive trims and deep cuts further down the road. A balance should be sought.

With the common advice to trim or clip our ends every six to ten weeks, and counter-advice suggesting to never trim at all, things can get confusing. Ultimately, how and when we trim our hair are personal choices that we must make. In order to grow black hair, trims should always be strategically factored into your hair care regimen. When hair trimming is properly synchronized with your personal hair growth rate, so that the hair removed is routinely less than the hair grown in, it is possible to grow hair longer.

Trimming textured hair serves three major maintenance purposes:

1. reactive maintenance to remove already damaged hair and ends.
2. preventive maintenance to remove old, worn hair at the ends regardless of condition.
3. aesthetic maintenance to even up hair that has overgrown and to give a fuller appearance to the hair's hemline (ends) regardless of condition.

Types of Hair Trims
Reactive-Maintenance Trims

Reactive-maintenance trims are usually the most aggressive and invasive maintenance trims. Here, we are reacting to damage already incurred. Regular reactive-maintenance trims can prevent textured hair from ever reaching its true length potential but are often a necessary evil, particularly at the start of a healthy hair care regimen to set the hair along a proper path for growth. These trims are also occasionally needed to fix hair after long periods of no trimming. Fortunately, the more we understand our hair and learn how to care for it, the less we will have to contend with reactive-maintenance trimming.

Preventative Maintenance Trims

As our hair grows, it naturally becomes worn and weathered near the ends. When damaged ends are not addressed in a timely manner, increased friction between neighboring fibers can lead to breakage. Hair should be maintained with light trims from time to time to reduce the tangling that can lead to unnecessary breakage. Preventive-maintenance trims are scheduled trims that are generally done on healthy hair. These trims, however, are notorious for toeing the gray area between trim and cut.

Dusting trims are an alternative trimming solution that preserves hair length. The term *dusting* was coined on Internet hair forums and is used to describe a preventive maintenance technique by which the hair is trimmed so finely that it resembles dust upon the floor.

Dustings serve as preventive maintenance against the advancement of split ends and the tangling that can lead to breakage. With these trims, only minute increments of hair are removed from the ends every few weeks, so that trimming does not jeopardize length retention. With dusting, hairs grasped with fingers are inspected under good lighting to detect splitting or knotted fibers. Dustings can be done two ways: 1) the ends of the hair are finely trimmed and removed together as a unit, or 2) single hairs are removed selectively. In the selective approach, single hairs are inspected for damage and trimmed one at a time. These types of trims are generally performed at home for general upkeep or maintenance between salon visits.

Aesthetic Maintenance Trims

Healthy hair grows and naturally tapers at the ends due to weathering. Aesthetic-maintenance trims even up overgrown hair at the ends and give it a nicer, fuller appearance. These trims are done primarily for aesthetic reasons and, depending on the look you are going for, are optional. These trims are generally for hair that has simply grown faster than other sections of hair around it, and not necessarily to remove damaged ends.

In healthy hair care regimens, it is important to keep in mind that problems may arise with

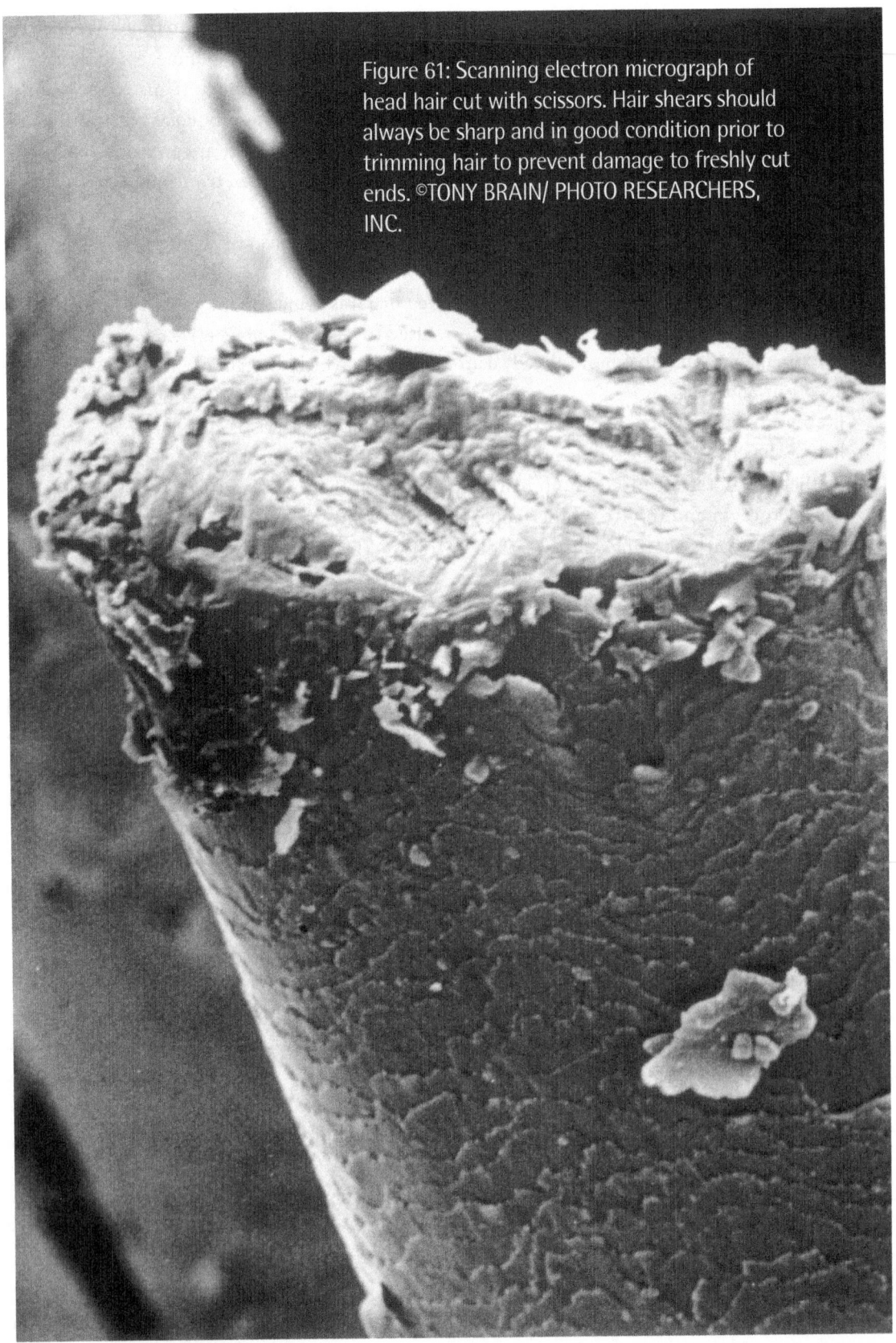

Figure 61: Scanning electron micrograph of head hair cut with scissors. Hair shears should always be sharp and in good condition prior to trimming hair to prevent damage to freshly cut ends. ©TONY BRAIN/ PHOTO RESEARCHERS, INC.

any type of maintenance trim when the amount trimmed equals or surpasses the growth rate of the hair. At the end of the day, we must decide whether length, appearance or a combination of these two factors is most important to us. This will determine the types of trims we do and the rate at which we employ them. If length is the goal, then less trimming should be done across trim types. If appearance is the goal, then maintenance trimming on a regular schedule works well.

Split Ends

When textured hair has experienced a great amount of trauma or simply has reached a certain age, split ends and single-strand knots can become a problem. While our hair will never be totally free of split ends, we can take certain measures to help keep them in check.

Splitting ends differ from *split* ends. Splitting ends are places along the hair shaft where the cuticle has broken apart and the cortex of the hair is exposed. These are the common V-shaped splits we tend to see on the ends of hairs, and these strands are still actively splitting. Splitting ends can occur at any point along the hair shaft but are most prevalent near the ends. Some say that splitting ends, left untreated, will continue to split up the entire shaft, but this is not exactly the case. Depending on the angle of the split, the tear can reach fairly high up the hair shaft, but a majority of splits simply peel away or break off not far from or right where they originate.

With split ends, on the other hand, the main split has already peeled away from the shaft. These ends are no longer splitting, they have already split and broken off. These ends are the thin, see-through-type ends that we are so used to seeing. Split ends can become splitting ends again if not treated with a sharp pair of shears.

Another type of "split" end is a kind of small break in the hair shaft known as trichorrexis nodosa. These are areas where the hair's cortex has swollen and exploded within the shaft as a result of heat styling, excessive brushing or use of chemical treatments. You can tell these types of splits by the white dot or node noticeable most commonly at the very end of the hair shaft. These nodes also can occur at mid-shaft and will result in a hard, angular, unnatural bend if the hair still has not broken off.

When split ends are present, the hair does not move well, and the hair tends to get caught up on itself. This type of hair also does not hold a curl well or straighten well with heat. Because of the slow breakage that has been allowed to take place over time, split hairs usually vary in length all over the head. Areas of dullness, redness or thinness (transparency) along your hair's hemline usually indicate a problem with split ends.

Hair breakage should always be monitored. Any time a hair breaks, the new end that is left behind has a great chance of becoming a new splitting end because most hairs do not break cleanly on their own. This is why it is best to trim splitting ends with sharp shears before they have a chance to simply break off. If left unchecked, these damaged hairs will tangle with healthy hairs and encourage more tangling and splitting.

The best way to check for split or splitting ends is by simply inspecting the hair shaft. Most splits occur along the lower half or third of the hair shaft, with the majority occurring right along the tips of the hair shaft.

Wet or Dry Trims?

Many stylists prefer to trim textured hair while it is wet. Unfortunately, this type of trimming may prove to be more damaging than beneficial for our hair in the long run. Imagine cutting a wet piece of paper and then cutting a dry piece of paper in the same way. You'll easily see that the cut on the wet paper is not a clean one. Your hair is really no different. Wet trimming can damage the new ends you create, leaving them more vulnerable to splitting later on. The damage is even more likely if you have your hair cut with a razor blade or if your shears need sharpening.

Hair Porosity Challenges for Trimming

When our natural or relaxed hair is wet, hair on different parts of our head will absorb water at different rates due to variances in hair porosity. Water causes our hair strands to stretch as much as thirty to forty-five percent of their normal dry lengths. Having each strand stretch exactly the same amount as every other strand every single time would be impossible. These differences in absorbency and porosity can be seen from strand to strand and from section to section in all hair types. If some sections of hair absorb more water (because they are more porous) than others, then assessing hair for trimming when it is wet is not likely to yield the desired result.

Differential rates of water absorbency are especially problematic for people who relax their hair in the same order at each application. When this happens, the area that is relaxed first each time always processes the longest and this area tends to be the most porous. For those with relaxed hair, the different absorbency rates in new growth and in relaxed length and ends also need to be factored in when trimming.

For those with curls and kinkier hair, portions of the hair with greater porosity will stretch and lengthen the most, while less porous areas will resist stretching to the same degree. Because tightly coiled areas may not fully release their curls when wet, if there are areas with looser curls or coils on the same head of hair, using wet hair as a guide for trimming can result in uneven sections.

Length Changes from Wet to Dry

Stretching of the hair while wet also contributes to our shock when trimming results in a shorter-than-expected final style length. As trimmed wet hair dries, it contracts to its normal, shorter length. Remember, hair that is wet trimmed will always appear longer than it really is—until it dries.

To reiterate, the ideal method of trimming depends on your finished style. If the hair is to be worn straight most often, trims should be done on dried, straightened hair. If the hair is to be worn in its curly or kinky state most often, the hair should be trimmed when dry or moistened (not wet).

How to Trim Split Ends

Always trim the hair straight across, at least 1/8 to 1/4 inch above the problem area. Never trim the hair at an angle. Trimming at a slant will expose more of the bottom and interior of your hair shaft to damage and increase its chances of re-splitting under pressure in the future. Notice how in figure 60, trimming hair at an angle exposes more of the cortex layer than hair that is trimmed straight across. This is not ideal. If you have a tiny knot or split hair where the end of the hair has already peeled off the main strand, cut ¼ inch above the knot or where the irregular angle begins.

For hair that is damaged and full of high-on-the-shaft split and splitting ends, you can use areas of hair transparency as a guide for where to cut.

Self-Trimming Relaxed or Straightened Hair

Textured hair can be trimmed straight or in its curly state. Relaxed hair should always be heat straightened prior to trimming to ensure an even cut. Trims should always be done after a relaxer, never before, to make sure that all new length is accounted for in the trim. Always start small, trimming away minute pieces of hair. This way, you won't cut off too much hair at once. Remember, you can always trim more if you haven't trimmed all of the damage in the first snipping—but once you've cut, you cannot go back!

Straight Hair Self-Trim Method 1

Standing in front of a mirror:

1. Gently detangle the hair, and comb it downward.
2. Create a center part that runs from your forehead back toward the nape of the neck
3. Comb both sides of the hair forward so that the hair rests in front of each shoulder.
4. Secure one side of the hair with a clip.
5. Grasp the ends of the hair on the free side, and hold the section down and taut with your index and middle fingers.
6. Scan the ends of the hair for thinness and unevenness, and trim slightly above where the hair begins to thin.
7. Repeat on the other side.

Straight Hair Self-Trim Method 2

The ponytail-guide method is great for lightly trimming longer, relaxed hair at home. Simply comb your hair and smooth it back into a low ponytail. Grasping the end of the ponytail, bring the hair forward in front of one shoulder and snip across the bottom to remove straggling hairs. Comb and ponytail the hair again, and then bring it forward over the other shoulder to trim straggling hairs.

Self-Trimming Natural Hair

Because natural hair does not provide length cues that indicate a need for trimming, such as areas of transparency along the hemline, those with natural hair must pay attention to manageability cues instead. When natural hair needs trimming, the ends are often drier, frizzier, sometimes straighter (from heat damage) and tend to tangle, snag and "catch" more readily.

Hair that is worn in its natural coiled and curly state can be trimmed in its finished style without straightening. In fact, trimming the hair in the style most frequently worn will ensure that any hair shrinkage or texture influences will be incorporated into the final result. Evenness is not as much a goal when trimming natural locks as it is for hair that is regularly worn straight. Instead, for naturals the idea is to simply create hair ends that do not readily catch or tangle. Straightening natural hair for trims when it will be worn curly a majority of the time not only carries the potential for damage but is counterproductive. Naturally kinky hair may be perfectly even while straightened, but once shrinkage and texture get involved, those perfectly aligned ends may end up producing a choppy and uneven Afro or wash-and-go style.

Self-trimming natural hair is simple. First shampoo and condition the hair. Style the hair in several braids or large two-strand twists. Air-dry the hair or use low heat to dry. Then, simply trim the very tips (1/4 inch or less) from each twisted or braided section. Trim any longer hairs on each twisted section that do not readily fit into the bulk of the twist, or hairs that simply taper off.

Night Care for Textured Hair

Sleep time is a time for rest and renewal not only for your skin, mind and other parts of your body, but for your hair as well.

Preparing Textured Tresses for Bed

Nightly application of a moisturizer to textured hair is extremely beneficial. As we toss and turn, our hair encounters considerable loads of tension. Moisturizer improves the elasticity of the hair and creates a layer of protection against dryness and breakage. For the best bedtime care, always moisturize your hair before retiring, and protect it by sleeping on a satin pillowcase at night or by wrapping it in a satin scarf or bonnet.

A satin scarf, bonnet or pillowcase is a must in any healthy hair regimen for nighttime protection. Not only does the satin surface protect the hair, it helps preserve and set styles for the following day. The barrier between your textured hair and bed coverings should always be a frictionless one. Satin or silk scarves, bonnets

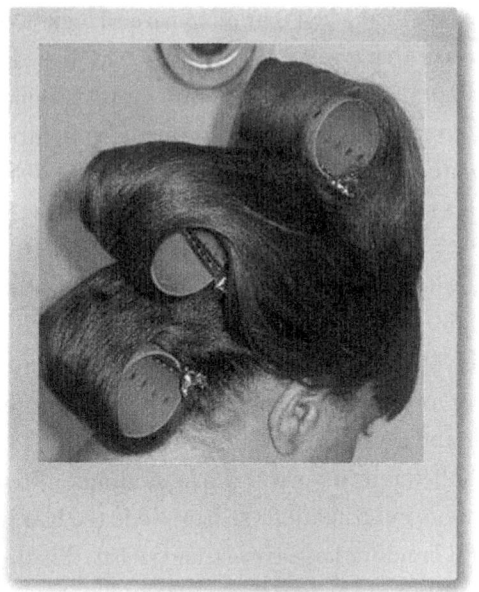

Figure 62: This modified rollerset helps refresh and keep curls bouncing for days.

and pillow covers are best for the hair because they allow free movement without harsh rubbing against moisture-absorbent bed fabrics, which can lead to breakage. The old familiar cotton headscarves or bandanas (which come in a wonderful variety of colors) are not recommended. Like cotton bed coverings, cotton head wraps absorb moisture from textured hair and create friction as the hair rubs against their rough inner surfaces.

Bonnets and scarves also provide an additional protective barrier against the moisture-stealing outside air and simultaneously protect your cotton sheets and pillow fabrics from moisturizer products. While you rest, satin scarves and bonnets allow your moisturizers to penetrate and condition your hair without unwanted evaporation into the environment. Moisturized hair kept under a scarf or bonnet during sleep is always well-conditioned hair the next morning.

Because satin scarves are so slippery, many women have trouble keeping them on their heads at night. Satin bonnets and pillowcases may be better options for those who fall into this category. Satin bonnets also work best for roller-set styles that require rollers to be worn in the hair overnight.

Night Styling

Nighttime hair styling should be minimal: just enough to keep the hair in place for the next day. Braid-outs and twist-outs can be misted, oiled and rebraided/retwisted for bedtime. Buns, twists, and braids can be moisturized, oiled and gently retwisted into shape for bed.

Ideally, sleeping in tight ponytails and wearing hair tools such as holders, bands, bobby pins, rollers and clips to bed should be avoided whenever possible. Wearing styling tools to bed can cause breakage and stress to textured hair fibers as you toss and turn.

If you must wear pins and rollers to preserve a style overnight, place pins, rollers and holders so that they do not receive pressure from the weight of your head while you sleep. Usually this means keeping pins and rollers at the top of the head. Pin curls should be carefully twisted and loosely placed and clipped so that they are not rolled on during the night. Any ponytails worn at night should be loosened and placed near the crown (top) of the head to avoid chronic night breakage to the nape, sides and edges.

To refresh roller sets, make a line of rollers down the center of your head from the front hair line back toward the nape for a fresh morning style. Keep rollers loose and cover with a satin bonnet or scarf. This "Mohawk" roller style is one of the best for sleeping with rollers without causing damage.

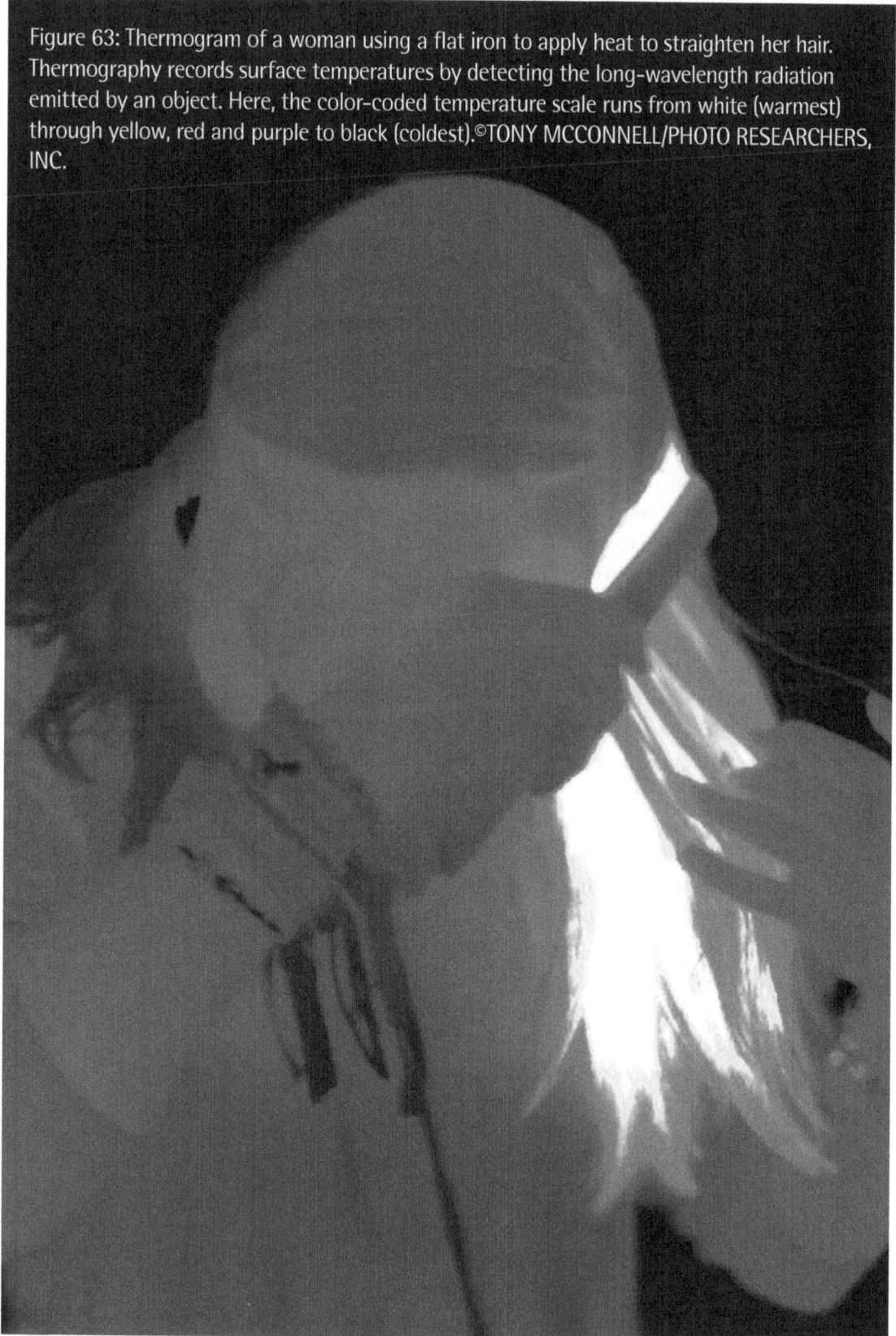

Figure 63: Thermogram of a woman using a flat iron to apply heat to straighten her hair. Thermography records surface temperatures by detecting the long-wavelength radiation emitted by an object. Here, the color-coded temperature scale runs from white (warmest) through yellow, red and purple to black (coldest).©TONY MCCONNELL/PHOTO RESEARCHERS, INC.

Healthier Heat-Styling Tools and Strategies for Textured Tresses

No one can deny that heat styling is a prominent feature in many black hair care regimens. From the smoke-filled days of grandmama's stovetop metal pressing comb to today's high- technology drying and straightening devices, many of us have continued to have intimate relationships with our blow dryers, hooded dryers, flatirons, curling irons, crimpers and steamers. Heat helps our deep conditioners perform, speeds up our styling routine and can take textured hair fibers from kinky to straight in no time flat. But heat can mean serious trouble for delicate textured hair fibers. Overuse of heated styling appliances can take a perfectly beautiful head of hair and completely destroy it in one bad drying, straightening or pressing. Once heat has damaged our hair, there is nothing that can be done to permanently repair it. Before another heated hair tool touches your precious mane, it is important that you understand the effects of heat use and proper methods for responsibly using heat on textured hair.

The hair's follicles determine the permanent shape of our hair and whether it is curly or straight. Any changes in the shape of the hair fiber must be accomplished from the outside through heat or chemical processing. If a hair-care regimen includes improper heat-styling practices, damage to the hair fiber will occur.

When hair is heat-treated, protein and moisture linkages are broken under the intensity of the heat. This bond breakage is the process by which hair is ultimately straightened through the use of heat. When determining an appropriate frequency of heat use in a hair care regimen, the hair's current condition, texture and general tolerance for heat are significant factors to take into consideration. Some black hair, despite the best conditioning efforts, will simply falter under a regular heat-styling regimen. It is important to know the implications of heat styling and the proper techniques for its use in a healthy hair-care regimen.

How Heat Affects Hair

Healthy hair burns at 233°C (451.4°F)—the same temperature that burns paper. If the hair has been damaged or compromised previously, burning can and often does occur at much lower temperatures. Research has shown that water first begins to exit the hair shaft at 50° to 120°C (122° to 248°F). Hair proteins begin to break and reform linkages at about 155°C (311°F). As temperatures climb toward 233°C or 451.4°F, our hair's keratin protein begins to melt. Any damage inflicted upon the hair shaft during heat styling is cumulative, and the negative effects build with each heat session. [1]

Typical flat irons and blow dryers operate within a 100° to 170°C (212° to 338°F) temperature range. Although these high temperatures fall outside of the burning temperature range, the hair's general condition ultimately affects its maximum heat tolerance and response to heat styling. Asian hair, for instance, primarily due to its many robust cuticle layers, is much more tolerant of high-heat extremes than our fragile coiled and dry hair types. Fine hair is also less tolerant of high-heat extremes than medium or thick/coarse/wiry hairs.

Temperatures should always be controlled, particularly when working with flat irons and curling irons. Effective temperature control, for textured hair, does not simply mean having an ON/OFF or HIGH/LOW switch. Similarly, randomly numbered temperature designations that have no direct correlation to actual temperature settings (i.e., dials with settings from one to twenty-five) on a heat-styling device are very unhelpful and should be avoided. Operating temperatures vary across styling tools and even with the same styling tool over its lifetime. All LOW settings are not created equal. These designations and settings tell us absolutely nothing about the temperature ranges being delivered through the device. A setting of ten, for example, could be 300°F on one device and 500°F on a different device, just as HIGH could easily be 250°F on one device and 450°F on another. You should always select flatirons with dedicated temperature dials that display heat ranges in either degrees Celsius or Fahrenheit. Although there may be some contention about whether the temperatures displayed even accurately reflect the actual heat being delivered by the heat-styling device, at least a temperature display gives us a logical scale with which to work. If nothing else, temperature displays give us the confidence to say that 200° is less than 300° on a relative scale.

How Does Heat Damage Our Hair?
Heat Decreases Moisture Levels

Textured hair is extremely sensitive to overall changes in its moisture content. Heat disturbs the moisture balance in the hair and stresses already naturally dry, porous ends. Heat appliances work by rapidly evaporating much of this desperately needed internal moisture from the hair's cortex. For this reason, it is critical that black hair be treated with a moisturizing deep conditioner, ideally one with hydrolyzed proteins, before heat is applied. Moisturizing deep conditioners reinforce textured hair by creating important crosslinkages deep within the hair fiber. The moisture received from regular conditioning not only helps maintain strong hydrogen bonding between keratin proteins, but also helps absorb and evenly distribute heat through the hair fiber.

Heat Affects Protein Structure

There is another reason why hair that is subjected to regular heat styling must be deep conditioned with adequate protein and moisture sources on a regular basis. In order to reshape our hair, heat must reform and disturb our hair's natural protein bonds. Without a strong protein backbone and structure, the hair cannot hold on to its own internal moisture. If textured hair is natural, heating it excessively may cause it to permanently lose its curl pattern. When the hair

is heat damaged or purposely "heat trained" to loosen the curl pattern, protein and moisture linkages deep within the fiber no longer remember their bonds and fail to reform. The result will be straight or loosely textured pieces that do not revert or curl in the presence of water.

Heat protection should start well before heat is ever applied to the hair. Hair is best protected from heat damage when it is properly conditioned and treated with a balance of moisture and protein conditioners. Black hair should always be clean and deep conditioned well prior to applying any heat source. The odds of damage increase dramatically when multiple heat sessions are inflicted upon the fiber. To protect the hair against the ravages of heat styling, avoid using heat-styling techniques such as blow drying and flat ironing back to back. If you are planning to flat iron or hot curl your hair, try eliminating the blow-drying step by allowing your hair to air dry fully or partially prior to heat styling.

How To Use Heat in a Healthy Hair Care Regimen

Heat does not have to be our enemy. In fact, if used sparingly, it can actually benefit the hair. For naturals who are prone to excessive tangling and knotting at the ends, using a bit of heat to roller set or "blow and stretch" the hair can provide relief from knotting during styling. (Of course, stretching can also be achieved through heatless methods as well.)

Selecting quality heat styling tools is imperative if you wish to incorporate heat use in your healthy hair care regimen. Again, all such tools—blow dryers, hooded dryers, flat irons, crimpers, etc—should have variable temperature controls. Always use your heat tools on the lowest setting that will still give you the results you desire.

How Much Heat Is Too Much?

The hair's condition and heat tolerance should dictate the frequency of heat use. Regardless of the hair's condition, heat should be restricted in any hair care regimen in which hair growth is the primary goal. As a rule of thumb, heat should be limited to no more than once per week on a cool setting. Regular heat use often means that frequent trimming will be required to keep up with the high level of splitting and breakage that occurs at the ends of heat-styled hair. Keep in mind that growing out textured hair using a moderate heat regimen can mean that length goals may be delayed. The risk for heat damage is greatest among those who chemically treat their hair because relaxing and coloring processes also destroy the protein and moisture linkages within the hair fiber.

Heat Breaks

At the start of a healthy hair care regimen, heat use should be eliminated entirely. Ideally, this initial heat break should last twelve to sixteen weeks. Heat breaks help to reestablish protein and moisture levels in the hair and may allow the hair to regain its natural thickness and strength. During the heat break period, heat use should be restricted to hooded dryer heat for deep conditioning and roller setting only. After the heat break, heat tools can be phased back into the regimen gradually, but should be used no more than once a week. Heat breaks should be reinstated during the course of a healthy hair regimen as often as needed to control breakage. The benefits of these breaks increase proportionally according to the length of time that heat is eliminated from the regimen.

Evaluate Your Hair

The very first consideration to make before using heat on black hair should be: *Is this hair up to heat styling at this time?* If the hair is breaking or dirty, it should not be straightened using heat. If the hair has already been heat styled in the previous day or so, heat styling may pose an additional risk.

Only Use Heat on Clean Hair

Never use heat on hair that has not been washed in the previous day or two. If product usage has been fairly heavy within that two-day time frame (particularly if gels, greases or hair sprays have been used), then the hair will need to be shampooed and reconditioned prior to heating. Heat appliances will simply bake salt-rich sweat, dirt, lint, oils and moisturizers into black hair, damaging its cuticle layers.

Control Heat Intensity

The safest way to use heat in healthy hair care regimens is at lower temperatures for longer periods of time rather than at higher temperatures for shorter periods of time. Research has shown that rapidly increasing the temperature of hair damages it and causes both protein and water loss to the fiber. Water loss is a primary concern, and we will get to why water is so vitally important for heat styling black hair.

Add a Protective Layer

To support healthy heating, thermal hair-protectant products should always be used prior to heat treating black hair. Ideally, heat protectants should have a low thermal conductivity, meaning they should be able to slow down the transfer of heat from heated appliances to our hair. Silicones, oils and water all play critical roles in healthy hair heating.

Silicones

Today's silicones are marvels of cosmetic science. Silicones are popular low-thermal-conductivity ingredients that slow down the transfer of heat from heated appliances to our naked hair strands. A material's thermal conductivity rate gives us an indication of its ability to buffer and protect the hair against heat. The lower a material's thermal conductivity rate, the better the heat protection qualities it offers. Silicones are routinely used in heat protectant sprays and serums to slow down heat transfer. Because their thermal conductivity is lower than oils, they are better equipped to slow the transfer of heat to the hair strands. Research has shown that silicones, compared to oils such as mineral oil and petrolatum, foster a more even transference of heat. Dimethicone and cyclomethicone are the silicone ingredients on the market with the lowest heat conductivity and are found quite frequently in heat protectant formulations.

Table 3 shows the heat conductivity rates for commonly used elements. Notice how copper, a metal, has a very high thermal conductivity rate! Oils in general have naturally low thermal conductivity and tend to transfer heat to the hair shaft slowly. Among the oils with the lowest rates of conductivity, some are better than others at protecting the hair from rapid temperature increases. Silicone has lower heat conductivity than paraffin (petrolatum), which is commonly used in pressing oils, creams and waxes. Mineral oil and olive oils are also preferable to petrolatum-based creams for protecting the hair against damage from rapid increases in temperature.

The Water Connection

Textured hair's internal water content plays a major role in how quickly the hair increases in temperature when heat is applied. Hair with low moisture content will heat more rapidly than hair that is adequately moisturized. Shampooing and conditioning the hair immediately prior to heat use provides important moisture support that allows the hair to be heat straightened with minimal breakage to the hair fiber. Give textured hair a moisture surplus by only heat styling recently deep-conditioned hair.

"Specific heat" is the amount of heat required to raise the temperature of a material one degree. Water has a very high specific heat, meaning that it takes considerable heat to increase its temperature one degree. When water is properly bound within textured hair, it acts as a buffer by absorbing the heat from styling appliances and controlling the rate and speed at which our

Blow Drying Tips

- Select a blow dryer with multiple temperature settings so that you can vary heat delivery as the hair begins to dry. Although straighter results can be achieved with heat, cold drying the hair from start to finish (or using the "cold shot" option) reduces dryness and split ends in textured hair.
- Use a warmer setting when your hair is most wet. As your hair begins to dry, switch to a cooler setting to help close the cuticle and protect against heat damage and dryness. Warmer settings can be used near the scalp end of the shaft because this hair is newer and stronger and therefore more tolerant of heat compared to the ends.
- Hold the blow dryer at least 8 to 10 inches from your hair and direct the airflow DOWN the hair shaft to help protect your cuticles.
- Avoid using the comb attachments on blow dryers to initiate the wet detangling process. If comb-attachment dryers are used, it is best to detangle the hair first with the fingers and then again with a larger personal comb. Because the teeth on comb-attachment dryers are usually very small and have serrated edges that can snag your hair, it may be preferable to remove the comb attachment and work with a smaller personal comb instead.
- Do not linger for too long on any one portion of your hair. If your hair is thick, section your hair beforehand and blow dry in an organized manner for faster results.
- Only blow the hair 80 to 90 percent dry. Allow the hair to air dry the rest of the way.

Table 3: Thermal conductivity

Element/Material	Thermal conductivity W/(m·C) at 25°
Silicone oil	0.1
Mineral Oil	0.138
Olive oil	0.17
Paraffin Oil/Wax	0.25
Water	0.58
Copper (metal)	401

Thermal conductivity of various materials. The lower the thermal conductivity, the better the material is at blocking rapid heat transfer to the strands.

hair increases in temperature. In essence, water slows the heating rate of the hair fiber. As the temperature of the water in our hair slowly increases, it allows the overall temperature of the hair fiber to increase as well. Without adequate moisturization of the hair fiber, the hair's temperature increases rapidly.

Silicone + Water

Together, silicone or oil and water work synergistically to safely heat the hair fiber with very little damage. Moisture increases the hair's specific heat capacity or the amount of heat required to increase the hair's temperature, while silicone and/or oils decrease the rate at which heat is transferred to the fiber in the first place. With silicone working on the outer hair strand to slow the transfer of heat into the hair fiber, and the hair's own internal moisture slowing the overall temperature increase of the strand, the hair is well protected from heat damage.

Dry It! Style It!

Once the hair is reinforced with internal moisture and heat protection, the hair may be dried safely and/or straightened with heat. Again, drying the hair at a low temperature for a longer period of time rather than at a high temperature for a shorter period of time is ideal. This is one of the reasons that hooded-dryer heat is easier on the hair than blow-dryer heat; essentially, it is a choice between applying a forty-five minute gentle breeze or a twenty-minute Category 5 hurricane to dry your hair! Indirect heat from hooded dryers is always less damaging for our hair than the direct forms of heat received from flat irons and curling irons. Hair drying rates depend on your hair's porosity, the products used, and whether the hair is air dried or heat styled. Highly porous hair dries more quickly than hair of low porosity, and certain products such as setting lotions can speed up the hair-drying process.

When black hair is wet, our hair's inner hydrogen bonds become more malleable and allow the hair to temporarily take on new shapes until the new bond arrangement is disturbed by re-wetting. This is the science behind wet setting. Wet hair is shaped while its hydrogen bonds are most elastic and malleable, creating a smooth rolled curl or style once dry. Unfortunately, if these wet hair bonds are allowed to reform in a less than ideal configuration, frizzing, tangling and breakage can occur. When drying our hair, we must control the shape and orientation of this hydrogen rebonding as much as possible to prevent hair breakage.

Blow Drying

Blow dryers work by 1) moving air to mechanically remove water from the exterior hair shaft and 2) heating the hair and evaporating internal moisture from the hair. In the early stages of blow drying, when the hair is wettest, most of the initial drying is done by physical displacement of water, not by heating. Once blow drying has displaced the water on the outside of the hair shaft, it begins to work on internally bound water to dry the hair. Hair begins to feel dry

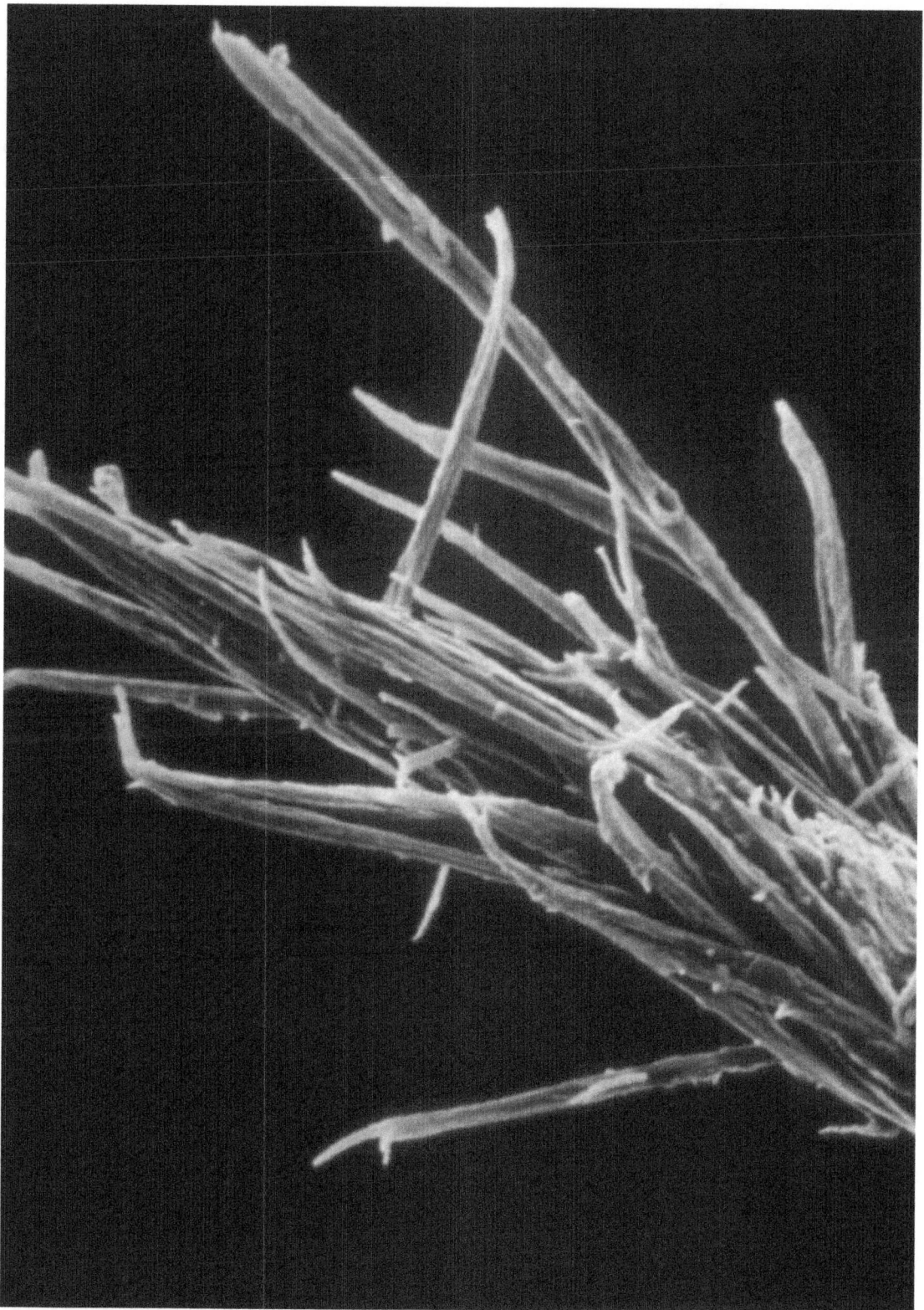

Figure 64: Scanning electron micrograph (SEM) of a human hair with a split end. Blow drying can cause cracking and peeling of the hair fiber which ultimately leads to splitting

once external moisture has been removed and internally bound moisture begins to evaporate. If you decide to blow dry your textured hair, use the hottest setting only while the hair is dripping wet. Decrease the heat intensity as your hair begins to dry.

Wet hair does not increase in temperature as quickly as dry hair does. Remember, water has a high heat capacity (specific heat). When the water inside the hair fiber absorbs heat, the temperature inside the hair fiber slowly increases. It takes quite a bit of heat to raise the temperature of water. Dripping-wet, well-moisturized hair can handle high heat better than hair that is starting to dry because there is more water available to buffer the temperature increase.

Blow drying depletes and removes moisture from the hair strands more violently and rapidly than hooded dryer heat drying. This drastic moisture loss increases the probability of splitting, cracking or peeling of the cuticle. Blow drying also results in increased levels of manipulation and added stress to the hair fiber since uncontrolled hot air is allowed to blow the hair around with very little order. Additionally, because blow-dried looks tend to be "unfinished," blow drying often opens the door for additional heat styling via flat irons and curling irons. When hooded dryers are used, they are often the last step in creating a style, and additional sources of heat aren't needed to complete the look.

Blow drying on cool is a great heat damage deterrent. Cold drying causes less damage because the hair fiber is heated to a lower temperature and moisture evacuates the strand at a slower rate than with heated drying. The hair can be gently stretched or lengthened to encourage the fiber's hydrogen bonds to dry in a new, straightened or lengthened state. Cold drying, unfortunately, takes considerably longer to complete than hot blow drying and does not make the hair as sleek and straight.

Ion Technology?

Many interesting claims have been made about the "ion technology" upon which "ionic hair dryers" rely heavily for marketing. Some claim that ions help to infuse moisture into the hair, speed styling time, and are healthier for the hair—but to date, none of these claims has adequate support in scientific literature.

Additionally, the true need for "negative ions" to improve the look of the hair is questionable, especially since research has found that damaged hair has a naturally high negative charge on its own. (Remember, positively charged (cationic) conditioners are able to bind to damaged hair more strongly and provide longer-lasting conditioning because the hair has a net negative charge when it has been damaged.)

For now, the claims of extra shine and hair health attributed to so-called ion technology appear to be manufacturer spin with no firm scientific basis. Until further research is done on the merits of this technology, the value of ion technology at this point appears questionable.

Hooded Drying

Have you ever wondered why black hair feels lighter, bouncier and much better moisturized after a hooded-dryer session than when it has been rapidly blown dry? How can thirty minutes to an hour of domed heat result in soft, luxurious hair, while less than fifteen minutes of blow drying leaves the hair feeling hard, swollen and thirsty?

Hooded dryers provide one of the safest forms of heat to our hair. Heat is diffused and evenly concentrated over a larger surface area under a hooded dryer. For those who set their hair on rollers, hooded dryers allow users to protect the ends of the hair from overwhelming heat. Because the hair ends are rolled and tucked underneath the other hair, only the hair that can best take it—the new growth and upper length—gets hit with heat. By contrast, hand-held blow dryers, unless used cold, attack the full length of the strand with more intense heat.

Hooded dryers also reduce the manipulation factor considerably because they are commonly used for "controlled" hairstyles—that is, styles in which the hair is usually set on rollers or rods or has been molded into shape already. Finally, the styles set by the hooded dryer tend to be longer lasting than those created with other forms of heat. This means that styles are worn longer and the actual use of the dryer is limited to once or twice per week.

Unfortunately, hooded dryers tend to be used less often than hand-held blow dryers in hair-care regimens. Most people who blow dry or flatiron their hair tend to do so pretty regularly. Some individuals fire up their blow dryers and curling irons every day or several times a week for styling. The same cannot be said for those who use hooded dryers. You would be hard pressed to find anyone who commits to whipping out a hooded dryer with that regularity!

Despite their relatively good reputation, however, hooded dryers are not without fault. With some lower-end tabletop models, heat may be concentrated at the back of the dryer unit, creating hotspots where the hair dries too quickly. For these types of dryers, alternating your position under them from time to time is a good practice.

Air Drying

Air drying is perhaps the simplest form of hair drying. It is quick, easy and perfect for those days when time is tight. Although with air drying the hair often takes longer to dry completely than with heated styling, it is the healthiest hair option. Air drying does not involve heat exposure, and this helps maintain the health of textured hair. If air drying is used for a style such as a wash-and-go, puff, bun or ponytail, the hair should always be moisturized and sealed with an oil to help smooth the cuti-

cles into a flat orientation. These products will keep the hair pliable and controlled as it dries. Never allow textured hair to simply dry on its own with no product or shaping support. Particular attention should be given to the ends of the hair when air drying because their natural porosity causes them to dry quicker than the upper regions of the hair shaft.

Occasionally, air drying can cause problems for those with highly textured hair—particularly if the hair is longer and is not guided or encouraged into a particular style before it dries. In fact, air drying any textured hair type (whether excessively kinked, curly or relaxed) with no styling direction or guidance can lead to excessive tangling and breakage. Outside of true wash-and-go styles, black hair should always be arranged, set and smoothed into place before the air-drying process is complete. Often this is done with hair rollers and rods, braids, or twists. Smoothed styles in which the ends are tucked under, such as buns or ponytails, are also good air-drying styles.

Smoothing the Hair with Air-Drying

Edges and new growth can be controlled by taking advantage of air drying and hydrogen rebonding. Simply smooth and tie down damp hair with a satin scarf to flatten and control edges and new growth at the roots. No gel is required. This method works because the hair is smoothed into place while its hydrogen bonds are most elastic and malleable. The satin scarf gently forces the hair to remember and retain the stretched bond configuration as it dries. Once dried, the hair maintains this straightened, flattened shape until the next time it is wet. This method works excellently for those wearing pulled-back styles including buns, ponytails and puffs. The style can be set in less than ten minutes and can be refreshed daily by simply misting the hair with water and retying the scarf to set.

Flat Irons and Curling Irons

Flat irons and curling irons are the heat tools of choice in many hair care regimens and are convenient for straightening textured hair. Frequent use of these heat-styling tools, however, can ravage textured tresses. Flat irons and curling irons should have well-made plates and hinges that will not snag the hair during the course of styling.

With flat irons and curling irons, temperature control is paramount. Flat irons and curling irons deliver a direct form of heat to the hair fibers that rapidly increases the temperature of the fiber on contact. Maintaining textured hair at constant high temperatures for extended periods of time damages the hair and drastically alters the moisture levels deep within the strand. Hair should not be left wrapped around or sandwiched within any heating appliance for longer than three to five seconds at a time. To safely use flat irons and curling irons, quickly pass over sections that are to be straightened and do not allow the iron to linger too long in one area, especially near the ends of the hair. The ends of the hair heat more quickly due to their naturally lower moisture profile; therefore, heat use should be minimized as much as possible at the ends.

Keep the pressure light as you move flat irons through the hair. Do not fully clasp and drag the hair down along with the heating appliance. This is particularly true once you reach the ends of the hair. The flatiron or curling iron should gently clasp your hair, and the plates should be held slightly open so as not to apply significant downward force to the strands. Allow additional plate separation as you reach the ends of the hair. Do your best to keep the hair well within the plates, even if this means using less hair per pass.

If your iron has been idle or at rest for longer than ten to fifteen seconds, test it on a cotton towel to discharge some of the heat that has accumulated before you introduce the heat implement to your hair again.

The Power of Ceramic

Have you ever had to preheat your flat or curling iron ten minutes in advance so that you could use it before you need to rush out the door—only to find ten minutes later that it still isn't as hot as you need it to be? Have you ever picked up an iron, only to have it start to cool as you use it on your hair? Have you ever flat ironed your hair and had it fall limp as soon as you walk out the door? Worse yet, have you ever run the flatiron repeatedly over a section of hair, only to find it was still puffed and definitely not straightened? If so, then you may need to consider upgrading your flatiron plate material to ceramic or tourmaline.

Ceramic irons are the current "it" technology on the hair market for heat styling. Ceramic irons heat evenly across the plate width and produce a flatter, sleeker press that lasts. Ceramic irons protect the hair by minimizing the need to iron the hair over and over. Unlike other irons, these irons do not produce hot spots or lose their heat over time. Once heated, ceramic irons maintain the heat temperature you set from start to finish. They heat up in a snap, and their straightening power is incredible. These are the same irons used by many high-end salons across the country and are safer than the conventional marcel irons we have come to know so well in many black hair salons.

Selecting the Best Ceramic Iron

Ceramic irons come in two varieties: irons with full ceramic plates and irons with several layers of ceramic coating on top of lower quality metals. Full ceramic plates are best for reaping the positive benefits of ceramic technology; however, these ceramic plates are soft and can be quite fragile. Dropping the iron or closing (clapping) the iron plates together abruptly can crack or damage the plates. The more popular and respected full-plate ceramic brands generally cost more than ceramic-coated irons. Farouk Systems, HAI, Sedu, FHI, GHD and Solia produce top-quality ceramic models. Most ceramic irons cost in the neighborhood of fifty to sixty dollars or more, and prices rise steadily as ceramic integrity increases. A thirty-dollar iron, for example, is most likely NOT a full, ceramic-plated iron.

Did You Know?
What is in a name?

The Farouk CHI® is a popular brand of ceramic iron that is known for its straightening and silkening abilities. However knock-offs of this iron abound in mass retail outlets. Keep in mind that the acronym CHI often only stands for Ceramic Heating Iron-- it is not a brand name. Any flatiron can be considered a "CHI" if it utilizes ceramic technology. Similar to how the acronym SUV is used to refer to all Expeditions, Navigators, and Yukons, the word CHI can be used to refer all irons that use "ceramic technology". Unfortunately, many drugstore flatiron products will use that acronym on the box to trick customers, because they know that consumers tend to associate the word CHI with the high end professional, *Farouk* CHI. So do not be fooled!

The vast majority of ceramic irons on the market are aluminum plated irons with several baked-on layers of ceramic coating. Unfortunately, the ceramic coating on lower-end irons tends to wear off within a few months of use. When this coating begins to peel, your hair can snag, and super-heated hotspots on the uncoated plate's surface may appear. Any iron with unconformities along the plate surface needs to be replaced.

Tourmaline Irons

Tourmaline is a semi-precious stone that can be finely ground and used to coat flat iron plates. Tourmaline irons are generally more economical than ceramic irons and offer some of the same even-heating capabilities. These irons may be good alternatives for those who have had little success with ceramic.

There are some claims that the shine that results from tourmaline flat iron brands is due to "ionic technology." Such shine, however, is likely due to the even heating surface and high temperature ranges these irons are able to reach. Similar shine results can be achieved with high quality ceramic-plated irons.

Why Won't My Hair Hold a Curl?

Even with the best quality heat-styling irons, our hair simply may not respond to heat treatment. In particular, the ends of the hair may exhibit certain signs of distress if they do not have a protein/moisture balance adequate to support heated styling or shaping. This usually occurs when the hair at the ends is very old, has been damaged, and is porous and split. Such hair is often reddish colored, stringy, swollen, frizzy or puffy looking near the ends. If you find that the ends of your hair do not straighten well, fall flat and do not hold a curl very long after styling, even when extensive heat is applied, these ends may have reached their styling limit and be damaged beyond repair. Ends in this condition need to be trimmed. Healthy hair will always respond to heat shaping or styling because the hydrogen bonding network within the fiber responds predictably to heating. Unresponsive hair is generally damaged hair that has been depleted of the moisture required to achieve various styles and shapes.

Maintaining Heat Styling Tools

Using a dirty flat iron is damaging to textured tresses and may cause your hair to snag on the rough surface created by burned-on hair product residues from previous uses. These residues can abrade the cuticle as the flat iron advances along the length of the strands during styling. All irons should be cleaned after every use. To clean curling irons and flat irons, simply rub the interior plates with a damp cloth to remove hair and product residue.

Putting it All Together: Sample Protective Styling Regimens

Now that you fully understand proper product selection, effective methods for balancing moisture and protein, and important low manipulation styling strategies, consider the following sample healthy hair-care regimens:

Sample Healthy Hair-Care Regimen 1 (With a Low-Manipulation/Conditioning Focus)

Shampoo and Conditioning

Hair is cleansed twice each week, for example, on Wednesday and Saturday. One cleansing session each week always features a heated deep conditioning. The mid-week Wednesday cleansing may be in the form of a conditioner wash.

Moisturizing products are used in the first two to three weeks (shampoo, conditioner, leave-in, moisturizer and oil.) (In some cases, the leave-in and moisturizer may be water or the same product.) After week two or three, protein reconstructing is added to the regimen.

Effective Regulation of Product pH

The hair's acid mantle is maintained effectively with acid-balanced products. Test all water-based products with pH strips to ensure their proper acidity between pH 3.5 and 5.5.

Product Layering

Effective product layering ensures that moisture hits the fiber before a sealant butter or oil product during styling. Hair may be moisturized daily or several times per week as the hair texture and style dictate, always with moisturizer followed by an oil/butter.

Heat and Chemicals Use

Heat use is restricted to hooded drying or light, cold blowing once a week, preferably less often. The more infrequent the heat, the faster and greater length-retention results will be.

The use of chemicals to alter the fiber is greatly restricted, with tradeoffs for one or the other common (i.e., no coloring if the hair is chemically relaxed, or no relaxing if the hair is colored).

Styling

Hair is styled protectively after each conditioning, for instance, in a bunned style. Long-term styles for which daily manipulation is not required are preferable.

Sample Healthy Hair-Care Regimen 2 (With a Low-Manipulation Focus)

Shampoo and Conditioning

Hair is cleansed once or twice a month, and is deep conditioned with both protein and moisturizing deep conditioners. For example, a cornrow or braid wearer might shampoo and condition with diluted products every ten days as needed.

Hair is treated daily with either a protein- or a moisture-based leave-in conditioning spray to retain suppleness. Moisture-based sprays are used daily to freshen hair; protein-based sprays are done every third day for strength.

Product Layering

Effective product layering ensures that moisture hits the fiber before a sealant butter or oil product during styling and arrangement of the hair. Hair may be moisturized daily or several times per week as the hair texture and style dictate, always with moisture followed by an oil/butter.

Heat and Chemicals

Heat use is restricted to hooded dryer heat to dry braided styles after cleansing/conditioning. Air drying is preferable. No chemicals are used.

Styling

Hair is braided, or in a long-term wear style such as a sewn-in weave.

unit 3

Working With Chemicals in a Healthy Hair Care Regimen

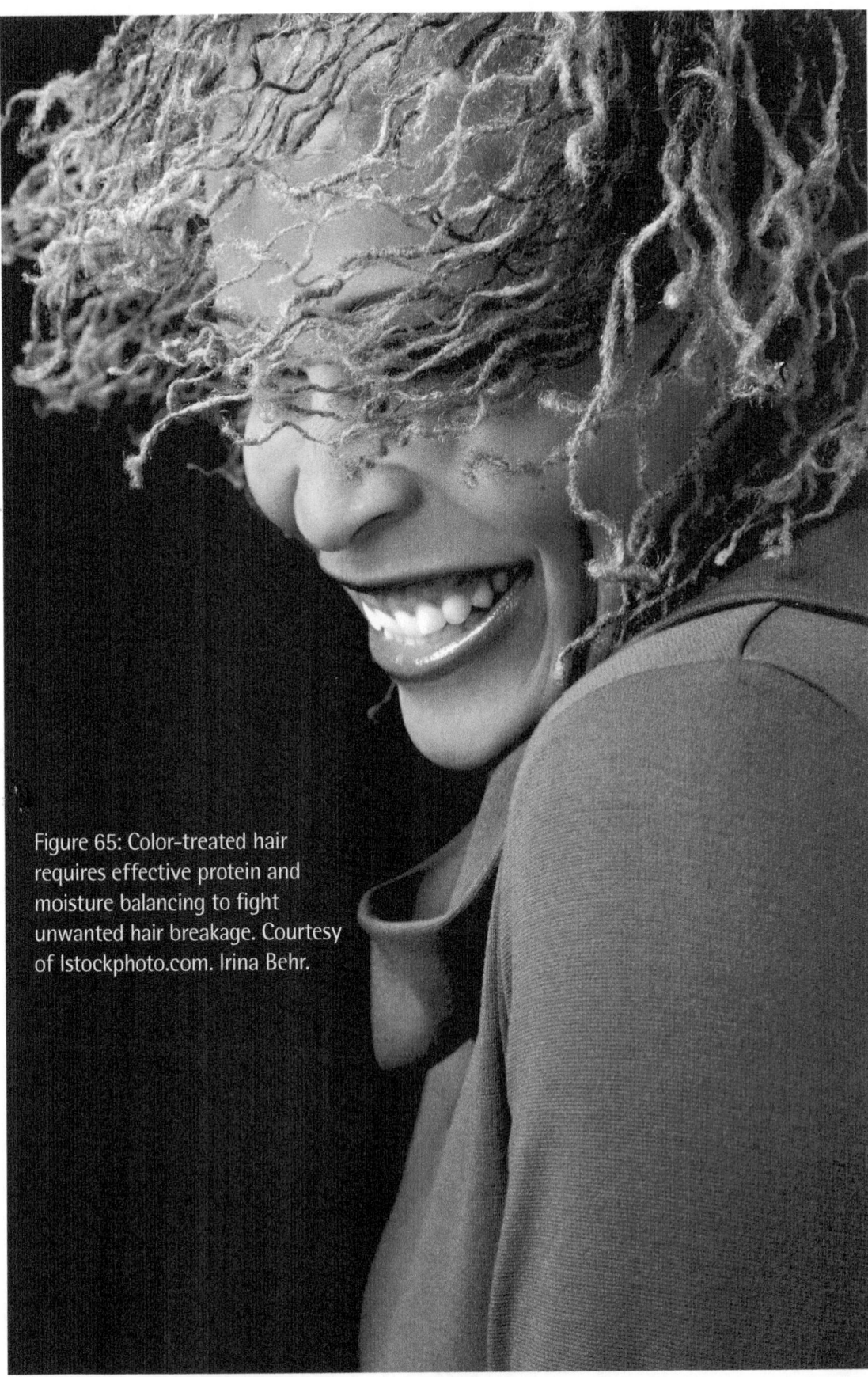

Figure 65: Color-treated hair requires effective protein and moisture balancing to fight unwanted hair breakage. Courtesy of Istockphoto.com. Irina Behr.

Chapter 9: Coloring Textured Hair

If you are reading this unit, chances are you have either taken or are considering taking the color plunge. Color can spice up a drab hair care regimen and can give you an entirely new look, but such hair moves often come with a price. Permanently coloring black hair weakens and changes its strong, natural cuticle architecture. With the hair's internal protein structure drastically weakened, colored hair is less supple and less able to accept and retain moisture. The chronic breakage problems that often result from the imbalance of structural moisture and protein in the hair is a major concern for those who are trying to grow out color-treated tresses. Whether you've used a simple color rinse or went all out on a permanent color, here are the key strategies you need to help your delicate, color-treated hair reach its maximum potential.

How Hair Gets Its Natural Color

Deep within the hair follicle, special cells produce three types of pigment: eumelanins, pheomelanins and oxymelanins. Oxymelanins produce yellow to red tones. Pheomelanin and eumelanin give our hair its dominant range of red-brown to black color tones. Specifically, eumelanins produce brown and black hues in the hair fiber, and are the dominant pigment in most textured hair fibers. The level of eumelanin pigment in the hair fiber determines the degree of black or brown color our hair will have. Pigment is produced only during the growing phase of the hair cycle, which explains why shed hair has a clear/white tip. (11)

Gray Hair

Hair grows in a variety of colors and in many different shades, but gray is not one of them! Gray hair is actually clear hair or hair that has no pigment at all. (11) The gray hair we see is actually an optional illusion that occurs when clear or white hair is contrasted against the remaining darker-colored strands on the head. Take a look at Figure 66:

This well-known color illusion is known as the Hermann Grid. No gray was used to create this black and white image, but if you glance at the image, you will see the color gray begin to fill the little squares at the intersections of the large black rectangles. If you stare at one tiny square at a time, the gray color will disappear and seem to become white. Try it! The same thing happens with your hair. If you focus on one particular hair, you will notice that it is not gray at all! It is indeed clear or white. This is the exact same optical trick our eyes play on us every single time we see a gray-haired person!

As we get older, usually between the ages of twenty-eight and forty, hair produces fewer and fewer pigment molecules. (12) Gray hair is simply hair that no longer produces melanin in the cortex. Since the cuticle is also colorless, gray hair is simply clear (see Figure 67).

Caring for Gray Hair

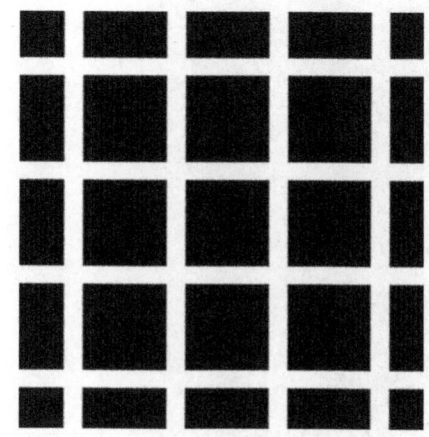

Figure 66: How our eyes see "gray" hair!

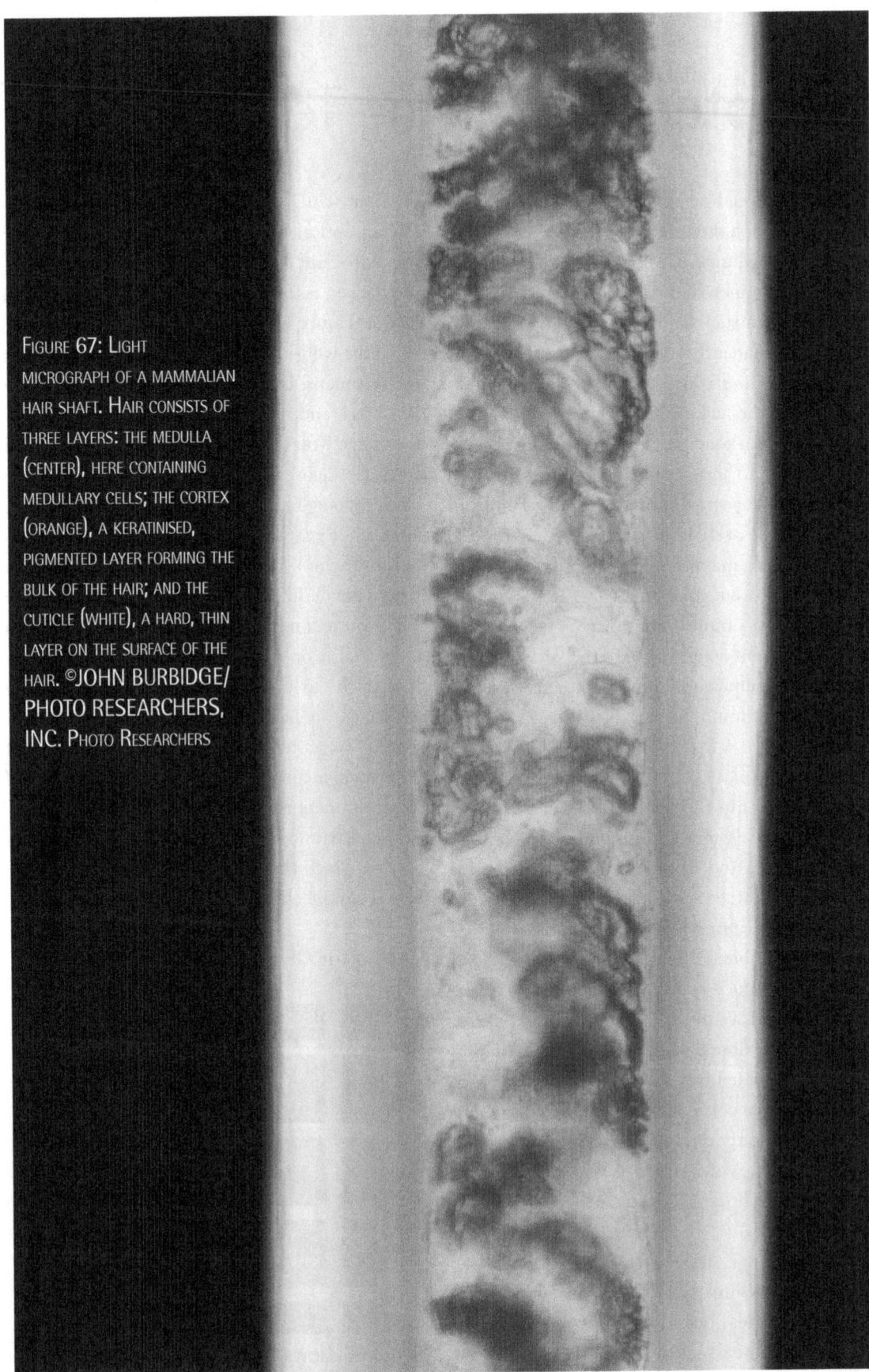

FIGURE 67: LIGHT MICROGRAPH OF A MAMMALIAN HAIR SHAFT. HAIR CONSISTS OF THREE LAYERS: THE MEDULLA (CENTER), HERE CONTAINING MEDULLARY CELLS; THE CORTEX (ORANGE), A KERATINISED, PIGMENTED LAYER FORMING THE BULK OF THE HAIR; AND THE CUTICLE (WHITE), A HARD, THIN LAYER ON THE SURFACE OF THE HAIR. ©JOHN BURBIDGE/ PHOTO RESEARCHERS, INC. PHOTO RESEARCHERS

Gray hair often feels drier and wirier than the hair of our youth. It is often resistant to chemicals and may be harder to effectively style with heat. Grays need regular moisturizing deep conditioning to keep their hair feeling nourished and moisturized. Shampoo gray hair with moisturizing shampoos and conditioners to keep it supple and restore its elasticity. Gray hair that is relaxed or color treated will need light protein reconstruction to reduce its porosity and support its moisture balance.

Healthy Hair Care for Color-Treated Hair

Changing natural hair color drastically affects the feel and appearance of textured hair fibers. Color-treated hair can often feel dry and weak and begin to look dull and lifeless over time. Maintaining a proper protein/moisture balance in color-treated hair is extremely important for managing both dryness and breakage. Because color-treating textured hair has the potential to seriously damage the hair fiber, black hair must be well maintained before, during and after any color treatment to ensure optimal results.

Ideally, chemical processes like coloring and relaxing should be left to professional stylists. While simple color rinses may be easy to apply at home with very little issue if things should not go according to plan, permanent colors and bleaching chemicals are not as forgiving of mistakes. Use your best judgment, and when in doubt, err on the side of caution. Consult with a professional if you are coloring for the first time, using a new product or are just unsure of your own skills.

To color effectively without jeopardizing our healthy hair, we must understand a few basics about hair color. There are three main types of hair color: permanent, semi-permanent and temporary. Each category of color has its own set of benefits and consequences for textured hair types.

Hair Coloring Options
Permanent Coloring

Permanent coloring is needed if you wish to undergo a drastic color change. The permanent coloring process involves using a hydrogen peroxide and/or ammonia-based product. These ingredients lift the cuticle layers to allow for color deposition. Once the tiny color molecules enter the hair shaft, they begin to clump and join together to become larger molecules that cannot be washed out. This process strips away some of the protein deep within textured hair strands and makes our hair weaker and vulnerable to breakage. Permanent color can and often does lose its intensity over time, but it will not wash away. Permanent coloring provides near 100 percent coverage for gray hair. Ideally, this type of coloring should be done professionally, but some women have no problems working their own magic at home!

Semi/Demi-permanent Coloring

Semi-permanent hair colors include partial penetration hair color as well as deposit-only color. Semi-permanent coloring does not last as long as permanent coloring because its color molecules are much too large to enter the shaft deeply. This group of colors covers hair that is up to 50 percent gray and can darken textured tresses easily. Semi-permanent colors are not effective at lifting or lightening hair color.

Partial-Penetration Semi-permanent Colors

Some advanced color formulas come with small, first-line (precursor) pigments that are small enough to enter the hair shaft. Once inside the hair shaft, these small pigments join with our natural hair pigments to create medium-size pigments that are slightly more difficult to rinse out than regular semi-permanent colors. Because the medium-sized pigments are harder to rinse out, the color they impart lasts longer than the color from rinses. Semi-permanent coloring usually ns its vibrancy for three to six months. Porosity enhances the penetration of these colors: the more porous the hair, the deeper the color penetration. Because the ends of our hair are naturally more porous, they process color much faster and allow deeper penetration of color compared to the rest of the hair shaft.

Deposit-Only Semi-permanent Colors

Henna, used to color hair since the days of antiquity, is an example of a plant-based deposit-only color. Its use, however, is only now gaining popularity in the textured hair community. Henna can be safely used by both relaxed and natural-textured individuals to give the hair a darker, reddish tint. Henna pigments bind to our hair's protein structure and have a protective, layering effect on the hair. Henna and its benefits for textured hair are discussed later in the color chapter.

Temporary-Color Rinses

Color rinses or glazes are the safest hair colors for textured hair types. These types of hair colors are derived from molecules that are too large to enter the cortex of the hair shaft. Instead, they simply coat the outside cuticle layers and are generally washed away in ten to fifteen washes. Because they coat the hair and cannot lift color, rinses and glazes can only enhance your current, natural color by making it darker, richer and glossier.

The great thing about rinses is that they do not damage the cuticle layers as more invasive types of color chemicals do. Because the colors only coat the hair shaft, your coloring options with rinses are quite limited. Although they come in a wide variety of colors including clear, these colors will not lighten your natural hair color. Rinse colors will enhance your own natural color but can only take you darker. In fact, unless a product contains ammonia or peroxide, you should not expect it to lighten your hair color at all.

Temporary color rinses are a good cuticle-protecting option for those with permanently colored or porous hair. When placed on top of a regular permanent or semi-permanent color treatment, they lengthen the life of these colors and protect the hair shaft against damage.

Rinses, due to their ability to deposit color on the exterior of the hair shaft, also temporarily thicken the hair strands. A colorless rinse could be a great option for those with fine or thinning hair who do not wish to add color but desire a fuller look. Because color rinses tend to behave very much like protein-based products, they can be drying for some individuals' hair. Diligent moisturizing and deep conditioning are needed to restore the hair's natural elasticity and pliability following a color rinse.

Rinses are effective at coloring hair that is 10 to 20 percent gray.

Henna, Cassia, and Indigo: Coloring Textured Hair Without Chemicals

Fortunately, coloring textured hair does not have to be a damaging process. In fact, some hair colorants like henna, cassia and indigo can actually benefit the hair with regular use. Unfortunately, these natural colorants are not widely used in black hair care, mainly because of misinformation about how they respond to chemically relaxed black hair. Henna, cassia and indigo colorants do not damage textured hair as synthetic dyes and colors do, and these treatments can be done as often as the user desires. True body art quality (BAQ) henna is very beneficial to textured hair types—relaxed, natural or previously colored by some other means.

Difficulties with Plant-Based Coloring

Compared to traditional, commercially available hair-coloring agents, the coloring process with plant powders such as henna, cassia and indigo can be quite time consuming. Powders often have to be ordered from a vendor and mixed; they may then need additional time to sit after mixing while the color develops fully. Application and processing times may take several hours, and overnight processing is not uncommon. With commercially available dyes, color selection may be as simple as choosing a shade on a box or a swatch, but colors and shades may vary with plant-based colors considerably. In fact, your desired coloring result may be several months and/or repeat applications away. Plant-based coloring can also be quite messy, and skin staining is common with some plant dyes.

Henna

Henna has been used as a hair colorant for millennia prior to the arrival of commercial hair dyes on the market. This plant-based powder is still used extensively as a coloring agent in many parts of the world including Africa, the Middle East, India and elsewhere in Asia. Henna adds color to textured black hair like any other deposit-only color—it just happens to be a natural

product rather than a carefully crafted product of modern chemistry. When henna is applied to the hair, some of its pigments migrate slowly

Benefits of Coloring?

Besides the wonderful changes in cosmetic appearance hair coloring offers, hair coloring has other benefits. One study found that coloring the hair offers protection from sun damage and degradation. Though the benefits translate throughout the gamut of colors in the color wheel, sun protection benefits are best realized in hair that is colored darker shades and with shades that deposit on the exterior of the hair cuticle. [2] While this is certainly impressive, and is quite a bonus for color rinses and glazes, it cannot make up for the increased porosity and other damage that permanent colors do the hair fiber.

Did You Know?

Plant-based colors can color textured hair, relaxed and natural, safely with no chemicals whatsoever. (29) These deposit-only colors take advantage of cuticle deposition, and pigment binding along the fiber gives the appearance of thicker, plumper strands. These treatments work well for those with extremely fine hair who need extra body and volume, and for those who are looking for a shine booster for their natural hair color but are not interested in taking a whirl on the color wheel. Plant-based colors also have been found, in some cases, to cause a loosening of textured curl patterns in natural hair over time—an advantage or a disadvantage, depending on your ultimate hair goals.

Because plant-based colors smooth wayward, ruffled cuticles and encourage them to lie flatter, the hair is better able to reflect light from its surface. Enhanced light reflection from the hair fiber surface contributes to a nice, healthy shine.

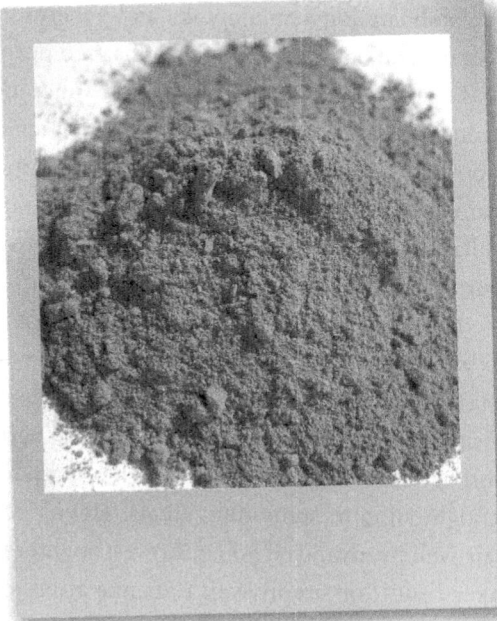

Figure 68: Pure Body Art Quality Henna (pictured here) is safe for textured tresses.

into the hair fiber and bind with the hair's natural proteins. Henna's pigments stain the hair fiber red. Color uptake with henna is cumulative. The more regularly the hair is hennaed, the deeper, longer lasting and more vibrant the color becomes over time.

There is quite a bit of misinformation surrounding henna coloring, particularly in the relaxed hair community. A bit of history explains the source of this anti-henna sentiment. Once natural, plant-based colors went mainstream and hit modern chemistry labs, they were supplemented with common synthetic dyes and chemicals to create additional hair color variants and characteristics. The addition of metallic dyes alters the way that natural colorants like henna respond to our hair. Henna, in particular, once "enhanced" in the lab with metallic dyes, becomes a death sentence for chemically-treated black hair, essentially melting the hair down to nothing. In their natural, unaltered form, however, these colorants can be safely used on all types of black hair: relaxed, colored or natural. Only body art quality (BAQ) henna should be used on textured hair.

Although limited in the scope of achievable shades, henna is an amazingly healthy hair-coloring agent. Henna behaves very much like a standard protein treatment. Because the pigments mostly adhere to the outermost cuticle layers, with some migration deeper into the fiber, henna is able to give our hair a nice gloss, reduce porosity and offer protective benefits to the cuticle. Henna increases the diameter of individual hair shafts, which gives the illusion of greater hair thickness. Henna can make textured hair feel stronger and perhaps somewhat coarse; therefore deep conditioning is highly recommended after coloring with henna. (29)

Henna powder is mixed with a low-pH (acidic) liquid such as lemon juice and only produces subtle red tones on black hair. The shade of red produced always depends on the natural pigment of the hair and the number of times the hair has been previously hennaed. *Any henna product that claims to produce a color other than red is not real BAQ henna and should never be used on black hair.*

IMPORTANT NOTE: "Henna products" that claim to produce colors other than red (including black henna and neutral henna) are not 100 percent pure body art quality henna and should be avoided. These colorful or "compound" hennas are often premixed solutions that contain artificial dyes and metallic salts that can cause severe damage to hair that has already been chemically treated. If you decide to try henna, only purchase BAQ henna from reputable dealers such as www.mehandi.com or local Indian stores.

Henna and Chemically Treated Hair

Body art quality (BAQ) henna can be safely and easily incorporated into a relaxed hair care or colored hair care regimen. It is the commercial compound hennas that have given this ancient coloring method bad press in modern cosmetology. In fact, chemically treated hair is a better candidate for henna uptake and penetration than natural hair because of its enhanced porosity. Deeper pigment penetration and adherence ensures a longer lasting color, as superficially deposited pigments will lift more readily upon shampooing. Henna users with chemically treated hair typically refresh their henna color every four to six weeks.

Henna may be used up to a week before relaxing the hair and as soon as a week following relaxer application. Note that henna's cuticle deposition action can act as a barrier to the penetration of relaxer chemicals and interfere with hair straightening in some individuals. Henna your hair well in advance if you desire a straighter relaxer result, or simply wait to henna after your relaxer service. Although much of the henna will survive the relaxer process, it is normal for some of the superficially deposited henna color to bleed into the relaxer cream, giving it a reddish tint. This is okay and nothing to worry about.

Cassia Obovata and Indigo

If a red henna color is not for you, then beautiful blacks and richer browns can be achieved by adding natural powdered plant dyes like *Cassia obovata* and indigo to henna.

Cassia Obovata

Cassia obovata, also known as senna, is a natural plant powder that conditions the hair without depositing color. (Although cassia dyes hair a faint yellow, these pigments do not show up on dark-colored hair.) On black hair, cassia is very similar to a clear rinse in that it simply enhances the shine of other colors without producing any color change. For individuals with lighter-colored tresses or gray hair, cassia adds a golden tone to colors. To prepare the cassia, water is slowly folded into cassia powder until a paste forms. Oils and conditioners can be added to the mixture at your discretion. (29)

Indigo

Indigo is another plant-based hair colorant that can be used safely on relaxed, permanently color-treated and natural black hair. Indigo is often paired with henna to produce deeper dark brown and black shades. Indigo (often incorrectly called *black henna*), like many plant-based hair colorants, has been used safely for thousands of years to stain the hair. (Indigo, in fact, is one of the main dyes present in denim jeans.)

Before mixing, indigo powder is not black but green. When combined with water, a dark-blue tint emerges. Any powdered indigo that appears black or brown before mixing should not be used.

For more information on henna, *Cassia obovata* and indigo coloring, along with suggestions about where to purchase BAQ henna to ensure healthy hair, visit www.hennaforhair.com. (29)

> ### Coffee Staining For a Natural Color Boost!
> A dark coffee rinse can provide a quick, natural color boost to brown or black hair. Simply brew a pot of dark coffee and allow it to cool. The bolder the blend, the more pronounced the color enhancement. Pour the rinse over your dry hair, just before a wash and allow the rinse to soak into the hair for twenty to thirty minutes. Shampoo the rinse and Voila! Alternatively, the rinse may be done as a post-conditioning final rinse.

How Coloring Affects Textured Tresses

Coloring black hair always changes the way the hair fiber looks and feels, especially if the hair has been colored or bleached. Changes in the feel and texture of the hair indicate that coloring causes modifications to the surface of the hair fiber. Because permanent color chemicals must break into the cuticle layers and disrupt their flattened orientation to introduce pigments, color-treated hair tends to feel drier and coarser than hair that has not been color-treated. When cuticles are lifted, uneven and chipped, they do not reflect light well. Hair also has greater difficulty maintaining a proper moisture balance.

Black hair that has been treated with bleach or other strong permanent-color treatments often loses "weight" due to the loss of internal sulfur bonds and the breakdown of critical proteins in the fiber. Hair that has been colored with rinses, glazes and plant-based colors tends to feel thicker than normal because these color pigments temporarily sit on the exterior of the cuticle. If the hair is already somewhat porous, color rinses and glazes also will find their way into deeper levels of the cuticle. Because of this increased ability to enter the shaft, color rinses, glazes and plant-based colors always last longer on porous hair types.

A majority of the damage to hair from coloring comes from permanent and semi-permanent coloring processes, which assault the hair's natural protein structure in order to deposit color deep into the hair. Research has shown that permanently coloring the hair leads to hair fiber swelling, cuticle detachment and eventually complete exposure of the cortex. (29) (30) (31)

Although perforations (holes) and chipping are common structural features of damaged hair that has not been colored, permanently colored hair tends to have more of these perforations in the cuticle layer. (32) Even when the hair's exocuticle appears to be normal, coloring produces damaging changes in deeper layers of the cuticle. The hair's sulfur-rich A-layer—which contributes significantly to the hair's overall strength—as well as the endocuticle—which supports the expansion and contraction of the hair fiber—are damaged by hair coloring. (33)

Maintaining Color-Treated Hair

Chemical processes always leave textured hair weaker and more compromised than it was before processing. Permanent coloring leads to dry, brittle hair that is breakage-prone and does not retain moisture well. Healthy color care regimens must always work to restore the hair's moisture balance by reinforcing the hair's damaged protein structure. In general, the best colors for textured hair are darker tones that deposit on the cuticle and do not damage the hair's proteins.

Double-Processed: Relaxed and Colored Hair

Hair that has been both chemically relaxed and permanently color-treated is especially vulnerable to damage. Porosity issues tend to be more extreme for those with double- processed tresses. Both chemical processes must breach the cuticle layers and damage the hair's natural protein structure in order to work. As a rule of thumb, color treatments should be applied no sooner than two weeks following a chemical relaxer treatment. The common saying is that you "color a relaxer, never relax a color." Any post-relaxer coloring treatment applied sooner than the safe, two-week window will irreparably damage the hair and drastically increase its porosity and tendency toward breakage.

Coloring Graying Tresses

Gray, textured hair can be quite a challenge to color and maintain given gray's natural resistance to chemical treatments. For those with minimal gray, it is best to spot treat rather than do full color treatments on the entire head.

If you prefer to return the hair to its natural, pre-gray color, most permanent hair colors will completely cover the gray; however roots will need to be touched up regularly to match the new hair color. Semi-permanent colors can cover hair that is 40 to 70 percent gray, but will fade over time. Gray hair can be safely colored with 100 percent coverage using natural plant-based colors like henna, cassia and indigo. Often, natural plant dyes such as henna will require several treatments or slightly longer applications on gray tresses due to fiber resistance.

Color Loss and Fading

All good things must come to an end, but you don't have to give up your awesome new hair color without a fight. There are many factors that lead to premature fading of new hair colors. What can you do to keep your hard color work from rinsing back down the drain?

Color-Application Steps

If heat is used to set your new hair color, allow your hair to cool for several minutes before rinsing the color from the hair. Hot hair leaches color, especially deposit-only colors and temporary rinses. Give your hair time to cool after heating.

The Water Problem

Once you have had your hair colored for a few days, the interaction between your new hair color and water may become an issue. Water in general is an enemy to long-lasting hair color but is also a requirement for the healthy maintenance and stability of the hair fiber. The water problem can be broken down into three major parts: water frequency, water type and water temperature.

Water Frequency

We all know that simply washing color-treated, textured hair will fade its color. No matter which type of hair color you have used (i.e., permanent, semi-permanent or temporary), each wash will pull a little color from the hair. Temporary colors are always lifted and pulled fastest.

Over-handling and frequently cleansing color-treated hair can stress the cuticle, encourage your hair color to fade and increase your hair's porosity. Keep it simple. Always make the most of your regular cleansings by treating the hair with carefully planned protein and moisture deep conditioning treatments.

For best results, allow your new hair color to settle at least a day or two after the initial color job before introducing water through the shampooing and conditioning process. For the first two weeks after a color job, aim to shampoo and condition every seven days. Beyond the second week, hydrate and condition the hair every four to seven days as your hair dictates. Lean toward the longer seven-day range between shampoos for optimal color preservation.

Water Type

Shampooing and conditioning your hair in hard water or water that is partially chlorinated will also strip your hair color. If your water is hard, or if you are a regular swimmer, consider purchasing a chelating shampoo for regular color maintenance. For longer-term results, a good water filter (although expensive) may buy you several more weeks of vibrant hair color. For swimmers, thoroughly saturating the hair in regular water prior to hitting the pool will help to keep pesky chlorine molecules at bay. Once in the pool, your hair won't be able to absorb as much of the chlorinated water. You will still want to shampoo and deep condition "pool hair" as soon as possible. Wearing a swimming cap is a better option.

Water Temperature

Avoid rinsing your hair in hot water. Hot water is drying to the hair whether it is color-treated or not. In addition, hot water (and hot oil treatments) has the opposite effect of cold water, which helps to close and seal the cuticles. Hot hair will release some of its color, and over time, your color will grow duller. Always cleanse and condition your color-treated hair in cool water. After conditioning the hair, do a final rinse in the coldest water you can stand. This final rinse will seal the cuticle and impart amazing shine to your strands.

Product Selection for Color-Treated Hair

Use color-safe shampoos and conditioners. Strong shampoos that are not formulated for color-treated hair can cause even the most vibrant color jobs to fade. Many color-safe shampoos and conditioners, particularly those that are geared toward a certain shade of hair color, will contain small bits of color and color enhancers to give your hair color a "pick-me-up" at wash time. They are wonderful for slowing the color fading process. Shampoos should always be sulfate-free. In addition to a good color-safe shampoo and conditioner, select supporting daily products that contain sunscreens and light oils. Keep your hair thoroughly moisture and protein conditioned! Regular conditioning goes a long way toward preserving hair color and keeping the hair radiant with little product!

Finally, use finishing products such as hair sprays, spritzes, mousses and gels sparingly. The alcohols used in these style-setting products help your hair dry faster and set your style but can fade your hair color prematurely. Some claim that volumizing product lines, or those for fine hair, also fade new hair colors quickly because they allow a slight lifting of the cuticle layers to provide the illusion of increased hair shaft thickness.

Kenra, Joico and Pantene offer great product options for color-treated tresses.

Other Styling and Handling Tips for Colored Tresses

Avoid over-drying color-treated hair with blow dryers and/or flat irons. These styling tools degrade the cuticle and can cause the hair color to become dull over time. The regular heat styling of colored tresses reduces moisture levels and can lead to extreme color damage, characterized by high porosity, dryness, breakage and often a dusty red coloration.

Avoid going outdoors with damp hair if it has been colored. The sun has powerful hair color fading effects, and this problem is exacerbated when hair is damp. (35) Swimming in pools and natural bodies of water introduces the hair color to chlorinated water, salts and other impurities that also leave hair colors looking dull.

Finally, for longer lasting color, try a temporary clear color rinse to seal in a permanent color. Applying a clear rinse over a permanent color will enhance your hair's shine and help preserve your permanent hair color for longer. Hair color rinses are also good low-maintenance shine boosters for non color-treated hair.

Hair Color-Maintenance Regimens

When textured hair is color-treated, getting maximum moisture into the fiber and holding it there are critical tasks. Whether the hair is color-treated, relaxed or none of the above, black hair needs moisture and plenty of it. Our color-treated hair also needs healthy doses of protein conditioning as well. To keep your freshly colored strands looking great, try the basic regimen template detailed below.

Before You Color

Before you attempt to jazz up your textured strands with color, a thorough hair evaluation is in order, particularly if you plan to take your color lighter. Those who are contemplating using color rinses and glazes should always remain aware of their hair's condition prior to rinsing, but the urgency is not as great. In fact, if the hair is lacking protein support, a rinse or glaze will actually improve the hair by reinforcing and protecting the cuticle.

For those who are permanently coloring or bleaching their hair, however, the hair's integrity should be taken into account prior to undergoing these processes. If the strands are damaged or breaking, or the scalp is shedding hair excessively, coloring may not be the best option at this point in time. Remember too that you should avoid coloring previously colored hair or hair that has recently been stressed from a chemical relaxer in the preceding two weeks. Never treat hair that is in questionable condition with permanent color. Stressed hair will simply fall out by the handful if additional chemical processing is inflicted upon the hair fiber.

To prepare textured hair for coloring, take two weeks before the scheduled service to deep condition the hair with heat using both a protein conditioner and a moisturizing deep conditioner. If you are shampooing and conditioning once per week, these two pre-coloring weeks should provide at least two opportunities for you to deep condition and treat your hair with moisture and protein. Emphasis should always be placed on the moisturizing component of this preparation. Hair can be treated with the protein/moisture conditioner combo at once, or by alternating each conditioner type at each wash. Hair that is thoroughly deep conditioned, with both moisture and protein intact, is better suited to undergo the coloring process.

Stick to the Basics

As previously discussed, if you have textured hair—color-treated or not—you should avoid shampoos that strip the hair of natural oils. This rule is even more significant for those with chemically-treated hair. Stripping shampoos are, of course, primarily sulfate based and will pull color from your hair with continued use. In the absence of sulfate-free shampoos, shampoos that are specifically formulated for color-treated hair are your best bet. These shampoos are generally more acidic and more conditioning than other shampoos and will help seal your cuticles, eliminating the rough, porous feeling so common with coloring.

Each shampoo should be followed by a fifteen to thirty minute deep conditioning with either a protein or moisture-based conditioner. The choice of moisture or protein depends on your wet-hair assessment analysis (See the Protein and Moisture Balancing section of this book). Unlike uncolored hair, color-treated hair is more likely to vary widely from one protein or moisture extreme to the next. Its high porosity causes it to feel limp one minute and rough the next. Wet assessing is key for chemically-processed hair. If the strands feel strong with little to no breakage, you will likely want to go with a moisturizing conditioner. If the strands feel weak, limp and mush-like, you probably need to add a protein conditioner.

If you are unsure whether your color-treated hair needs protein or moisture, simply mix the two types of conditioners.

Color-Day Regimen for Self Colorists

If you have coloring services done professionally, a stylist will ensure that all proper services and treatments are performed during your visit. For those who apply their own color, these steps will ensure that your hair receives proper support. Product suggestions are listed in the Regimen Builder, and all are suitable for pre- and post-color care.

1. Before coloring your hair, perform strand and allergy tests. These two tests are usually done two days prior to coloring, and are quite important! Allergy tests ensure that you won't develop a skin rash, peeling or irritation after using the color product. Strand tests confirm your expected processing time and final color results. Follow the manufacturer's guidelines for performing these tests.

2. It is very important that you read (and re-read) the manufacturer's instructions prior to using coloring agents. Methods for color application vary widely. Gather all tools and products needed prior to color application to streamline the process.

3. Since the ends of textured tresses are more porous than the rest of the strand, and because our scalp's natural body heat speeds up color processing near the roots, color application should begin mid-strand. Start the color application mid-shaft, work up toward the roots, and then back down toward the ends of the hair for even processing.

4. After textured hair has been color-treated, you should immediately follow the color with a slightly acidic, pH-balanced shampoo. Ideally, the shampoo should be sulfate-free to ensure that it is color safe. Check your shampoo's pH with test strips to confirm.

5. Follow the sulfate-free, color-safe shampoo with a simple, diluted apple cider vinegar (ACV) rinse to close down the cuticle layers further. (This cuticle-constriction step is completely optional.) This old-fashioned homemade rinse is a great way to control porosity, especially for relaxed and color-

treated hair. Simply mix ¼ cup ACV with 2 cups cool water in a large cup. You can use an applicator bottle or pour the rinse from a cup slowly over your strands. Because ACV has a pungent smell, you may need to rinse the hair for several minutes to lift the smell. Both the ACV mixture and the rinse water should be cool or cold to ensure tight cuticle closure.

6. Deep condition your hair for twenty minutes with a mild protein reconstructor mixed with a moisturizing conditioner. If you decide to use two conditioners and prefer to apply your protein and moisture conditioners in succession, always apply the protein conditioner before the moisture conditioner. You want to give your hair a chance to accept the protein so that when you introduce moisture, the hair shaft will present a sound structure for the moisture binding. Additionally, the last product applied should help support the detangling process. Moisturizing conditioners give the hair more slip than protein conditioners, which drastically improves textured hair's manageability and the comb-out process.

Post-color Treatment Plan

Caring for color-treated hair day to day can be challenging. Hair breakage and dryness are common battles for those with color-treated tresses. Managing color-treated hair really requires that you get a true understanding of protein and moisture balancing. Putting together a dedicated regimen of regular moisture and supplemental protein products in the early weeks following a hair coloring session is important. Once this healthy hair tool is in your hand, navigating the often unpredictable personality of colored tresses will become second nature.

Week 1

In Week 1, shampoo and condition the hair with a sulfate-free shampoo, and select a mois-

ture-based conditioner to use once or twice a week to address your moisture balance. Deep condition the hair with heat. For daily moisture as needed, stick with water-based moisturizing products. If you sense that your hair's balance is becoming too burdened with moisture, substitute a protein-based moisturizer or leave-in conditioner for the moisture products.

Protect the Cuticle (Optional)

The extreme lifting of the hair cuticle that is necessary to properly deposit permanent color can leave color-treated hair feeling dry, rough and flat. Closing the cuticle and restoring its tightness will not only protect your color but will support the integrity of the hair. Applying a clear color rinse over a permanent color a week or two after the color job will help protect the cuticle and prolong the life of your color.

Week 2

In Week 2, continue with the sulfate-free shampoo and opt for a protein-based conditioner or reconstructor product, followed by a brief ten minute heatless conditioning session with a moisturizing conditioner.

Again, as previously discussed, be flexible. If you feel at Week 1 that your hair needs additional protein structuring, then do not hesitate to do your protein conditioning then. You can always mix protein and moisturizing treatments in any week to give your hair a personalized level of conditioning for your specific situation. As long as you meet both its protein and moisturizing needs, your color-treated hair will thrive.

Week 3 and Beyond

Conditioning from this point should concentrate on your individual moisture and protein conditioning needs.

Chapter 10: Chemically Relaxing Textured Hair

If you ask the average black woman why she chooses to relax her hair, you will hear one response time and time again: convenience. The convenience of chemical relaxing, however, does not come to us without great consequence. Relaxing is by far the harshest process a hair strand will encounter in its lifetime. Compromised from the start, relaxed hair is a challenge to keep in tip-top shape— but it can be done! Like color-treated hair, chemically relaxed hair has an inherent element of damage to it and must be given much more diligent care than unprocessed fibers. If we consider the trauma textured hair endures upon relaxing, we can better understand its enhanced fragility. During the relaxer process, the cuticle is raided and the bonds within the hair strand are seized, broken apart and physically rearranged. A healthy hair care regimen must address both the increased protein and the increased moisture needs that must be met if chemically straightened hair is to thrive.

Chemical Relaxer Basics

The use of relaxers in black hair care is so widespread that little introduction is required. Chemical relaxers are high-pH, strongly alkaline products that are formulated to quickly straighten naturally kinky, coily and curly hair. The pH of relaxers ranges from a low of 9 to a high of 14, with higher pHs translating into stronger formulas with faster, more intense straightening powers. As relaxer formulas increase in pH and move up the strength scale from mild to super, hair fiber swelling and cuticle lifting increase. The more the shaft swells, the more damage the cuticle endures. In summary, as the relaxer pH increases, the strength of the relaxer formula, degree of cuticle swelling and cuticle lifting all increase as well.

Repeat applications of relaxers should only be made to the new growth of textured hair from just above the scalp to the *line of demarcation*. The line of demarcation is the line that separates new growth from previously processed hair. This juncture is one of the weakest points along the hair shaft and must be treated with extreme care. Combing relaxers through the hair is discouraged to prevent stress and breakage at this delicate hair fiber junction.

Although chemical relaxers are often referred to as "perms" in common conversation, this terminology is incorrect. *Perm* is short for *permanent wave*, a chemical process with the exact opposite effect (and chemistry) of a relaxer. Permanents make straight hair curly; relaxers start with curly hair and make it straight. Regardless of intent, both chemical processes cleave disulfide bonds to achieve a new, permanent hair configuration.

Types of Relaxers
Hydroxide relaxers

Hydroxide relaxers are the most commonly used chemical relaxers in black hair care. These relaxers include products based on sodium hydroxide, lithium hydroxide, potassium hydroxide and guanidine hydroxide. Hydroxide relaxers can be broken down into two basic formulations: those with and without lye. The major difference between lye and no-lye formulas is simply the chemical compound responsible for breaking the hair bonds. In lye relaxers, this bond-breaking compound is usually sodium hydroxide. In no-lye relaxers, the active compound is generally guanidine hydroxide. The general public often incor-

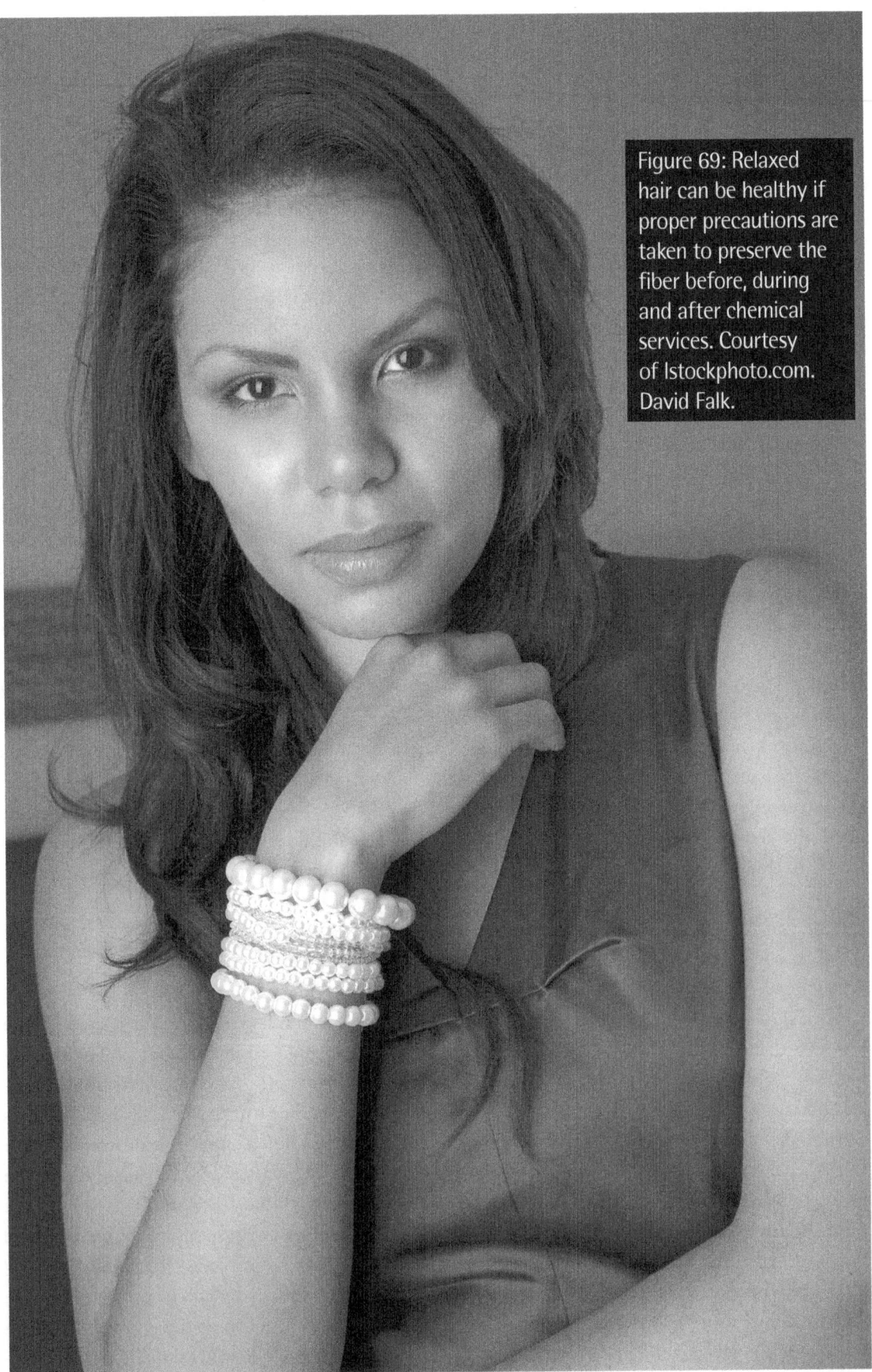

Figure 69: Relaxed hair can be healthy if proper precautions are taken to preserve the fiber before, during and after chemical services. Courtesy of Istockphoto.com. David Falk.

rectly assumes that a no-lye designation means that a relaxer is not as dangerous or is safer to use than a lye relaxer; however, this is simply not the case. The active elements guanidine, lithium and potassium hydroxide found in no-lye relaxers are in the same chemical family as sodium hydroxide, and no-lye products are just as dangerous as lye products if mishandled.

One way to determine whether a relaxer formula is lye or no-lye is by the presence of an activator. No-lye relaxers generally include an activator step: a secondary component to be mixed into the main cream. Lye relaxers typically come premixed in a tub and ready for use. Furthermore, lye relaxers are generally only available to licensed cosmetologists, though the Internet has made them increasingly available to the public.

Lye Relaxers

A hallmark product of black hair salons, the lye relaxer has taken a prominent position in black hair care. Lye relaxers are the preferred chemical relaxer formula of the salon industry. These sodium hydroxide-based relaxers are stronger than no-lye relaxers and are generally formulated at a much higher pH. Lye relaxers can easily approach the 13 and 14 pH range.

Lye relaxers are said to be easier on the hair and harder on the scalp. This is because they do not leave drying mineral deposits on the hair fiber, and so are more likely to leave the hair with a softer, silkier result without further treatments. Lye relaxers' high pH, however, can cause considerable scalp irritation and burning if they are used incorrectly.

Hair straightening quality and processing time are more functions of the relaxer's pH than of the type of active ingredient. Compared to no-lye relaxers, lye relaxers are more likely to provide a level of disulfide bond breakage that still allows the hair to retain its natural strength and elasticity. This lower degree of bond break-

age tends to produce moderately straight results compared to no-lye relaxers, despite the generally higher pH. Disulfide bond breakage may be reduced in lye relaxers because its chemical aggressiveness tends to put time constraints on the straightening process.

Because they are able to lift the cuticle layers more forcefully and breech protective layers of petroleum base more quickly, lye relaxers must be applied carefully and quickly to avoid damage to the hair fiber and scalp. Lye relaxers are best for individuals with coarser, resistant hair types who need higher-pH relaxers to open the cuticle, those who prefer professional applications at salon establishments and those who desire a moderate degree of straightening. Since lye relaxers are stronger and composed of more aggressive chemicals than no-lye relaxers, most lye formulations have traditionally been unavailable "over the counter" for general consumer use. However, with the advent of the Internet and online product retailers, anyone can get their hands on their favorite lye relaxer brand for at-home application: *for better or worse.*

No-Lye Relaxers

No-lye relaxers are hydroxide relaxer products that include guanidine hydroxide and other metal hydroxide formulas such as potassium or lithium hydroxide. (21) Although guanidine hydroxide relaxers or "box relaxers" come in boxed kits that must be mixed to activate the formula, both lithium and potassium hydroxide no-lye relaxers may be sold as "no-mix" formulas sold in tubs.

For years, no-lye relaxers have had a bad reputation in the hair industry, and for good reason. While the product chemistry of no-lye relaxers is satisfactory and generally results in acceptable straightening, the threat of damage from these formulas increases handily as the level of skill of the applier decreases. While some members of the consuming public are quite skilled at relaxer application, others who are not as adept at the proper techniques for chemical use often commit to self-relaxing despite this. Unfortunately, the potential for overlapping, overprocessing, and general misuse increases significantly when chemical applications are placed in the hands of untrained consumers.

No-lye relaxers are often considered to be extremely drying to textured tresses. The common saying that no-lye relaxers are "harder on the hair and easier on the scalp" speaks directly to this common observation. (1) (33) In guanidine hydroxide relaxers, the chemical reaction between guanidine carbonate and calcium hydroxide leaves stubborn, dulling calcium deposits on the exterior of the hair shaft. Calcium deposits decrease the hair fiber's ability to absorb new moisture: the same problem that we see in hard water mineral cases. No-lye relaxing can be continued successfully if proper calcium chelating takes place to lift the deposits as needed. Cleansing the hair with a chelating shampoo after the relaxer can help remedy calcium buildup and dryness within the hair fiber. No-lye relaxers are considered gentler on the scalp because they tend to be less irritating than lye relaxers. This is why most sensitive-scalp relaxer products are no-lye formulas.

No-lye relaxer mixes are good for only one application and must be used the day they are mixed. Any leftover relaxer cream cannot be stored and must be discarded because the active ingredient in most no-lye relaxers, guanidine hydroxide, does not remain stable for very long once it has been created by mixing the activator and the cream. The two chemicals, guanidine carbonate and calcium hydroxide, that are combined to create the relaxer are stable in the mixture for about twenty-four hours.

No-lye relaxers tend to take longer than lye relaxers to process the hair but often make textured hair straighter than lye relaxers. Ultimately, however, a relaxer's ability to straighten the hair fiber is more a function of the relaxer's pH than it is of the relaxer type or brand. (21) Because many people understand the classic relaxer tingle or burning sensation experienced with lye products to be their rinsing point, no-lye relaxers, which may not cause this sensation on the scalp right away, can give users a false sense of security with their processing time. This greater degree of comfort in no-lye chemical processing often encourages users to leave these relaxers in the hair longer than they should—and certainly for longer than would ever be possible with a lye relaxer. Lengthier processing time translates to increased disulfide bond breakage in the fiber and therefore straighter hair. Unfortunately, this straighter turnout can be a double-edged sword. The straighter hair produced with no-lye relaxers is generally dry, severely overprocessed, limp and lifeless hair that is more prone to breakage.

If using a no-lye relaxer, invest in a trusted, professional relaxer brand. If mineral buildup on the hair fiber is a source of dryness when using no-lye relaxer formulas, chelate the hair in the first shampooing several days after the relaxer service or select a brand that contains lithium or potassium hydroxide. Keep in mind that lithium and potassium hydroxide tend to be more aggressive than guanidine hydroxide and can easily burn and irritate the scalp.

Thioglycolate Relaxers

In addition to traditional high-pH relaxers for straightening textured hair, mildly alkaline, low-pH chemical straighteners are also available. Like lye and no-lye relaxers, thio formulas also work by breaking disulfide bonds in the hair. These products use a thiole, most commonly ammonium thioglycolate, to straighten the hair. These "thio" straightening products have pHs ranging from 6 to 9 and come from the same chemical family as permanents that curl straight hair. For permanent waves, the formula is applied and the hair is rodded to produce curls. For straightening curly hair, the product is simply combed through and the hair is smoothed to straighten it. Thio relaxers are not compatible with any form of hydroxide relaxer and cannot be applied to hair that has been previously relaxed with lye or no-lye preparations.

Unfortunately, thio relaxers rarely produce impressive straightening results and are extremely hard on black hair. Some forms of these relaxers are used to texturize or loosen the curl in black hair without making it straight. Soft-curl perms use a combination of thio relaxer and thio permanent waving to loosely curl the hair. Hydroxide relaxers are by far the most popular relaxer types and will be the basis of discussion in this chapter.

Which Relaxer Type Is Best?

Regardless of its type, a relaxer is only as good as the person applying it AND the person maintaining it afterward. In the wrong hands, all relaxer formulas can lead to extensive, irreversible damage to textured tresses including hair breakage and complete baldness. Unfortunately, there are just as many damaged and breaking heads of hair relaxed with lye relaxers as with no-lye products. This truth underscores the very important point that application and maintenance, not relaxer brand or type, are the true determining factors governing the health or demise of chemically relaxed hair.

Just because a certain form of relaxer is easier on the scalp or easier on the hair does not mean that it won't damage the scalp or hair. Relaxers by their very nature damage the hair and scalp if they come in contact with them. Chemical burns, irritation and hair loss can result from any kind of chemical relaxer. Both lye and no-lye relaxer brands must be evaluated on their own merits. Personal hair straightening results will always have much to do with the condition of your hair and your smoothing technique.

How Relaxers Straighten Textured Hair

Chemical relaxers straighten black hair in four basic steps. First, relaxer chemicals swell the hair fiber and gain entry into the hair's inner cortex. Second, the relaxer's active chemical ingredient breaks the disulfide and polypeptide linkages that are responsible for the hair's strength and natural texture. Third, with key bonds broken within the fiber, the hair is smoothed into a straightened shape. Finally, the pH of the hair is reduced and the hair is fixed into shape permanently by a low pH shampoo or rinse.

Step 1: Gaining Entry

As mentioned in previous chapters, pH levels affect black hair in several ways. Low pHs close, constrict and tighten the hair cuticle, while high pHs swell the hair shaft and cause a disruption of the hair's normal, flat cuticle orientation. Because relaxers are formulated at some of the highest pH levels of any products used in cosmetology, they are able to swell and force open the cuticles to expose the inner layers and workings of the hair. Lye relaxers are formulated near the pinnacle of the pH scale and therefore swell the hair shaft quickly and more significantly than other relaxer types. Research has shown that hair fibers can swell as much as 60 to 80 percent of their normal diameter during the chemical-relaxing process. This swelling stresses the hair fiber and can result in extensive cracking and fracturing along the length of the hair fiber.

Step 2: Cleaving Textured Hair Bonds

Relaxer chemicals migrate within the swollen hair fiber and dismantle the millions of cross-linked disulfide bonds that make up the hair. (Remember: The hair's disulfide bonds are responsible for our natural curl patterns.) Hydroxide relaxers break disulfide bonds and create new, weaker bonds in a process known as lanthionization. (34) (7) Disulfide bonds contain two sulfur atoms, whereas lanthionine bonds contain only one sulfur atom. The newly created bonds are weaker because a sulfur atom is lost in the lanthionization process. In addition to the disulfide bonds, the chemical relaxing process also affects the hair's protein linkages and hydrogen bonds, making both protein and moisture supplementation and balancing vital. Some "natural relaxers" use terminology such as weaken, loosen and soften to describe the bond-breaking action of their products. Do not be fooled. These products are not natural, and the process of "softening" bonds is the same as breaking bonds.

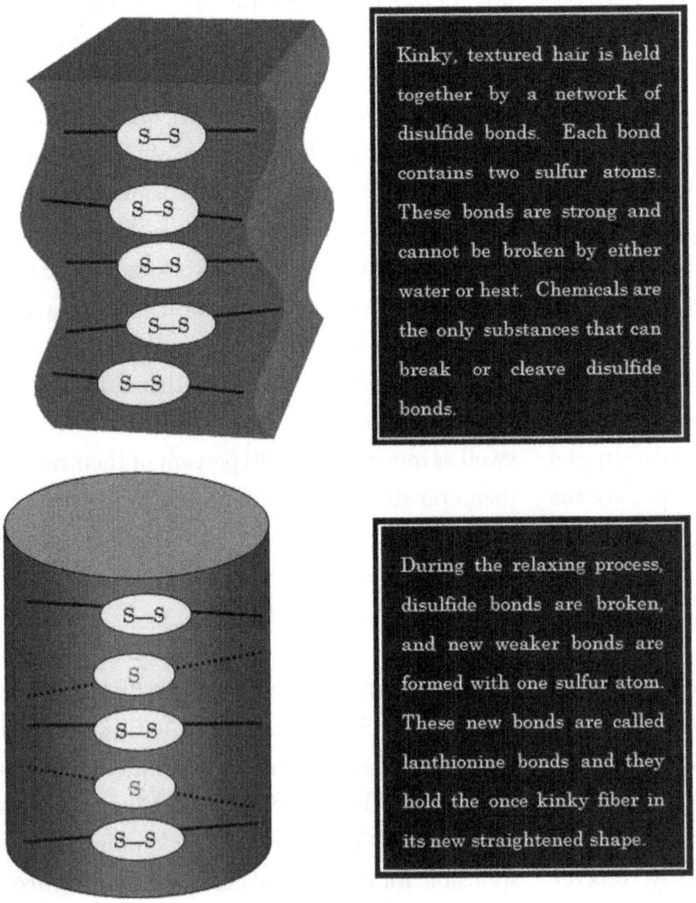

Step 3: Final Arrangement and Shape Fixation

Contrary to popular belief, the chemicals in the relaxer cream are not responsible for the physical straightening of black hair; rather, it is the mechanical smoothing process with gloved fingers that is responsible for rearranging the relaxer-broken bonds into the desired straight form. The alkalinity of the relaxer simply swells open the shaft and breaks the hair's disulfide linkages so that they can be manipulated into shape. Kinky hair is weakest and thinnest in diameter at the points where it naturally bends and curls. During the relaxer smoothing process, these bends and curls are elongated and bent sharply in the opposite direction to keep them smooth and aligned in a new straightened configuration.

The relaxer cream's consistency also aids in the straightening process. Most relaxer products are thick, heavy creams. These paste-like products keep the hair immobile while coils and curls are extended for straightening. This process is highly damaging to textured hair fibers and great care must be taken during the smoothing stage to ensure that as little damage as possible is inflicted on the fibers. Although combs can help ensure even relaxer coverage and a straighter result, relaxer chemicals should never be combed through the hair during a relaxer application. Combing stretches the fiber while it is in its most vulnerable state and causes irreparable damage.

Kinky, textured hair is held together by a network of disulfide bonds. Each bond contains two sulfur atoms. These bonds are strong and cannot be broken by either water or heat. Chemicals are the only substances that can break or cleave disulfide bonds.

During the relaxing process, disulfide bonds are broken, and new weaker bonds are formed with one sulfur atom. These new bonds are called lanthionine bonds and they hold the once kinky fiber in its new straightened shape.

Figure 70: The chemical relaxing process.

Step 4: Neutralization

The application of an acidic, neutralizing product lowers the pH environment created by the alkaline relaxer cream and brings the chemical relaxing process to a close. Neutralizers may come in the form of lotions, conditioners or shampoo products. These low-pH neutralizing products help fix our hair's sulfur bonds in their new permanent shapes.

Healthy-Hair Relaxing Strategy
Preparing Textured Hair for Chemical Relaxing

Relaxing textured hair is serious business. This chemical process, when poorly or even expertly executed, can take relatively healthy black hair and destroy it in one application. Proceeding with a relaxer application on compromised hair is taking a huge gamble with your hair's condition and health. Unfortunately, many of us use relaxers to try to solve common hair problems such as breakage, dryness or shedding. Never EVER relax textured hair to solve a problem. The underlying hair problem should always be investigated, treated using the strategies presented in this book, and corrected prior to chemical relaxing, coloring or any other major hair service. Even if you have no major hair issues, keeping textured hair in top physical condition prior to the relaxer service ensures that better results will be achieved with the finished product. If your hair is healthy, and you are ready to proceed with chemical relaxing, follow these critical relaxer prep steps:

> Relaxing on top of a hair problem will only aggravate the condition by weakening the hair fiber and making it more vulnerable to further damage post-processing.

Step 1: Clarify the Hair

Approximately three to five days before your relaxer treatment, the hair should be clarified to remove product buildup. As discussed in the Shampoo Basics Chapter, any shampoo with sodium or ammonium lauryl sulfate will be strong enough to clarify the hair and remove stubborn product buildup that may get in the way of the straightening process. If you do not wish to have a bone-straight look and prefer some texture, then you may forgo the clarifying session and simply cleanse with a sulfate-free shampoo to lift light product debris.

Step 2: Treat Textured Hair with Protein

Give the hair a protein treatment at the last shampoo and conditioning three to five days before your relaxer. Rebuilding the hair in the days leading up to the relaxer service gives the hair a bit more protein to work with going into the relaxer process. This prevents the relaxer from completely compromising the strength of textured hair when the inner protein bonds are manipulated.

To determine the best protein conditioner to use prior to relaxing, consider your hair's current condition. If there is minimal to no breakage, go with a Zone 1 protein conditioner. If breakage is moderate, use a Zone 2 protein conditioner. DO NOT proceed with the relaxer application if you are experiencing Zone 3 breakage or if your Zone 1 or Zone 2 breakage still has not improved with the application of light to moderate protein.

Follow up the protein treatment with one of the moisturizing deep conditioning treatments from the Regimen Builder.

After this point, do not wash, comb, scratch or do anything to disturb your scalp before undergoing your relaxer service. Avoid sensitizing the scalp with scalp-stimulating products such as essential oils, heat and other heavy product use. DO NOT shampoo or condition the hair in the next seventy-two hours leading up to a relaxer service.

Step 3: Protect Textured Hair Fibers

On the night before, and the day of relaxing, you should pay special attention to the ends of the hair. The previously relaxed length of the hair shaft and the ends are especially vulnerable to the relaxing process. Keep the hair moisturized, oiled and styled very simply in the days preceding a relaxer service.

Step 4: Perform a Strand Test

Always perform a strand test according to the relaxer manufacturer's instructions before applying relaxer or hair-coloring chemicals. The hair should be strand-tested twenty-four to forty-eight hours prior to relaxing, even if you have previously used the chemical in question. (Alternatively, you may decide to perform a strand test as part of relaxer-preparation Step 1.)

Why perform a strand test? *Because, things change!* A chemical that may have worked well for years may suddenly fail to give the desired effect, product manufacturers may change or modify relaxer formulas, or you may develop a sensitivity to an older formula. Performing a strand test will always let you know where you stand. If you are having your hair professionally relaxed, your stylist should perform a strand test with each relaxer service. Be proactive and request a test if the stylist doesn't schedule one.

Relaxing Strategy

If, after preparing the hair in the previous week with a strand test, clarifying shampoo, protein treatment and deep conditioning, you have determined that your hair is relatively breakage and shedding free, you may proceed with the relaxer application. Always follow your relaxer's instructional guide for application to the letter. The following tips can be incorporated alongside those basic instructions to help clarify and improve the relaxing process.

Self-Relaxing Support Guide

Ideally, chemical relaxers should be applied by licensed professionals. Often, though, circumstances may not permit a professional relaxer service. When this happens, it is imperative that proper self-relaxing techniques be employed to ensure the healthiest possible head of hair. Before attempting to self relax the hair with chemicals, always practice your technique with your favorite conditioner to get the timing down and to work out any application issues. If you overlap or take longer than expected to complete the application with conditioner, your hair won't suffer but will benefit from the lengthy conditioning.

In your conditioner trial run, be sure to apply the product in the exact manner and under the same conditions that you would apply the real relaxer. Be mindful of your available timing and take care not to overlap the conditioner onto previously relaxed hair. Apply the conditioner to the most resistant areas of the head (where the hair is thickest, tightest and/or coiliest), saving the hairline for last.

Gather Your Materials

Having everything you need for your relaxer application ready beforehand will enhance efficiency and save precious time. Before you begin your relaxer application, gather all of the products that will be used from start to finish in one accessible place. Take inventory. Ensure that each and every bottle, towel and treatment is accounted for prior to introducing the relaxer cream to your hair. Always follow the manufacturer's directions for the use of each item.

Gloves

Gloves should be worn during the relaxer application to protect your hands from the relaxer chemicals. Relaxer chemicals can irritate your hands and weaken and/or discolor fingernails—which, like your hair, are composed primarily of keratin protein.

Base or Oil

Apply a rich petroleum base or oil to the hair to protect the hair and scalp from chemical processing.

Check Relaxer Compatibility

Select a relaxer strength that is compatible with your hair. Those with thick, coarse hair should use regular-strength relaxers. Fine to medium hair needs a mild strength formula. Super-strength relaxers are formulated at the highest pHs possible: a highly corrosive pH 13 or 14. The high pHs of super-strength relaxers are much too high for most textured tresses and can cause considerable damage to the hair fiber. Remember that straightening power is all in the smoothing stage of the relaxer application. Poor or inadequate smoothing will result in decreased hair straightness. Be sure to carefully observe processing times for your chosen relaxer, and try to work within that window. If you ever feel tingling or burning, you have waited too long to rinse the relaxer.

Towels

You may need as many as five towels (four large, one small) to support the relaxer process. A small hand towel should be used for your face. The four large towels should include one to drape over your shoulders during relaxer application, one to drape during rinsing stage, one to dry the hair and one extra just in case!

Timer

Use a timer to keep track of time during the relaxer application.

Comb (optional): After your initial four corner partings, using a comb during the relaxer process is optional. A comb can inadvertently scratch or irritate your scalp during the relaxer application, so they are not recommended. Using the fingers to section and smooth new growth is preferable.

Neutralizer

Select a neutralizing shampoo with a color alarm that changes color according to pH.

Conditioners

Choose a mild protein treatment or protein conditioner for the optional mid-relaxer protein step. Select a thick, creamy moisturizing conditioner for following up the relaxer application.

Clips

You will need four clips to keep loose hair controlled as the relaxer is applied.

Gloved Finger Method	Applicator Bottle Method	Applicator Paintbrush Method
• Hands are gloved and relaxer is smoothed onto sections with the fingers or the back of a comb. This method offers less control for neatly applying the relaxer.	• Relaxer is placed into a plastic applicator bottle, squeezed onto the new growth, and smoothed with a gloved finger. This method allows for more control of the relaxer application	• The hair is parted and relaxer is "painted" or smoothed onto the new growth with the applicator brush. This method gives the user more control over the application and prevents overlapping.

Figure 71: Relaxer application techniques and methods

Step 1: Base the Scalp and Hair

Basing the hair and scalp with a light coating of oil or a petroleum-based product is the all-important first stage of the chemical relaxer application process. Although some relaxer types do not require pre-basing, it is a good practice to base the hair and scalp anyway.

Often, we base the scalp to the exclusion of the hair—but hair receives protection from oiling just as the scalp does. Because new growth is typically short and compact, it is virtually impossible to avoid chemical overlap onto the scalp and previously treated hair without this protective layer. Oil should be applied to the previously relaxed hair from the point of new growth all the way through to the ends. This protective oil coating prevents previously relaxed hair from being reprocessed during the final rinsing of the relaxer.

NOTE: If a professional stylist performs the relaxer application, it may be beneficial to base the hair prior to arriving for your salon appointment to ensure thorough, even base coverage. Stylists are usually short on time. By getting this essential basing step out of the way, you will ensure that you have protected yourself against burning and damage from overprocessing.

Step 2: Section Your Hair

Divide your hair into four quadrants using a comb of good quality. You may adjust this number as you see fit. Many individuals have success relaxing their hair in two or three sections. Always relax your hair in an organized manner, working through one section of hair at a time. Use your clips to tie back the other hair sections while you concentrate on one.

Step 3: Take Note of the Time

Start timing your relaxer from the moment you apply it to your hair. The general processing rules of thumb, WHICH SHOULD NEVER BE EXCEEDED unless directed by the product packaging, are:

- Thirteen (13) minutes or less for fine or previously damaged (porous) hair.
- Fifteen to eighteen (15 to 18) minutes for slightly damaged (porous), normal hair.
- Twenty (20) minutes for coarse, resistant or minimally damaged (porous)hair.

Note that these time constraints are guidelines and may vary depending upon the relaxer brand and the texture and condition of the hair. "Damaged" in this case refers to the hair's porosity.

Step 4: Choose Where To Begin

Always begin working on the most resistant section of hair first. After putting on gloves, make a ½- inch parting with your comb (or index finger) in this section and generously apply the relaxer to the front and back sides of new growth for that small section. You want to part, lift, apply, part, lift, apply. Be sure that you coat both sides of the sectioned strands with your relaxer. Keep the relaxer confined to the new growth only. Do not overlap the relaxer cream onto the previously relaxed areas, and keep the relaxer away from your scalp. Continue to make ½-inch partings throughout the section, smoothing the new growth down as you go. When the section is complete, unpin another section and repeat with ½-inch partings until you have completed it. Proceed in this way until you have applied the relaxer cream to all of the hair's new growth. Once application is complete, continue to smooth and work the cream into the new growth without overlapping.

Step 5: Rinse Out the Relaxer.

Head to your sink and gently and thoroughly rinse the relaxer cream from the hair in warm water. Use gloved hands to gently agitate the hair to remove the physical traces of the relaxer.

Step 6: Apply a Mid-Relaxer Protein Conditioner

Relaxers disrupt the same protein-bonding structure that is responsible for our hair's strength and elasticity. When the hair's protein architecture is diminished, the hair is more susceptible to breakage, splitting and fracturing. The most critical point in the relaxing process occurs at the point after the relaxer is rinsed and just before the hair's pH is brought down via neutralization. It is at this point that the cuticle layers are most permeable and receptive to treatments. The purpose of the mid-relaxer protein step (MRPS) is to neutralize the hair and deposit protein deep within the ravished cuticle while the hair is in the state that will allow for maximum penetration.

One common misconception about the relaxing process is that a shampoo is required to begin relaxer neutralization, and that relaxed hair continues to process until it is shampooed with a neutralizing shampoo. Relaxer neutralization, however, is simply a shift in the hair's pH from a highly alkaline state back to the hair's naturally acidic state. Each product applied to the hair after a relaxer is rinsed out contributes to the gradual decrease in pH, and has a neutralizing effect on the hair fiber.

Compared to the extreme alkalinity of the hair post-relaxer, all other products are acidic. The initial warm-water rinsing of the relaxer cream has a neutral pH of 7. This water alone helps to bring down the pH of freshly relaxed hair from a high 11 to 13 pH range to a lower, alkaline range of 8 to 11. This lower pH range is still higher than the hair's normal acidic pH of 5, but relaxer chemical reactions cannot continue full force at these lower pH levels. Conditioners are formulated at normalizing (acidic) pHs of 3 to 5, which further neutralize the hair after the rinse stage and bring the hair's alkaline pH level under control. Protein conditioners are a common feature in most professional lye relaxer systems. They help rebuild the cuticle and return

the scales to their normal flattened orientation after the cuticle lifting and swelling damage induced by the relaxer. This optional conditioning step can be successfully incorporated into no-lye relaxer systems as well.

Protein conditioning should take place immediately after the relaxer is rinsed and just before a normalizing or neutralizing shampoo is used. Simply apply the protein conditioning treatment to the hair after thoroughly rinsing the relaxer. Allow the conditioner to remain on the hair for three to five minutes, then rinse. Remember that uptake of conditioner products is improved in hair that has been damaged. Since the cuticles and shaft are swollen following the relaxer and the shaft will readily absorb product, this conditioning step takes only a few minutes to work on the hair. Immediate strengthening effects can be felt from this conditioning phase.

Pump it Up!

Freshly relaxed hair often can feel limp and flat. If you have decided to do the Mid-Relaxer Protein Step (MRPS), you will find that the protein makes the hair feel very strong and gives the hair a nice "weight" almost immediately upon rinsing. The MRPS increases the body, strength and thickness of relaxed hair immediately following a relaxer, with results that linger for weeks.

Step 7: Apply an Acidic Normalizing Shampoo.

The critical neutralizing step is one of the most misunderstood phases of the chemical-relaxing process. Unfortunately, the neutralizing step is where many self and professional relaxer applications go wrong. Often during relaxer application sessions neutralization may occur too quickly to bring the pH of the hair down sufficiently. If the hair's pH is not properly reduced or neutralized, the relaxer will continue to work on the bonds within the hair strand. If the amount of relaxer residue in hair strand is still significant after you have performed the neutralization step and moved on, permanent hair loss and thinning will result. Whether you follow a multistep neutralization process or simply use a neutralizing shampoo or conditioner, the neutralization process should be the lengthiest part of the relaxing process.

Once a neutralizing product—conditioner or shampoo—has been applied to the hair, you should allow it to remain undisturbed on the hair fiber for three to five minutes before rinsing. The product must be given sufficient time to penetrate the hair shaft and change the hair's pH environment. Proper relaxer neutralization cannot be achieved in a few lightning-fast latherings and quick rinses because the deep penetrating relaxer chemicals are not always easily removed from the hair shaft. Gentle scalp agitation during the neutralizing process often lifts additional traces of high-pH relaxer.

Finally, it is always important to know where you stand in the neutralization process. Insist on using a neutralizing shampoo with a color indicator with all relaxer applications. If you neutralize your hair in less than five to ten minutes with one or two quick lathers, there is a strong possibility that the neutralizing process will be insufficient to bring down the pH enough to halt the action of the relaxer. If the relaxer is insufficiently neutralized, the fiber will become extremely dry, porous and weak and will be prone to chronic breakage over time.

Step 8: Deep Condition

Once the hair is properly neutralized and rinsed, moisturizing deep conditioning must take place immediately. Deep condition the hair with heat for fifteen minutes, and rinse the hair in cool water to encourage the cuticles to constrict. Applying an apple cider vinegar (ACV) rinse to the hair after shampooing and conditioning will help to further adjust the hair's pH to acidic levels. Hair can remain at slightly elevated pH levels and porosity for several days following a chemical relaxer service. You may decide to include an ACV rinse for pH adjustment for the next two to three conditionings following a relaxer service.

Science of Black Hair Street Interview

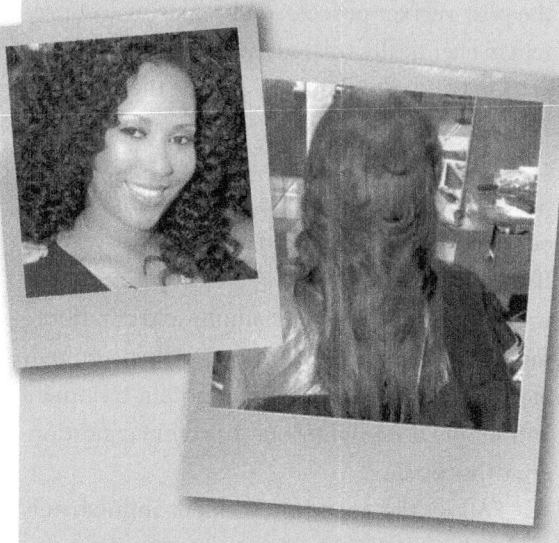

Name: Kimberly
Occupation: Photographer CEO/K's Photography in Eunice, LA

Q: Is your hair relaxed or natural?

A: *I actually tried to go natural once, but that only lasted for about six months. I relax my hair about every four months, and most of the time I do it myself.*

Q: How often do you visit salons for your hair care?

A: *I normally do my own hair, but I may visit a salon when I want a cut and style or when I just want to get pampered.*

Q: What is your hair regimen/routine?

A: *My normal routine is to wash and condition on Saturdays with Paul Mitchell shampoo and conditioner, and then I use Nexxus Mousse, Paul Mitchell Heat Seal and Paul Mitchell Super Skinny Serum. After all of that, I comb it through and then set it. My sister-in-law, who is a beautician, recommended these products, and they work well for me.*

Q: Tell us about your nighttime hair regimen?

A: *All I do is wrap my hair and wear a satin night-cap.*

Q: How do you keep your hair moisturized?

A: *Honestly, the few times that I do moisturize my hair, I use Paul Mitchell Super Skinny Serum.*

Q: What are your must-have hair products?

A: *I absolutely love Paul Mitchell products. They make my hairstyle long lasting and healthy looking.*

Q: Have you always had great hair?

A: *Well if you consider it great, then yes, as long as I can remember.*

Q: What is your go-to style—the style that you know looks great no matter what?

A: *Well, because my hair is long, I think I can really rock a ponytail, whether dressy or casual, but my absolute favorite hairstyle is the natural wave look. After washing, all I do is simply braid my hair in four large braids starting from the crown of my head adding a roller at the end. I then either sit under the dryer or let it air dry. Once my hair is dry, I just separate the parts with my fingers, and I'm done. This style normally lasts a week because I start off with it down then the second day I pull the sides up, day three I wear a high curly ponytail, the fourth day I rock my wavy top with a low curly ponytail, and the fifth day I pin it up in a corn roll. No curling irons!*

Q: What is the number one challenge you face with your hair?

A: *I would have to say that my biggest challenge is its thickness, which makes it very hard to dry while under the dryer.*

Q: What was your biggest hair mistake?

A: *Sometimes I get in that mood where I want a change ASAP. I look in the mirror with a pair of scissors, and I cut. I always cut the front way too short, and I normally end up going to a salon to have the damage repaired.*

Q: What do you like best about your hair?

A: *The thing that I like best about my hair that it is easy to manage, and it grows really fast.*

Q: What hair-care tips or advice would you share with others?

A: *I am often asked how I get my hair to grow so long. After reminding people that it has a lot to do with genes, I simply tell them that I try to stay away from flat irons and curling irons as much as possible. Also, when I get that strong urge to cut my hair really short, I go out and buy a short wig, wear it for about a week, and then realize how tired of the style I am. Last, I think that keeping my ends clipped helps a lot. The longer you wait to clip the ends the higher they will split, and that means that you will likely have to clip more than you really want.*

Post-relaxer Hair Care

Protein supplementation is a critical part of the post-relaxer process, and replacing lost protein in chemically treated hair is a top concern. A protein treatment should be done at the follow-up shampoo and conditioning session after a relaxer service. Ideally, this treatment, and the first post-relaxer cleansing and conditioning, should occur no later than seven days after your relaxer. If you applied an MRPS, or if heavy protein was used in the preparatory shampoo and conditioning prior to your relaxer service, then you may elect to skip the post-relaxer protein treatment and simply use a light Zone 1 protein conditioner at this wash.

Follow the protein treatment immediately with a heated, moisturizing deep conditioning treatment. Monitor the hair's protein/moisture balance carefully as post-relaxer hair may shift between its need for one or the other very quickly.

Relaxer Application Tips

*   Attempting to perfectly part through the hair with a comb or back end of a paintbrush, especially several weeks post-relaxer, can lead to breakage. Finger parting works just as well for applying a relaxer, particularly for self relaxers.
*   With any subsequent relaxer applications, begin applying the relaxer product at a different part of your head. For instance, if with your first relaxer application you begin with the back left section of your hair, the next time you relax, choose a different starting section. If you consistently relax a particular section first each time, this section of your hair becomes compromised because it is always exposed to chemicals for the longest periods of time. Years of relaxing the same section first may begin to thin it out. Switch your starting point from time to time so that no single section is overexposed.
*   Keep your eye on the clock. Relaxer timing depends on the texture of your hair and the look you want to achieve. You should follow the time frame stated in your relaxer's instructions. Speed is the key to a successful application.
*   Rinse the relaxer from your hair in the same order in which you applied the relaxer cream. This will ensure that each section is processed for the full, suggested processing time.

Common Relaxer Problems
Irritation and Burning

How many times have you felt that familiar relaxer tingle on your scalp? How many times have you run to the water bowl with a head burning with white chemical fire? How many of you have used this burning or tingling as the end point or gauge of the straightening process that lets you know it is time to rinse out the relaxer? Many of us have been raised to believe that the relaxer is working when it begins to tingle. This is a costly mistake and a sign of incorrect, unskilled relaxer application. Chemical burns are not the cost of acquiring straightened hair. They should never happen, period.

Relaxer tingling means that the relaxer has breached and broken down the protective-base barrier that was placed on the scalp, and is now in contact with the scalp skin layers. Some "fast burners" may have a naturally high scalp or body heat that causes the relaxer to process at a faster rate. At other times, the relaxer strength is simply too high for a given person's hair. Whatever the cause of chemical irritation, strand testing, proper relaxer-strength selection and adequate basing can help prevent unnecessary burning and scabbing from relaxers.

Relaxer Reversion

The straightening success of a relaxer service cannot be gauged until after the first or second wash following the process. When textured hair is introduced to water following a relaxer service, it will occasionally revert or reproduce some of its original texture. Reversion is simply the consequence of inadequate disulfide bond breakage during the relaxing process, an inadequate smoothing procedure, or an insufficient processing time that ultimately becomes revealed in the presence of hydrogen re-bonding (wetting).

Minimizing Relaxer Damage

Despite the challenges that chemical relaxing presents, proper hair maintenance can help relaxed tresses thrive and reach greater lengths. While a relaxer-free approach is certainly best in terms of working toward improved hair health, textured hair can be maintained quite well with a relaxer if additional regimen steps and precautions are taken. In order to maximize the health and vitality of chemically relaxed tresses, it is important to understand the primary health and risk drivers for chemically altered hair. There are two main healthy hair tenets that taken together, will improve the condition of chemically relaxed hair:

1. Controlling the degree of texture release and straightening achieved through the chemical relaxing process, and
2. Managing the chemical relaxer application frequency.

Controlling texture release greatly enhances the hair's elasticity and leaves the fiber more robust and strong. Reducing relaxer application frequency decreases the opportunities for overlapping and reduces stress points along individual textured hair fibers. If both health drivers are addressed and included together within a broader healthy hair care regimen, then chemically relaxed hair will have a better health and growth outlook.

The Benefits of Controlling Texture Release

While the goal of chemical relaxing is to straighten hair fibers, black hair thrives best when some texture is allowed to remain within the fiber. Completely eliminating the natural texture in relaxed hair greatly reduces its elasticity—a necessary quality for breakage resistance. In addition, relaxing the hair bone straight increases the likelihood of overprocessing the fiber in subsequent relaxer applications because some overlap onto previously relaxed parts of the strands cannot be avoided even in the most careful chemical applications. If relaxing to the brink of straightness continues, textured hair simply thins out over time.

When texture remains in the hair fiber, chemically relaxed hair holds natural moisture better and retains much more of its original strength. For maximum protection against breakage, black hair should never be relaxed to the point of complete straightness. Instead, the healthy hair aim should be for roughly 80 percent fiber straightness. If straighter hair is desired, temporary styling tools should be used.

Black hair relaxed to 80 percent straightness is able to resist breakage and dryness better than bone-straight hair that has had much of its natural protein strength removed by the relaxing process. The straighter the hair, the more internal bond breakage was required to achieve that result. A high degree of bond breakage not only ensures a straighter hair fiber, but a weaker, more fragile hair fiber as well.

Texlaxing?

"Texlaxing" is a term that was coined on Internet hair care forums to describe a relaxer service that is intentionally underprocessed in order to create volume and texture in the hair strands. (Note that the word *texlax* is not a term used or recognized in cosmetology; rather, it is a play on words used to describe a process that mimics two very real chemical services: texturizing and chemical relaxing.) In short, *texlaxing* describes a chemical relaxing process in which bond breakage is minimized and hair straightening is controlled to 80 percent or less.

What's the Difference Between Texturizing, Relaxing and Texlaxing?

Texturizing (Soft Curl)

A texturizer is a chemical process that is formulated to loosen the natural curls and kinks of textured hair types. Texturizer formulas typically use thioglycolate chemicals, and are generally used by individuals who wish to wear their hair curly a majority of the time, but prefer a looser, defined curly look.

Relaxing

A relaxer completely straightens the kinks and curls in textured hair. It is typically worn by those who wish to wear straighter hair styles on a regular basis.

Texlaxing

Texlaxed hair straddles the fence between relaxing and texturizing and seeks to provide the best of both worlds. Texlaxing—or deliberately underprocessing a relaxer—imparts many of the benefits of full relaxation but enables the hair to retain much of its natural, unprocessed strength. Depending on the degree of underprocessing, texlaxed hair can allow much of the original texture and curl to remain in the hair while still allowing it to straighten easily in the presence of heat. Although this textured look is achieved with a straightening relaxer, the underprocessed hair often looks similar to texturized hair—hence the term *texlaxed*.

Depending on the level of processing, it is often very difficult to differentiate between texlaxed hair and relaxed hair if the hair is heat styled. Texlaxed hair shows its texture best when the hair remains unmanipulated and is air dried after a wash.

Methods for Controlling Texture Release

There are many methods for texlaxing the hair, and most involve reducing initial disulfide bond breakage in the hair fiber. An alternative texlaxing method involves simply skipping the official disulfide bond straightening process. Texlaxing methods can be used alone or in combination to achieve various degrees of textured relaxed-hair results.

Why Control Straightening and Curl Release?

When black hair has texture along the relaxed length, the transition from the new growth emerging from the scalp to the older relaxed length along the fiber is less pronounced. This gradual shift in textures reduces stress at the juncture between the processed and unprocessed hair. When black hair is relaxed bone straight, the contrast between the new growth texture and the relaxed fiber is so pronounced that a hard demarcation line is created. Breakage and tangling are common at the line of demarcation: the juncture where the natural and relaxed textures meet. Relaxing the hair to roughly 80 percent straightness creates a softer demarcation line that is less prone to breakage.

1.) Downgrading Your Relaxer

Reducing disulfide bond breakage by downgrading the strength of your relaxer is the easiest method for texlaxing the hair. Reducing your relaxer strength from a super or regular formula to a mild or sensitive scalp formula (or even going from lye to no-lye) will increase the amount of time required for full processing. This will give you more time to quickly apply your relaxer and then rinse before enough bond breakage has occurred to really straighten the hair.

2.) Diluting Your Relaxer

Similar to downgrading the actual relaxer formula strength, adding oils or conditioner to your relaxer formula also decreases the strength of the relaxer and increases the processing window. This texlaxing dilution method also works by reducing the viscosity (thickness) of the relaxer cream.

The relaxer cream's thick, pasty consistency helps the hair remain fairly straight after the disulfide bonds have been broken during chemical application. Oils and conditioners reduce this straightening power by making the cream thinner, so that the curls are not weighed down and flattened as easily by the relaxer. If you decide to add oil to your relaxer, add a little at a time and check the consistency of your formula. Do not make the formula too runny or soupy; some thickness is desired. (For a basic relaxer mixture, about 1/4 cup oil works well with a small (7.5-ounce) single-use relaxer tub.) Also avoid using essential oils (like peppermint and rosemary) in the relaxer. You don't want anything tingling or stimulating your scalp while the relaxer is present. Instead, opt for traditional oils like olive, almond, or jojoba.

A variation of relaxer dilution is possible with no-lye relaxer formulas that come with a separate activator that must be added to the relaxer cream. Adding only half or three quarters of the activator to the formula automatically reduces the relaxer's strength. Remember, no-lye relaxers are inert (not active) and cannot work on the hair until they are mixed. Portions of the relaxer that are not mixed with activator will not process your hair.

3.) Putting Up a Barrier

Applying a thick cream or oil barrier to the hair prior to relaxing will protect it from damage and slow down the action of the relaxer. By slowing the relaxer down with a heavy protective base, you can still relax your hair for the normal suggested time period for your hair type without fully straightening the hair. Reducing the relaxer's contact with the hair reduces overall bond breakage and helps the hair retain a little natural texture.

4.) Decreasing Relaxer Contact

One of the easiest methods for texlaxing the hair is simply decreasing the relaxer's contact with your hair. Simply reduce your processing time! This method works when all other texlaxing methods fail. In fact, this method is perhaps the number one cause of unintentional texlaxing and underprocessing. Processing the hair for less than the recommended time will always texlax your hair.

5.) Skipping Disulfide Bond Straightening

Contrary to popular belief, hair straightening does not begin and end with the application of the relaxer. The relaxer chemical simply breaks your hair's disulfide bonds; the smoothing step is where your hair and its bonds are straightened into their new, permanent position. A texlaxing method that takes advantage of this concept would simply involve applying the chemical relaxer and allowing it to process without physically manipulating (smoothing) the hair into place. Skipping the smoothing step of the relaxer application prevents the disulfide bonds from fully setting into a new, permanently straight configuration.

Final Considerations

After texlaxing your hair, the results may not be apparent at first. Some hair properties including texture take a few washes to bring out because of the various levels of deep bond breakage that take place during the relaxing process. Texlaxed hair may appear almost bone straight and even limp and flat immediately after processing, but replacing your lost/broken hydrogen bonds through washing and deep conditioning will return some of the original thickness and texture.

Texlaxing is not for everyone. Before texlaxing your hair, decide on the level of texture you wish to maintain. Allowing too much texture to remain when you are used to dealing with much straighter hair can cause manageability problems which can lead to breakage.

Some individuals also experience uneven textures, dryness and shedding when they texlax. Each person is different and will have a different experience with this procedure. For a vast majority, however, when done correctly, texlaxing

can be extremely beneficial to the hair because it preserves some of the hair's natural bonds—the bonds that make our hair naturally strong.

Relaxer Deferment or Stretching

Relaxer deferment, or relaxer stretching, refers to going without a chemical relaxer for any length of time beyond your normal set relaxing interval. For most people, this translates to more than nine weeks after a previous relaxer service. Relaxer deferment greatly improves the condition of chemically relaxed hair fibers, and those who regularly stretch their relaxer services often observe increased hair thickness as the primary improvement. Stretching relaxers benefits the hair and scalp by decreasing exposure to harmful chemicals. The less often textured hair is exposed to relaxer chemicals, the better.

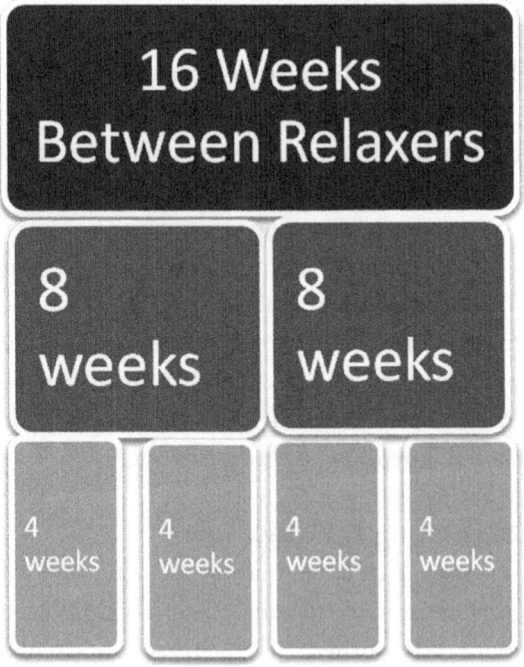

Figure 72: Chemical Relaxing Schedule and exposure rate based on relaxer frequency. Unfortunately, no matter how careful the relaxer application, some relaxer will find its way onto the scalp and previously relaxed hair, especially during the smoothing phase of the relaxing process.

Eight to ten weeks between relaxer touch-ups is usually an acceptable interval between services from both a hair condition and an aesthetic point of view. Ideally, incoming new growth should not be touched up before eight weeks post-relaxer unless the hair is maintained in a short, cropped style that can handle high frequency chemical processing with little damage.

Benefits of Relaxer Deferment
Deferment Decreases Chemical Exposure

One benefit of relaxer stretching is the personal reduction in exposure to harmful relaxer chemicals that can take their toll on both the hair and scalp over time. When the hair is relaxed every six weeks, the scalp and hair are exposed to strong relaxer chemicals eight or nine times per year. Add years and years of faithfully relaxing at this rate, and the chances of hair damage and permanent scalp problems increase over time. Conversely, if you stretch your relaxers to ten to twelve weeks or more, you will expose your hair to as few as five or six relaxers per year. Consider the exposure rate for someone who stretches and relaxes their hair every sixteen weeks versus an individual who relaxes every four weeks (see Figure 72). The individual who relaxes every four weeks will have relaxed four separate times by the time someone who stretches relaxers to sixteen weeks has a second processing.

Deferment Decreases Overlapping

Overlapping new relaxer applications onto previously relaxed strands is a primary cause of overprocessing and hair breakage in black hair care. Relaxing strips away cuticle layers, and chronic overlapping leads to weakened hair and cuticle degradation over time.

In a perfect world, overlap would never happen. Chemicals would be confined to new growth areas, and previously relaxed or chemically treated hair would never reprocess with future relaxer applications. However, the compact nature of our textured new-growth hair renders some relaxer overlap onto older relaxed strands unavoidable, despite our best efforts. The amount of new growth present at the four-, six- or eight-week mark is just not enough to prevent relaxer overlap of some degree onto the scalp or previously relaxed hair. Stretching out relaxer applications reduces the likelihood that hair will be overprocessed from overlapping by providing more tangible new growth to work with at the time of your application.

The ends of the hair pay the ultimate price for overlap. As relaxer is rinsed from the hair, the alkaline cream passes right back over the ends of the hair before finally heading down the drain. The fewer times you put your hair through this process, the thicker and healthier your hair will become over time. Again, although the new growth can appear quite thick in the four-to-eight-week window, the hair is simply not long enough to substantially decrease the chances for overlapping.

Deferment Decreases Potential Stress Points

Each time the hair is relaxed, the potential for overlapping onto previously relaxed hair is high. Unfortunately, the points where the relaxer has overlapped create new weak points along the hair strand (see Figure 73). The distance between the stress intervals is dependent on new growth length and the degree of relaxer overlap during application. These stress points can occur at variable distances along the hair fiber. If the hair is relaxed every four to twelve weeks with minimal overlap onto previously relaxed hair, then stress points would most likely be present at intervals of ½ to 1½ inches along the length of the fiber. These points of weakness present challenges for protecting the hair fiber and curbing breakage. The more often the hair is chemically relaxed, the more stress points there will be along the strand from relaxer overlap. When applications are stretched out, the stress intervals along the fiber are further apart and breakage potential decreases along the length of the fiber.

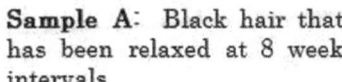

Sample A: Black hair that has been relaxed at 8 week intervals.

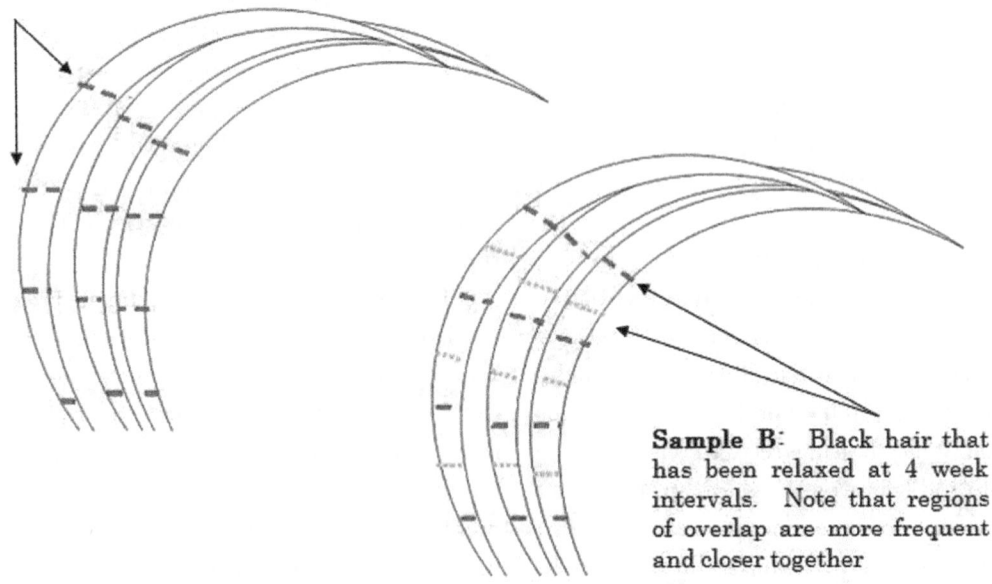

Sample B: Black hair that has been relaxed at 4 week intervals. Note that regions of overlap are more frequent and closer together

Figure 73: Diagram showing relaxer overlap stress points along the hair fiber.

Getting Through a Stretch

Successful relaxer stretching takes time and patience but grows progressively easier with practice. Many find it is difficult to stretch their relaxer more than two or three weeks beyond their regular relaxing schedule in the very first attempt. This is normal. It is always best to set small, attainable goals for the first few deferment attempts. The length of the relaxer deferment is up to you. Whether your relaxer stretch is twelve days, twelve weeks, or twelve months—it is always a matter of personal choice. The keys to successful relaxer stretching are simply decreasing heat use, reducing combing and styling manipulation as much as possible and developing a bit of patience.

Managing Relaxer-Stretched Tresses
Reduce Combing and Handling Manipulation

Overmanipulation of the hair during a relaxer stretch can lead to breakage. Because relaxer-stretched hair is fragile near the line of demar-cation, combing the hair frequently can cause unnecessary breakage and stress at this fragile point. Long-term wear styles such as braids, protective weaves, simple curly sets or buns work well for reducing the rate of combing and other handling during a stretch.

Be mindful that under-manipulation or hair neglect can also be a problem during relaxer stretching. Always keep your hair fully detangled to avoid inadvertent matting or creation of locs. Relaxer stretching is a time to make good use of your fingers and hands for preliminary detangling, arranging and styling the hair. Follow the steps for detangling and preparing textured hair for combing described in the previous chapters. Only comb relaxer-stretched hair while it is slightly moisturized, damp or wet. Dampness improves the hair's elasticity and allows the comb to glide through the two textures for detangling with minimal resistance. DO NOT attempt to comb through air-dried hair as this will lead to breakage.

Keep Protein and Moisture Balanced

Breakage is one of the most common complaints among those who choose to stretch out relaxer applications. Most hair breakage during a chemical relaxer stretch occurs as a result of too much hair manipulation and an imbalance of protein and moisture in the hair. One-size-fits-all treatments rarely work well for hair on a relaxer stretch; therefore, it is imperative that individuals monitor their hair to track breakage and dryness trends between the natural and relaxed textures.

Protein and moisture needs may vary significantly between the two types of hair texture, and each has its own set of needs. New growth tends to crave moisture conditioning more than the chemically relaxed length which tends to waver between needing moisture and protein conditioning. Relaxed hair in general has a tendency toward dryness. Weekly deep conditionings are the key to keeping the moisture balance in check for both new growth and the relaxed length. Incorporating conditioner washes between regular deep conditionings can also keep moisture levels high.

To keep the protein balance in check, use a mild protein conditioner or reconstructor every two to three weeks with your moisturizing deep conditioner as your hair dictates. As you progress through a relaxer stretch, it is not uncommon to find that the hair needs less protein than before.

Keep Heat Use to a Minimum

As the weeks progress after a relaxer application, we face increasing opposition to our attempts to flatten our new growth so that it once again resembles fully relaxed hair. The more time that has passed since the last relaxing, the more tempting it becomes to use heat to blend the natural and relaxed hair textures. In fact, many people think that cutting back on the frequency of relaxer use means that they can now use heat more often to style their hair. This is not the case!

Unfortunately, relaxer-stretched hair usually requires more heat to keep styles tamed than hair that has been freshly relaxed. Since new growth is so close to the scalp, any perspiration at the scalp level will lead to reversion of heat-straightened hair. This can result in the new growth needing to be flat ironed on a daily or weekly basis just to keep up with a style. Unfortunately, a routine like this simply trades one detrimental styling tool for another, defeating the purpose of stretching: protecting textured hair by giving it a rest from chemicals and manipulation.

Rocking Smooth Styles

A satin hair scarf is a powerful styling tool, particularly during a relaxer stretch. When applied to damp, moisturized hair, the scarf has the potential to tame and flatten new growth in just a few minutes. The tighter the scarf is tied, the smoother and flatter the end result will be. For buns and pulled-back styles, simply misting the new growth and edges and tying the hair down with a satin scarf works very well to flatten and smooth the hair. Using light styling gels, butters, and moisturizing pomades adds shine and control to the smoothed look.

Going Curly

The less the relaxed length of the hair and the incoming new growth have to contend with one another texture-wise the better. It is much less damaging to make the kinky, coiled new-growth hair blend into curly hair than it is to blend into straight hair. That said, textured-looking styles like spiral rod sets, straw sets, braid-outs and twist-outs are the best styling options for relaxer-stretched hair that has progressed many weeks past its last relaxer service. Beyond ten to twelve weeks post-relaxer, it may be in your best styling interest to place the hair in longer-term-wear styles such as braids and weaves to further reduce manipulation.

Common Relaxer Deferment Issues

When your hair has been relaxed for some time, it can be quite overwhelming to deal with what seems to be an unmanageable amount of hair that just does not behave like your normal relaxed hair. Often, relaxer-stretched hair does not respond to the same products as freshly relaxed hair and opposes attempts to flatten it. Relaxer stretching can even make relaxed ends look thinner and shorter due to the natural shrinkage in the unprocessed new growth. Shedding and breakage can cause additional stress. Despite the temporary discomfort, once relaxer stretching has been successfully practiced for a few cycles, the reward is longer, thicker tresses. Common issues faced by frequent relaxer stretchers are shedding, demarcation line breakage and the appearance of hair loss.

Contrary to popular belief, the simple act of extending a relaxer application is not enough to cause shedding or hair breakage on its own. Rather, hair loss from relaxer deferment comes from a combination of improper styling techniques, unrealistic hair expectations, hard demarcation lines from bone-straight relaxing and some causes beyond our control such as natural shedding. Most often, it is an individual's post-relaxer care techniques that stress the hair, not the absence of harsh relaxer chemicals! A lack of knowledge or experience in dealing with textured hair during a relaxer stretch causes many relaxer stretchers to inadvertently inflict damage on their tresses while trying to make them healthier. If relaxer stretching is executed with techniques that simply do not suit the stretcher's hair, then hair breakage problems can arise.

Shedding

Shedding is perhaps the first reason most people end long-term stretches and transitions to natural hair. The cause of shedding during a relaxer stretch is not really known and has been hotly debated. Shedding tends to occur in phases and could simply coincide with the time when a relaxer would have been applied on the most common six-to-ten-week schedules. Shedding does eventually subside, but the tangling, breakage and stress those falling hairs can cause often usher stretchers back into the relaxer chair before the end of the shedding phase arrives.

The best approach to shedding is to simply wait it out. Some shedding is normal, and occasionally we all enter periods of heavy shedding as our hormones fluctuate and the seasons change. Relaxing the hair to cure shedding is not advisable. Chemical relaxing is the harshest process either the hair or the scalp will ever endure. If anything, the chemicals will encourage and aggravate the process of dropping hair. Shedding cycles will come and go, whether the hair is relaxed or not. Because shedding is an internally controlled process that is aggravated by trauma to the follicles and scalp, the application of an external relaxer or any other chemical or product will not solve it.

Never relax the hair to solve the problems encountered during a relaxer stretch. Correct the issues (breakage or shedding) with the proper treatment first, and only proceed with relaxing once the problem has subsided.

Hard Demarcation Lines

When incoming new growth and the relaxed portion of the hair strand are of significantly different textures, a hard demarcation line is created that causes the hair to be more susceptible to breakage at that point. This differential occurs when the hair has been relaxed bone straight or if the incoming new growth is highly textured and kinky. In this situation, the difference between the natural new growth and the chemically altered portion is too stark and highly incompatible. When the demarcation line is strongly defined, stretching out the relaxer can prove more difficult. The practice of relaxing the hair to only 80 percent straightness produces a softer demarcation line and allows individuals to stretch out their chemical relaxers with greater ease.

Where is My Hair?

When a relaxer application has been stretched for several weeks and considerable new growth is present, the hair's ends will seem thinner than the hair closest to the scalp. The appearance of thinner ends is especially marked if the hair has been air dried or is naturally fine. Even without actual damage to the hair fiber, the ends of relaxed hair appear thin or ratty because the natural hair near the scalp simply has much more volume than the straightened ends. The dense network of kinks and coils at the root can draw up tightly and appear much thicker than straightened ends, even if the amount of hair is the same. The longer a relaxer is stretched, the thinner the ends will appear compared to the new growth at the top near the scalp. Many stretchers are tempted to trim the hair at this time, but try to hold on. If the hair ends still look thin after heat straightening or relaxing, then a trim is in order. By reserving hair trimming until after a relaxer or heat straightening, you will avoid the unnecessary removal of healthy hair ends.

Bringing Deferment to an End

Over the course of relaxer deferment, a point may come when a decision will need to be made about next steps. Deciding whether to continue or end a relaxer stretch often becomes an issue when the battle between straight and natural textures simply becomes too much and breakage along the demarcation line begins to occur. Several months out from the most recent relaxer application, new growth will begin to become the dominant texture on any head of hair. The incoming new growth is vastly stronger than the relaxed length, and the relaxed ends can begin to falter. Breakage problems may intensify at this point, and this is a natural progression.

Relaxed hair and incoming natural growth are not compatible with one another, and simply cannot be maintained together on the same head for long periods of time with success. You may decide to end a relaxer stretch by relaxing the hair or by simply removing the relaxed hair and wearing your hair natural. If you decide to relax the hair again after a long-term stretch, always be sure to resolve all breakage problems FIRST by restoring the protein/moisture balance in the fiber. Never relax breaking hair.

Chapter 11: Transitioning from Relaxed to Natural Hair

Transitioning relaxed hair back to its natural, unprocessed state can be a liberating experience. While the decision to forgo relaxing entirely has gained popularity in recent years, the process is often not for the faint of heart. Whether the decision to transition to natural hair comes out of necessity due to previous damage, breakage and hair loss from chemical relaxing or is simply a matter of conscious styling choice, transitioning the hair can greatly improve its health and growth potential.

Transitioning relaxed hair to natural hair often requires a mental investment in the process. Transitioning can be quite personal—even emotional—for some. Our society places a premium on straight, flowing locks, and hair that does not fit this profile is often shunned and vilified in the popular media and in our everyday lives. Wearing natural hair, in many places, is simply not the norm. Oftentimes, some barrier-breaking and educating of individuals in our environments may be required. In addition to the mental preparation, a whole new set of styling skills may be required to manage natural hair as it grows and its needs change. When your hair has been chemically straightened for much of your adult life, your old tried-and-true approaches to hair care may require tweaking and adjusting to support newly natural tresses.

Since hair texture is determined at the cellular level deep within the scalp, relaxed hair texture cannot be stripped from the hair to return it to its natural state. Natural hair must be grown in slowly, and relaxed hair must be trimmed away. In other words, the hair must be transitioned. There are several ways to transition relaxed hair, and the transitioning process can take anywhere from one day to several years, depending on personal preferences and goals. Relaxed hair can be cut off in one sitting or trimmed over the course of time.

Science of Black Hair Street Interview

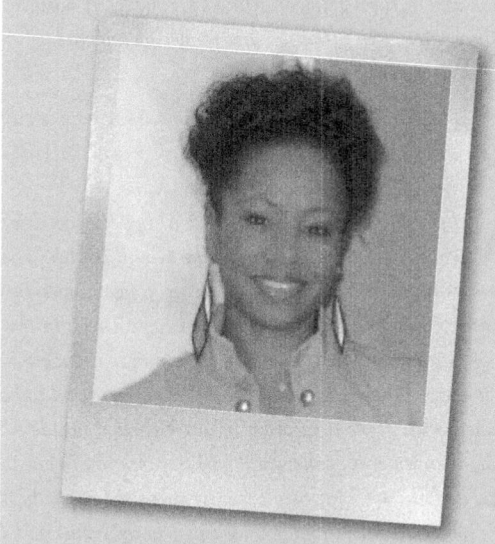

Name: Felicia
Occupation: Communications Specialist/PR

Q: Why have you decided to transition back to your natural texture?

A: *I was tired of my damaged relaxed hair. No matter what I did, it just never seemed to be healthy and long at the same time (and I had great hair habits). Plus, I wanted the freedom that comes with natural hair.*

Q: Is your family supportive? Friends? Coworkers?

A: *Yes, everyone is supportive. They don't have a choice. As you can tell, I'm very vocal about things I believe strongly in, so my family and friends were well aware of my plans to go natural long before I started my transition.*

Q: How long do you plan to transition? How close are you to your goal?

A: *My plan is to transition for one year, but if things continue to go well (or if I haven't met my hair-length goals), then I may go longer. I'm approximately eight months into my transition.*

Q: What is your hair regimen/routine?

A: *I keep it fairly simple. I wash with a sulfate-free shampoo [SheaMoisture or Wen] and deep condi-tion with a moisturizing conditioner once a week [Shea Moisture or Jane Carter Solutions]. I do an apple-cider-vinegar rinse twice a month, and I apply a pH-balanced moisturizing leave-in after I shampoo and condition [own home mix]. Daily, I lightly mist my hair with water and moisturize with Shea Moisture's Coconut and Hibiscus, seal with Jane Carter's Nourish and Shine or EVOO, add a little Eco Styler Gel to smooth my edges and wear my hair in a bun.*

Q: What is your detangling strategy? How do you manage the two very differ-ent textures?

A: *My hair is tightly coiled. During the week, I do not comb through my hair. It's already slicked into a bun and was detangled on shampoo day, so I just moistur-ize with my hands. On shampoo day, I prep my dry hair by saturating it with either olive oil or an inexpensive condi-tioner. I put on a plastic cap and let it sit for about fifteen minutes. I then run water over my hair and detangle with my fingers. The conditioner or olive oil allows for easy de-tangling and removal of shed hairs. Once I've finger combed my hair, I then continue running water over my hair and use a large-tooth comb to further detangle and remove loose hairs. I gently comb from tips up to the root. I then proceed with my shampoo and conditioning routine.*

Q: Tell us about your nighttime hair reg-imen.

A: *I apply my daily moisturizer, put my hair in a loose bun and tie up with a satin scarf.*

Q: How do you keep your transitioning hair moisturized?

A: *An all-natural daily moisturizer like Shea Moisture or Jane Carter and seal with a light natural oil.*

Q: What are your must-have hair prod-ucts?

A: *Shea Moisture is my go-to brand for hair products right now. I've had great success with almost every-thing in their line of products. Jane Carter Solutions and Eco Styler hair gel are also favorites.*

Q: What is your go-to style for transition-ing—the style that you know looks great, no matter what?

A: *My bun. I purchased some Jamaican braid hair because the texture of it looks like a braid-out. I put my hair in a small bun and wrap the extension hair around my bun for fullness. I prep the braid hair by soaking it in warm water and vinegar to remove the alkaline base on it. I let it dry, and it's good to go.*

Q: **What is the number one challenge you face with your transitioning hair?**

A: *I still experience some breakage because my relaxed hair was overprocessed before I began my transition. I trim my relaxed ends monthly and will continue to do so until my relaxed hair is gone.*

Q: **What was your biggest hair mistake?**

A: *I love henna! But I do not think it's a good idea to henna transitioning hair. Henna can tend to function like a strong protein, and your hair may feel stiff on the initial rinse. Stiff hair combined with transitioning hair is not good! I could barely get my fingers through my hair. It was a disaster, and I know I caused some breakage trying to detangle and get rid of the knots. This was early on in my transition, when I still didn't know what I was doing.*

Q: **What do you like best about your hair? Least?**

A: *I love my waves and the spiral curls that are popping out. I enjoy thinking about the potential for my hair.*

I don't worry about humidity or ruining a style while working out. My least favorite thing about my hair is that I may have several textures going on. Once I'm completely natural, it will require extra attention and tender loving care.

Q: **What hair-care tips or advice would you share with others who are thinking about taking the natural challenge?**

A: *I think everyone should give it a shot. It's good for your hair, your scalp and your overall health. The chemicals in relaxers are not good for us. Some women believe they can't do it because they don't have a certain texture of hair. Those are the women I encourage the most to give it a try. We've been taught to hate our hair and to be ashamed of it. If we take pride in our hair and decide we love it, then the rest of the world will have no choice but to accept it. Plus, you may be pleasantly surprised at the hair that grows naturally from your scalp. I know I am, and I was one of those little girls who was told that she had awful hair and "had to" have a relaxer to make it "better." But like so many other little girls, I had straight, overprocessed hair, broken off by chemicals and heat damage and weighed down by hair grease. Not a good look, but still somehow "better" in the eyes of our families and communities. Today there is a new awareness and better/healthier products available for kinky/coily/curly Afro-textured hair. These products bring out the beauty of our natural hair by defining our curls, giving our hair shine and increasing its health and elasticity.*

Transitioning Methods
The Big Chop

The "Big Chop" is one way to quickly transition from relaxed to natural hair. This method involves cutting all relaxed hair from the head in one session. It's fast. It's bold! Depending on how long the new growth is, a Big Chop can result in hair as short as a low fade or longer. Big Chopping is best for those who want to be completely natural right away and do not want to bother with handling relaxed and natural textures together. Keep in mind before chopping that the straight, relaxed length of hair, while still attached, stretches the new growth slightly, so that it appears longer and often wavier. Once the straight hair is removed, the new growth often curls up and draws back tighter against the scalp, making the remaining natural hair appear shorter than the wearer may have anticipated. This hair shrinkage is normal, and is a part of kinky, coiled natural hair's character.

A Big Chop often reveals and brings out the beauty of our facial features that longer hair often hides. Use this time to play up your eyes, lips and cheekbones. Earrings are an accessory that may become indispensible to you after a major chop. The right pair of earrings can add pizzazz and interest to any short look.

Long-Term Transitioning

Keeping relaxed hair throughout a long-term transition to natural hair without a Big Chop is another transitioning method. Long-term transitioning is best for those who prefer not to part with their hair in one big event. A long-term approach gives individuals the time they may need to transition their mindsets to natural as well. If you decide to transition over the course of time, use that time to educate yourself about natural hair care and prepare family and friends for the change. Visit natural hair care blogs and online hair communities like www.blackhairscience. com to get the latest information on natural hair care and trends.

The best transitioning styles are typical protective styles such as buns, braid-outs, twist-outs, braided styles and sewn-in weaves. Braids, extensions and sewn-in weaves that are carefully done to keep breakage and manipulation low will allow the hair to grow out quickly and are great for longer-term transitions. Buns work best at the start of a transition, but caution should be exercised as the transition progresses. Slicking and smoothing transitioning hair back into a style can lead to breakage along the edges as new growth attempts to grow up and out against the pull of ponytails.

Maintaining Transitioning Hair

Many of the same tips for standard relaxer deferment apply to transitioning relaxed hair to its natural state. Heat use should be minimized as much as possible to prevent damage to natural tresses. Obsessive heat straightening to blend natural and relaxed textures during a transition can have a permanent effect on natural hair, causing it to lose its precious curl pattern. Conditioning efforts will need to be stepped up to ensure a healthy moisture balance is maintained between the two textures. Demarcation breakage is also a major concern for transitioners. Always use great care when manipulating transitioning hair. Please review the Relaxer Deferment section of this book for additional tips and information on handling a head of hair with two very different textures.

Get motivated, and Set Clear Goals

Goal setting is an important part of the transitioning process. Write down small, achievable goals and work toward them one day at a time. Examples of hair goals could be making it to a certain number of weeks without relaxing or improving your hair's thickness. Cross off each goal as it is completed successfully. Each week post-relaxer is a milestone and reason for celebration. Visualize your end goal, and continually press toward it. When the transitioning process becomes overwhelming, remind yourself often about your reasons for transitioning to natural hair. Each day will bring new challenges, and some days in the transition will be easier than others. Transitioning may bring out a flood of emotions and in-between moments of excitement and anticipation. It is normal to feel unmotivated, unattractive, discouraged, upset and frustrated as well. When you reach a hair goal, be sure to treat yourself to something nice. You've earned it!

Monitor Protein and Moisture Levels

Maintaining the proper protein/moisture balance is critical during a transition to prevent unnecessary hair breakage. Increase deep-conditioning efforts as you progress along past the date of your last relaxer treatment. Like those who are simply stretching out relaxer applications, many transitioners find that conditioner washing improves their moisture profile significantly and cuts down on breakage.

Customize Hair Care to Each Hair Texture

As a relaxer transition progresses and the natural texture becomes dominant, customizing the product regimen to the two types of hair—natural and processed—may become necessary. Hybridized hair (relaxed and natural hair together) was never intended to be maintained simultaneously on one head, and each type has its unique needs and challenges. For example, natural new growth tolerates frequent hydrating and conditioning better than relaxed hair. Similarly, the regular protein treatments that relaxed hair thrives on may prove to be too much for natural new growth over time. Remaining attentive to the hair's needs as they change for each texture therefore is very important.

Work With Damp Hair

Damp hair styling is best both for those transitioning to natural hair and for those deferring relaxer treatments. Water softens the texture of the natural new growth and allows it to be arranged and smoothed into a style with less breakage.

Embrace Curls

Besides braided styles, curly styles are the best styles for transitioning and managing multiple textures on one head. Curly styles easily mask awkward or drastic texture changes between natural new growth and relaxed hair. In addition to offering a welcome break from day-to-day styling manipulation, curly styles also prepare you to envision yourself with hair that closely frames and hugs your face.

Seek the Company of Others

You do not have to endure transitioning from relaxed to natural hair alone. The ability to connect with and follow other transitioners in real time via websites such as www.youtube.com (video) and www.fotki.com (photo albums) has changed the transitioning game. Online communities like the one at www.blackhairscience.com/forum are great for those who do not have the family support to endure a transition to natural hair. These communities are also great resources for learning about new products and techniques to manage the hair during this time. Always use discretion when following techniques learned online, and don't allow yourself to become overwhelmed by the vast amount of conflicting information out there. Listen to your own hair, and select a few people who have similar hair types, textures and goals to follow for inspiration.

unit 4

Children's Hair Care

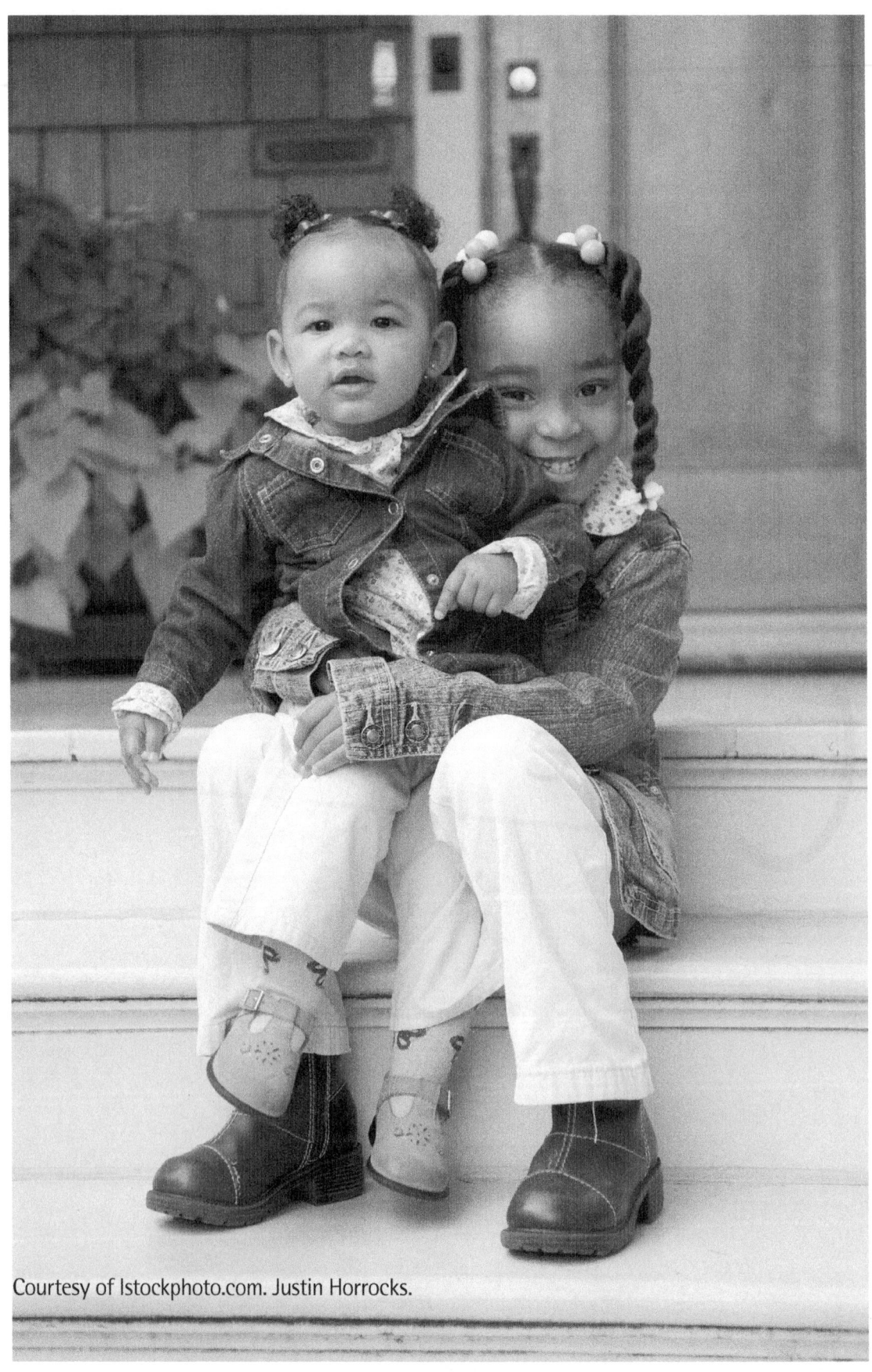

Courtesy of Istockphoto.com. Justin Horrocks.

Though this book focuses on hair care strategies for adult heads of hair, many of the techniques presented here are also applicable to children's hair care. Simple regimen building should begin with your child at birth and should evolve as your child's lifestyle dictates. Children with textured tresses should learn the basics of caring for their hair just as they learn to care for their teeth, skin and the rest of their bodies. Developing a simple healthy hair care regimen now will instill great confidence in our children and help them make their own informed decisions about their hair care going forward.

Chapter 12: Regimen-Building Considerations for Kids

Birth to Two Years

Hair care for newborns and toddlers should be minimalist. Children's scalps are extremely tender and sensitive at this age, and the hair fiber itself is undergoing rapid development and change. At birth, many babies are born with very little texture or curl to their hair, and in the early months of life their hair is often fine, wavy or curly. As your child grows and matures, his or her hair will begin to pick up texture.

Basic Regimen

Quite commonly, newborns and infants are born with hair patterns that are not conducive to traditional styling. They may be born with full heads of hair or come into this world with none at all. Still others are born with patchy hair growth and may have very little hair in the front, along the sides, or in the back. This variation is normal, and hair will eventually fill in.

The important thing to note about hair in this age group is that the hair is rarely damaged. In the early months of life, a simple rinsing with warm water at each bath is sufficient. Shampoos are not necessary for children in this age range. As the hair begins to pick up texture and thick-

ness, adding a light conditioner product and leave-in conditioner may be beneficial for keeping the hair moisturized at wash time. Light moisturizers may be used daily to nourish the hair and aid in styling. As the hair thickens and increases in texture, hair may require thicker, creamier moisturizers followed by a light oil product to retain its moisture.

Because newborns and young babies spend quite a bit of time on their backs, many develop a bald "rub spot" on the backs (and sometimes on the sides) of their heads. Babies' fine-textured hair is simply rubbed out from the friction caused by tossing and turning on harsh cotton fabrics in cribs and car seats. The scalp may begin to feel tough, scaly or leathery in the affected area as the hair begins to fall. To remedy this issue, apply a bit of coconut oil to the hair and scalp in the region affected by rubbing to protect it.

Putting the child down on a simple sateen or satiny blanket will also prevent this hair loss. Blankets with appropriate "slip" are often sold as reversibles, with soft cloth on one side and a slippery satin fabric on the other. These blankets can also be placed behind the baby in car seats and bouncers to prevent the rubbing that leads to hair loss.

Toddler Years and Beyond

Once a child's hair texture matures and the hair thickens, the hair fibers will require more moisture to keep them pliable and supple. If the hair remains without adequate moisture supplementation, the hair will dry out and break. All products used on textured hair should complement and support the hair's moisture profile. Any shampooing should be done with moisturizing sulfate-free shampoos, and conditioners should be creamy and rich. To grow out children's hair, low- manipulation styling must be instituted at an early age. Introducing heat, color, chemical relaxers and weaves at an early age, while fashionable, can retard healthy hair growth in children.

Hair Products, Styling and Care Methods
Hair Products for Textured-Haired Kids
Shampoos

Many young children use "no-tears" baby shampoos to cleanse the hair, but these products tend to be problematic for black hair. Although no-tears shampoo formulas are considered gentle, they are just as strong and drying as adult shampoos due to the high level of surfactant detergents many contain. These shampoo formulas may be easy on the eyes but have very little conditioning power. Textured hair by its very nature leans toward dryness, and baby shampoos strip already fragile textured hair types, leaving the hair shaft unprotected. Young children typically do not need to use shampoo of any kind on their textured hair unless it is heavily soiled (sandbox, swimming, food). A shampoo-free regimen is best for those under five years of age. No-shampoo or conditioner-only regimens insure that moisture is infused within the strand and is not lost to the harsh stripping action of a shampoo.

Conditioners

Children's conditioners should always be moisturizing formulas. Because very young children's hair is rarely damaged, they do not need high-powered reconstructing conditioner products. A light instant conditioner or traditional moisturizing conditioner is sufficient for most hair care needs early in life. The exception is when a child's hair has been chemically treated. In this case, more substantial conditioning will be required to maintain the hair, and the recommendations for handling chemically relaxed hair in previous sections of this book will be necessary.

Moisturizers, Oils and Butters

Moisturizing is one of the most important parts of any textured hair care regimen, and selecting quality moisturizers, oils and butters is important in children's hair care in particular. The proliferation of hair greases in children's hair care, unfortunately, has resulted in fragrant but dry, weighed-down tresses for many of our children. Ultimately, the type of moisturizer selected depends upon the individual's hair type, thickness and choice of style.

Water and water-based spray and cream products are the ultimate moisturizers for children. These types of moisturizers come in the form of detangling sprays, leave-in conditioners, creams, custards—and even simple homemade half water + half conditioner concoctions. They are great for softening the hair and preparing it for detangling and styling. With children, as always, avoid mineral oil and petrolatum in moisturizers whenever possible.

The choice of oils and butters for children's hair is also important. Baby oil, composed of 100 percent mineral oil, is a much better oil for the skin than for the hair. Nourishing butters such as avocado, cocoa, mango and shea—or even rich oils such as coconut, olive or almond—are better healthy-hair options than mineral oil or petrolatum-based grease products. Remember: Oil and butter products should be used on the hair only after adequate moistening with either water or a water-based moisturizer. Oil sealants and butter

Butters!

Butters and putty-like moisturizers are great slicking products for textured hair. Combined with a bit of water, a nice weighty butter can add shine and sleekness to textured strands around hairlines where frizzing and puffing can be an issue. On finer-textured strands, butters can be used in the place of gels for smoothing the hair. Butters and putty-like products are much more conditioning to the hair fiber than most gels, and add a nice weight to the strands.

lubricants will help the hair fiber retain moisture and will add to the hair's softness and shine.

Product Layering by Hair Type

The advice for adults about product-layering with moisture plus an oil seal also applies to children's hair—with the exception that often, much less product is needed.

For fine-haired children whose hair is easily weighed down with product (and for younger children whose full texture has not yet emerged), creamy moisturizers and oils may add too much weight to the hair strands when used in succession. Therefore, children with finer or looser-curled hair types often do better without the traditional layering technique of a creamy moisturizer plus an oil. Variations of this product layering method may work better for this hair type. For the finest hair types, the dampness remaining in the hair after simply wetting or shampooing/conditioning may suffice for moisturization. Spray-type moisturizers and light, creamy leave-in conditioners are also great options for fine hair. Depending on how fine the hair is, water, detangler or leave-in conditioner can either be sealed with a creamier moisturizer product OR with a light butter or oil as needed.

Children with thick, coarse, curly or dry hair also benefit from the layering of cream-based moisture plus an oil seal. Sprays and light

leave-in conditioners may not be enough to keep these types of hair moisturized and supple on their own. These types of products are simply not substantial enough. Those with relaxed or straightened, natural hair types also fare better with cream-based moisturizers to maintain their styles as liquid and spray-type moisturizers can lead to rapid reversion. Depending on the hair type, both forms of moisture—spray and cream-based—may need to be used together for better results. As with adult hair care, products may be added or subtracted from the regimen as the hair's condition changes and dictates.

Hair Tools

Combs and brushes for small children should be well made. Large, wide-tooth, seamless combs are preferable to cheaply made plastic combs. Combs with longer teeth are great for detangling textured tresses with little damage. Brushes should be soft and used only to smooth the hairline very gently. Avoid working brushes down the length of textured hair; this is unnecessary and will lead to considerable breakage.

For young boys, brushes with a harder set of boar bristles work well if the hair is kept short. Gently mist the hair with water and apply a bit of moisturizer, oil or butter to soften the hair before brushing. Massage the products into the hair to ensure even coverage, and gently brush the hair in short strokes with the grain of the hair.

Shampooing and Conditioning Methods

Frequent hydration will keep the hair and scalp moisturized and supple. Babies and small toddlers should have their hair rinsed and lightly conditioned at bath time as time permits. Older children's hair should be hydrated and conditioned every three to seven days. The general hair cleansing process for older children is: detangle, rinse, (shampoo/optional), condition, detangle, moisturize, seal and style. Babies and toddlers should use a modified version of this technique as hair length and thickness permit.

Hair length plays a role in the frequency of hair washing. Shorter, cropped hair lends itself more easily to frequent washing, while longer hair may present a manipulation challenge. Most small children's and boys' hair can be rinsed and conditioned daily in the shower or tub. Older children and those with longer hair may find it easier to go a full three to seven days between conditionings. If hair is cleansed and conditioned less often than every three or four days, the hair should be moisturized through regular water misting.

Hair Cleansing Process for Textured Hair

Detangling

Textured hair should be detangled prior to rinsing or conditioning whenever possible, regardless of hair type. Never start the detangling process at the roots of the hair, and always have a sectioning plan in mind. Freeform combing of long or textured hair will always lead to unnecessary breakage. Follow these steps for simple detangling of children's hair:

- First, moisten the hair with either water or a moisturizer.

- Next, carefully section the hair into four manageable parts using your fingers or a large comb.

- Carefully detangle the hair using your fingers. Any large sections of hair that have attempted to mat or clump together should be carefully worked apart with the fingers.

- If the hair is tightly coiled, gently smooth and stretch it with your fingers to remove additional knots and tangles.

- Then, starting about 1 inch above the ends of the hair, carefully detangle the hair with your large, seamless comb. If a tangle is encountered, redirect the comb back toward the bottom of the hair section.

- Once fully detangled, loosely braid or twist the hair and clip it out of the way. Repeat on small sections of hair until the entire head of hair has been detangled.

Refer to the steps outlined in the Protective Shampooing and Conditioning chapter for detailed information on how to detangle textured hair.

Fine Hair Moisturizing Method

- Detangle
- Rinse
- Shampoo/Condition
- Dry
- Apply Leave In Spray/ Detangler
- Seal with Oil or Butter
- Style

Thick/Coarse Hair Moisturizing Method

- Detangle
- Rinse
- Condition
- Dry
- Apply Leave In Spray/ Detangler
- Apply Water-Based Moisturizer
- Seal with Oil or Butter
- Style

Figure 74: Hair Cleaning Process for Textured-Haired Children

Conditioner Washing

Unless your child is extremely active or swims, the best method for cleansing children's hair—especially the hair of under-fives—is conditioner washing. Most conditioners contain small amounts of cleansing agents in them, so getting hair clean is never an issue with this method. A conditioner wash works the same way a regular wash does, except that the shampoo stage is skipped. The hair is rinsed with warm water to remove any topical debris, and then a conditioner is placed in the hair for five to ten minutes while the child plays or takes care of other business in the tub. During the final rinsing of the body, the conditioner is rinsed from the child's hair as well.

Shampoos

Remember, all shampoos used in a child's hair-care regimen should be sulfate-free. If you must use shampoos with stripping ingredients, add a couple of tablespoons of olive or almond oil to the bottle. These oils will make the shampoo much gentler for your little one. If the child has been particularly active or needs more cleansing, the hair may be clarified with a slightly stronger shampoo every two to three weeks. Clarifying will help lift any product buildup or debris.

Conditioning

Because children's hair is generally very healthy, heated deep conditioning is not mandatory. Quality conditioning products, however, are still required. If the child has chemically-treated hair, a moisturizing deep conditioner should be used on the tresses every seven to ten days. A protein conditioner may be added to the moisturizing deep conditioner every other week or as needed to maintain the child's protein/moisture balance.

Drying Children's Hair

Children's hair should be dried using the hands in a soft squeezing fashion to release excess water. The hair should then be dabbed carefully with a microfiber towel or T-shirt to absorb any additional water. Rubbing and scrunching through the hair with a regular cotton towel should be avoided.

Healthy Hair-Styling and Care Strategies
Preparing Children's Hair for Styling

Textured hair should always be managed in several small sections for easier handling. If the hair is approached without a plan, parental frus-

tration will set in, and the styling process will likely be painful for both parent and child. Begin preparing the hair by gently misting it with water, detangler or a moisturizing leave-in solution. This moisture will soften the hair and aid in detangling. You should always detangle moistened hair with your fingers in small sections first to remove any large knots, and then proceed to detangle the hair with a large-tooth comb (ten to thirteen teeth). You may move to combs with smaller teeth after the hair has been sufficiently detangled with the fingers and larger comb.

After the moisture spray and preliminary detangling, apply a water-based moisturizer to each hair section, concentrating on the ends. (Again, the need for an additional water-based moisturizer is dependent on the child's hair texture. Fine hair may be thoroughly moisturized at the moisture-spray-/detangling phase, with no further need for product support. Detangle the hair again using the technique described above. Once the full head of hair is detangled, seal the hair with a light oil or butter, and proceed with the style of your choice.

Always concentrate moisturizing and sealing efforts on the ends of the hair: the last two to three inches from the bottom of the strands. If your child's ends and ponytails have a reddish tinge, these ends are in desperate need of moisture and protection. Red-colored ends, a common hair feature in the summer, are a sign of sun damage or overprocessing with relaxers.

Kids' Styling Considerations

Childhood is the premier time for protective styling because the temptation to chemically relax, color and use heat on the hair is relatively nonexistent. Children's hair can be styled in many of the same protective, low-maintenance styles as adults' hair. Braids, cornrows, two-strand twists, buns, ponytails, puffs, locs, spiral/rod sets, straw sets—the choices are endless. Many of these styles can be re-moisturized daily and worn, with a few fixes and tweaks, throughout the week. Avoid styles that require heavy greases, hard gels and sticky spritzes to maintain them as these can cause both dryness and breakage. Whenever possible, children's textured hair should be worn in its curly state. Heat straightening should be a rare event.

Heat Styling

If a child's natural hair will be worn straight at some point, it should be loosely braided in several large sections and air dried to loosen the curl and lengthen the hair. Heat protectant should be applied to protect the hair from unnecessary damage. After the hair has been partially air dried, it can be gently blown dry on the lowest setting. If time does not permit air drying, the hair can be blown completely dry on a low setting. Simply section the hair and blow it dry in those small sections. If the hair dries out, simply add a bit of water-based moisturizer or water to the section. Once the hair is dried, twist up and pin the completed hair section, and then continue drying with another small section. If a flat iron is used, make sure the iron's surfaces are clean and smooth. Protect the hair with a bit more heat protectant and use the lowest heat setting possible to achieve the desired results. Only use heat on clean, freshly conditioned hair.

For more information on heat styling textured hair, see the Heat Styling unit.

Ponytail Rules

Ponytails are a staple of childhood and are perhaps the simplest, most manageable style for active little girls. These hallmarks of childhood can spell trouble, however, if they are not properly done. Although nice, slick ponytails and parts look gorgeous, ponytails should never be made too tightly.

If you have a newborn or young girl with very short hair, avoid the temptation to force her short, fine hair into hard barrettes and ponytails.

Opt instead for pretty satin or elastic bands, ribbons or matching, soft clip-on bows to accentuate the hair. If the child's hair is too short to make a ponytail comfortably, do not force it! The tension placed on both the scalp and hair when short hair is manipulated into a ponytail holder or barrette can stress and damage both the hair and the hair follicles. Thinning edges and missing nape areas are the consequences of ponytails gone wrong.

Always be sure that the hair underneath the ponytail holder has freedom to move by performing a tension test. Have the child tilt her head to the side until it touches her shoulder on one side. Ask her if she feels any tightness, discomfort or pulling. Tilt her head to the other side and repeat. Have her lean her head forward and touch her chin to her chest. If she notes any tension, loosen the ponytail holders.

Next, gently grasp the ponytail holder between your thumb and index finger, and move the holder from side to side. If the hair does not move under the holder, or if the holder does not have enough slack to move on its own, then the holder must be loosened to prevent hair damage. Ponytails should always yield as you gently tug them, and there should be gentle bunching between the holder and the scalp as you tug and push the ponytail back toward the scalp. You should also be able to insert a finger, or part of a finger, underneath the holder with ease. Visually inspect the hair, especially at the nape and hairline for signs of tension and stress. If the scalp looks shiny, red or tender—or if little bumps are visible along the child's hairline or partings—then ponytails should be loosened to relieve tension on the scalp. The child's hair should never be pulled to the point of "buckling" at the scalp when multiple parts and ponytail segments are present. This kind of extreme tension will not only cause discomfort for the child but stress the follicles and lead to breakage if not properly managed.

Try to limit the number of ponytails to no more than five or six. The more ponytails in a style, the smaller the individual ponytails will be. Numerous small ponytails increase the opportunities for breakage, especially around the delicate edges. Larger ponytails in general are much easier on the scalp.

Pay attention to the types of holders used on the hair. When using ball-type holders, be sure that the elastic is in good condition and that there is no metal crimp in the center to break the hair. Never use rubber bands, or any elastic bands, with glued or metal clasps to secure a child's delicate hair. These types of holders place too much stress on the hair strands and can damage and degrade the cuticle with regular use. If end holders or barrettes are used, always seal the hair ends with a bit of extra oil as a finishing touch prior to securing the end holders.

Braids

Like ponytails, braids and cornrows can create high levels of stress along the hairline and temple areas in small children. Always keep braids around the frontal hairline relatively loose so that the style places no tension on the hair when the child plays, sleeps or moves her forehead muscles to make facial expressions. Damage to the child's hair follicles from tight braiding can affect her ability to grow and maintain a healthy head of hair in her adult years. Braids and cornrows should be misted daily with a spray moisturizer and sealed with oil for shine. Never allow braids to dry out: Dry synthetic braid or weave hair is stronger than our hair and, when intertwined with delicate children's hair, can abrade the cuticle and lead to terrible breakage. Children under the age of seven should always have their own hair braided without adding extensions.

Night Care

Leaving children's hair styled overnight can make getting ready the next morning a breeze. However, this practice—no matter how time efficient, often leads to hair problems later on. Have you ever seen little girls with short pieces of hair sticking up around the rim of the hairline and nape? Or others whose short hairs around the head no longer fit into the main ponytail? This rim or "halo breakage" is a common symptom of sleeping in ponytail holders.

At night, it is best to remove all hair accessories, bows, barrettes and holders from your child's hair. These hair ornaments can snag and snap your child's hair while she tosses and turns at night. Even loose ponytails can cause breakage to the edges of the hair during sleep. Preserve your child's style overnight by simply removing the holders, moisturizing and oiling the hair, and rebraiding or retwisting each section of hair. The braids and twists will keep your child's hair together, preserving her style until morning. Styling without holders will also prevent the holders from contributing to breakage at stress points along the hair fiber. If your child's hair is short, or a type that will unravel overnight, place a small, oil-dipped terry cloth holder on the ends instead.

It is best to get your daughter in the habit of preserving her hair by tying it at night. If your daughter is old enough to understand the use of a satin scarf and doesn't toss so much that she will lose it during the night, go ahead and try one to protect her hair. If she cannot keep up with a scarf, a satin bonnet may suit her better. For active little ladies who will have no part of a scarf or who are simply too young, opt for a satin pillowcase. One, or a combination of these night preservation methods will protect your little one's hair at night and prevent excessive hair rubbing that can lead to nape- and side-hair breakage.

Chemicals and Kids

Once your child enters her teen years, she may decide to express her creativity and independence with her hair. This creativity might lead to a new haircut or style, or could bring the chemical discussion into the picture. While haircuts and styles can be managed relatively easily, hair coloring and chemical relaxing greatly alter and change the basic strength and moisture characteristics of black hair. The moment that chemicals become a part of your child's hairstyling routine, a new level of hair care should be ushered in for both you and the child. Too often teens—and even some smaller children—are relaxed and/or colored and left to fend for themselves against dryness and breakage. If you have chosen to relax or color your child's textured hair, give her hair the same care you would give your own. Chemically altered hair requires regular conditioning and protective styling in order to reach its greatest lengths. It is never self-maintaining.

Chemical Relaxers

Relaxing children's hair is a hot button issue in the black community. All of us, no doubt, want to teach our daughters to love and appreciate the hair that God has given them, but there is considerable debate about the way in which this teaching is done. Whether it is right or wrong to chemically alter our children's hair—or even our own hair—ultimately is an individual call. The older the child is at the time of the first relaxer service, the better. Relaxing children younger than ten or twelve is generally not recommended.

Relaxers formulated for children contain the same ingredients as those formulated for adults. They are simply repackaged, mild-strength adult relaxers. Compare the ingredients lists, and the only difference between kiddie relaxers and adult relaxers is the colorful packaging and the smiling third or fourth grader on the front of the box. Relaxers for children are simply the manufacturers' marketing ploy to appeal to the nurturing side of parents and thus tap into a younger, more impressionable consumer market: our young daughters.

If relaxer chemicals come into the picture, protein and moisture conditioning should take a more prominent role in the child's hair care regimen. Ideally, children should be of an age where they can appreciate the care that must go into maintaining relaxed hair.

Vitamins for Hair Growth?

It is not advisable to give children growth-enhancing vitamins or hair products in the absence of a medical directive. Childhood is when the hair grows the fastest, so if your child's regimen is solid, the length will come. General healthy maintenance is all that is required to see fast hair growth and improved condition.

If you decide to use dietary supplements, a simple one-a-day multivitamin formulated for the child's age group is more than sufficient. Vitamins never should be emphasized strictly for hair growth reasons. Incorporating them within a healthy hair care regimen is useless if the hair is not well taken care of once it does grow out. If the hair is cared for, not only will its condition dramatically improve but added length and thickness will become evident.

With patience, love and knowledge of proper hair care principles, working with our children's hair can be significantly rewarding. Our little girls should never be afraid or ashamed of their kinky-textured hair, whether in the form of emerging new growth or worn as a full head of curls and coils. Remind your daughter that she and her hair are beautiful—long, short, thick, fine, straightened or not. Avoid speaking negatively about her hair, even if it is damaged or seems to present a unique styling challenge. Hair is hair, and it comes in all colors, shapes and sizes. All types should be celebrated and are as beautiful as the people to whom they belong.

unit 5

The Hair-Total Body Connection

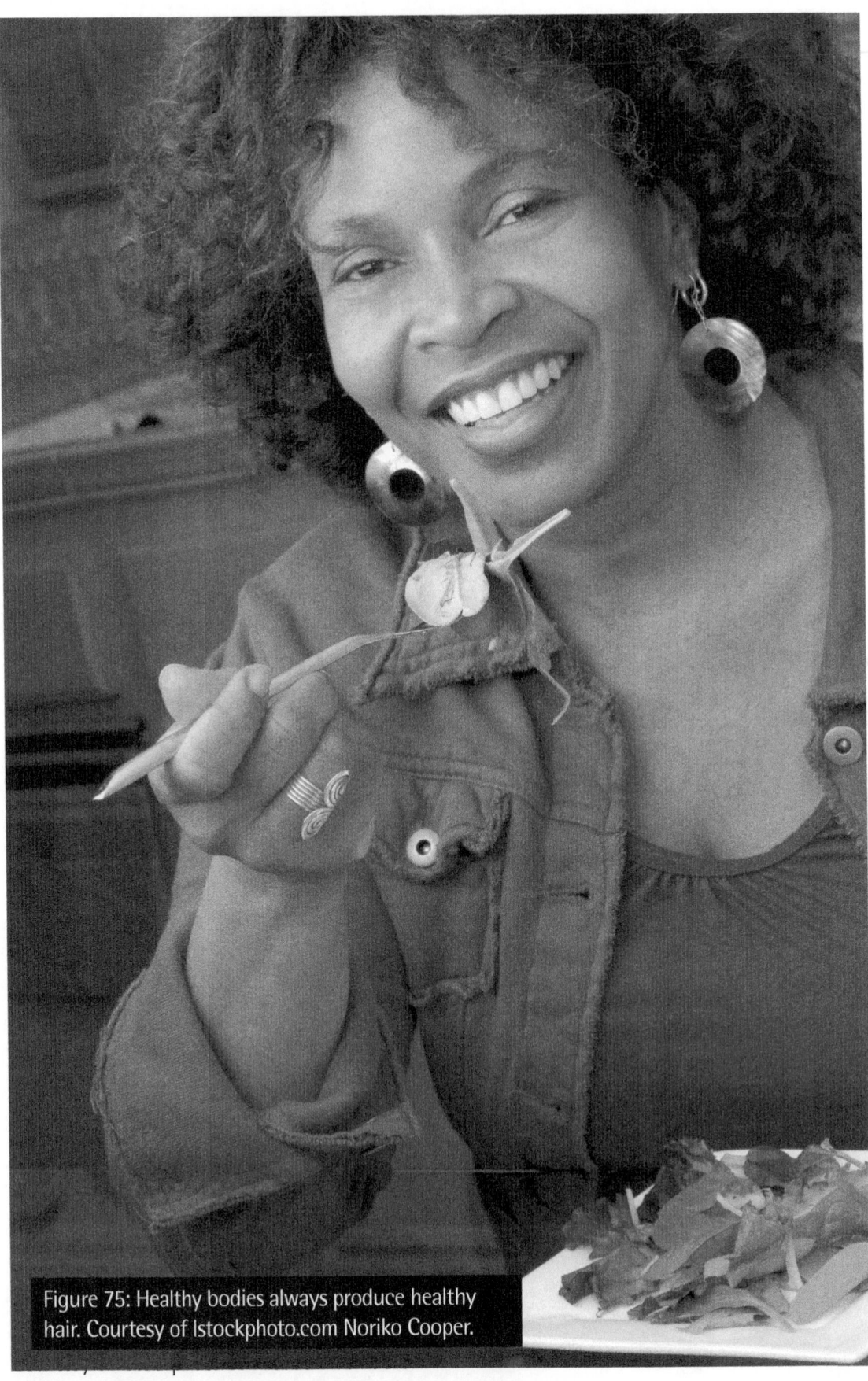

Figure 75: Healthy bodies always produce healthy hair. Courtesy of Istockphoto.com Noriko Cooper.

While the perfect shampoo and conditioner can work wonders for improving the look and feel of black hair, healthy black hair growth starts from within. From the moment textured hairs exit the protection and nourishment of the scalp skin, these hairs are on their own to battle our combs, dryers and chemicals. At the follicle level, emerging hair is fortified with as much strength and robust infrastructure as it will ever have. If hair is compromised from the start by ill health and an unhealthy diet, the hair will be weak and will eventually languish from a lack of nutrition. Our hair, along with our skin and nails, are direct reflections of our internal bodily conditions.

Chapter 13: Our Health Affects Our Hair

The cells that reproduce within the hair follicle are among the fastest-growing cells in the human body. When our bodies are under stress from nutritional deficiencies, thyroid conditions, illness, medications and hormonal shifts—or simply from day-to-day life—energy is redirected from growing hair to reinforcing more critical bodily processes. Hair follicles are very sensitive to these shifts in attention and are programmed to respond by slowing down growth rates, producing thinner, less vibrantly colored fibers, and shedding hairs altogether.

Thyroid Problems

The thyroid is a butterfly-shaped gland located at the frontal base of the neck. The thyroid gland produces hormones that regulate how our body's cells use energy and directly affects many of our body's organs and organ systems. Hair growth is one of many things regulated by the thyroid. (35) When the thyroid releases too many hormones, or too few hormones, our hair suffers. With an underactive thyroid (hypothyroidism), hormone release is inadequate and the shortfall results in thin, brittle nails and hair. Weight gain, fatigue and feeling cold are other common symptoms of underactive thyroid. Overactive thyroid (hyperthyroidism) may result in actual hair loss. Weight loss, nervousness, excessive perspiration and menstrual irregularities are other common symptoms of overactive thyroid. (35) (36) If you suspect you have thyroid problems, consult your doctor for expert diagnosis and treatment.

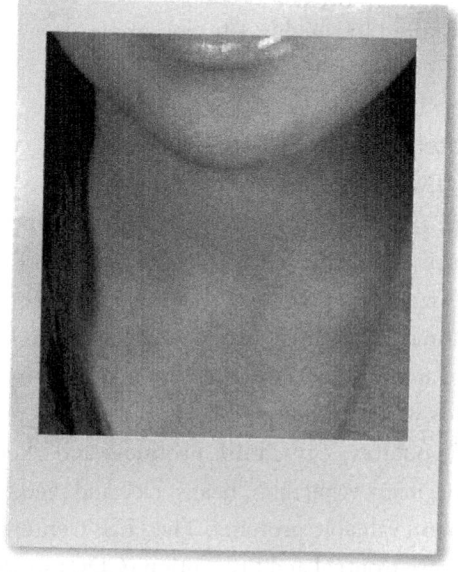

Figure 76: Thyroid problems can affect hair quality and are common among women.

Diet

Poor quality diets produce poor quality hair. Eating a rainbow palette of healthy fruits, nuts, seeds, grains, lean meats and leafy vegetables will ensure that you receive the full suite of vitamins, minerals and antioxidants that your body needs to produce quality hair. Vegetarians should carefully plan meals so that they can ensure that they are getting the nutrients typically found in meats from their vegetables, seeds, nuts, fruits, grains and supplements. (37) Finally, giving your body the hydration it requires by drinking water regularly will not only improve the moisture content of your tresses, but will improve the look and feel of your skin and scalp as well. Experts at the Institute of Medicine recommend that women consume 2.2 liters of liquids each day (men, 3 liters) to keep the hair and body properly hydrated.

Smoking and drinking work against hair health by hindering the positive effects of the good foods we do consume. Alcoholic beverages should be enjoyed in moderation, and smoking should be eliminated entirely in any healthy regimen. Reduce the amount of sugars, sweeteners and salts in your diet. Salt or sodium intake should be limited to roughly 1 teaspoon per day.

Healthy Hair Dietary Guidelines
Proteins

Every single cell in our body contains protein, and our hair is comprised almost entirely of this substance. Although the body produces its own basic proteins, there are key proteins (known as essential amino acids) that the body does not make. These must be provided by the foods we eat. These proteins are found in meat, fish, poultry, eggs, milk products and cheese. Tofu, many vegetables, beans, rice and seeds also contain valuable proteins. The U.S. Centers for Disease Control and Prevention (CDC) suggests that 10 to 35 percent of all daily calories should come from protein sources. The recommended

daily allowance for protein in women aged nineteen to seventy is 46 grams and for men in the same age bracket 56 grams. (43)

Our bodies digest and break down food proteins into amino-acid components that in turn replace proteins lacking in our own bodies. Given that our hair is protein, it is no surprise that research on both animals and humans has shown that low-protein diets produce weak, protein-deficient hair shafts. These protein-deficient hair shafts were found to be more brittle than normal hairs, and they also lacked the color, natural curl pattern and texture of normal hairs. In addition to color changes, a decrease in the diameter and size of hair follicles was also observed with protein-deficient dietary regimens. Once hair follicles shrink or miniaturize, hair texture and color changes soon follow. Eventually, a total disappearance of the hair's growth phase occurs. Adding adequate protein sources to the diet can reverse negative hair follicle trends. (44)

L-lysine

Because it is an essential amino acid, the body cannot make L-lysine and must take it up in the foods we eat. L-lysine helps support the uptake of calcium and iron in the blood. L-lysine, an essential amino acid, has shown some promise as a dietary remedy for shedding. Although the science is emerging, one double-blind study found that L-lysine, when combined with iron supplementation therapy, helped reduce the rate of hair shedding in women. Natural sources of L-lysine include chicken, beef, lentils and beans. (42)

Vitamins and Minerals

Vitamins are organic substances that are produced by plants and animals. Minerals, by contrast, come naturally from the earth's soil and water and are taken up by the plants we eat. While numerous vitamins and minerals are beneficial for total body health, a select few have great hair health benefits.

Occasionally, vitamins like biotin or Vitamin E are used in hair products. However, their inclusion in products is nothing more than marketing hype. External applications of vitamins and minerals are always temporary solutions and are generally rinsed directly down the drain. Vitamins and minerals work on the hair best from inside, where they can travel through the bloodstream and interact with the body internally at the cellular level.

Iron

We need iron to accomplish a variety of cellular tasks throughout the body. Iron's primary roles are to carry oxygen from our lungs to destinations around the body and to help our muscle tissues manage and store oxygen. Iron deficiency can be devastating to the hair. Research has shown that iron deficiency leads to dry, brittle and dull hair. When iron is deficient in the blood, hair shedding rates may increase and an overall thinning of the hair may occur. (39) (40)

> ### CDC-recommended Iron Needs for Females Across Age Groups
> - 14-18 years old = 15 mg/day
> - 19-50 years old= 18 mg/day
> - 50+ years old =8mg/day

Iron deficiency is the most common nutritional deficiency in the world. (38) In women, menstruation and pregnancy are major causes of iron deficiency. Iron needs are higher for women in general, and are greatest during adolescence and the child-bearing years. (42)

The best natural sources of iron supplementation include dark green leafy vegetables, kidney beans, egg yolks, soybeans, raisins and bran. Iron can also be found in red meats, poultry and fish. According to the U.S. Centers for Disease Control and Prevention (CDC), plant-based iron is not absorbed by the body as well as iron from meat sources such as poultry and fish. Studies have shown that iron absorption can be improved in the body by eating foods rich in Vitamin C, or by pairing meat sources of iron with plant sources of iron during meals. Coffee, tea and calcium-rich foods such as dairy products should be taken several hours after eating as they can inhibit the absorption of iron in the body. In addition, research has shown that when levels of zinc and iron are the same in a multivitamin, iron uptake is substantially decreased. To prevent absorption interference, iron:zinc ratios should be roughly 3:1. (38) (41)

Vitamin A

Vitamin A is beneficial for healthy, growing hair because it supports healthy cell division—the primary means by which hair is formed and exits the follicle. Research has shown that vitamin A supports a healthy scalp environment for hair growth by keeping the scalp-scaling (dandruff-forming) process under control. (42) Although vitamin A deficiency is rare in the United States and in the rest of the industrialized world, it must be monitored and carefully balanced in our diets. Too little vitamin A can lead to dry hair and scalp, as well as to a condition called *follicular hyperkeratosis* (or phrynoderma) which is characterized by overproduction of keratin in the hair follicles. This overproduction of keratin creates plugs that occlude or block hair follicles, stunting hair growth. Too much vitamin A in the body, however, is toxic and can lead to thin, coarse, brittle hair. (45) Natural sources of vitamin A include meats, carrots, milk, cheese, eggs, dark leafy vegetables, apricots, papayas, watermelon and mangos. (46) (47)

Vitamin B -Complex

The vitamin B-complex consists of eight interdependent vitamins, each working to improve the look and feel of our hair as it emerges. These "blockbuster vitamins" are very popular in healthy hair circles for their amazing hair and scalp benefits. These vitamins are all found in the same foods, and sufficient amounts of each B vitamin are needed for the others to work well. Together, the B vitamins play a major role in protein metabolism and in cell growth and repair: all necessary internal processes for better hair growth.

Research has shown that together the B vitamins—found primarily in eggs, rice, milk, whole grains, poultry and organ meats—help prevent hair loss, hair thinning and loss of hair color (graying). B vitamin deficiency can lead to dry scalp and excessive dandruff. In particular, biotin (B7) deficiency has been linked to severe cases of dermatitis and hair loss. Folic acid (B9) supports red blood cell development as well as tissue growth and repair in the body. B6 and B12 are especially important for hair health because they support the iron-carrying capability of blood.

B Complex Vitamins
Vitamin B1 (thiamine)
Vitamin B2 (riboflavin)
Vitamin B3 (niacin)
Vitamin B5 (pantothenic acid)
Vitamin B6 (pyridoxine)
Vitamin B7 (biotin)
Vitamin B9 (folic acid)
Vitamin B12 (cyanocobalamin)

Vitamin C

Vitamin C is important for maintaining strong, healthy hair and follicles. This important vitamin is a collagen builder that helps our bodies absorb iron: another important mineral for healthy hair maintenance. Vitamin C is an antioxidant, which means that it helps protect our body's cells from damaging stressors. A lack of vitamin C in the diet can cause bleeding under the skin, especially around the hair follicles. Vitamin C deficiency causes hair shafts to grow in

weak, brittle and dry and often results in a dry, flaky scalp as well. Common sources of vitamin C include citrus fruits, broccoli, cauliflower, bell peppers and tomatoes. (48)

Developing a Vitamin Regimen

Experts agree that the best source of dietary nutrition is directly from consumed food sources. In today's fast-paced world, however, healthy eating often takes a backseat to other demands. Even those of us who demand a higher eating standard and seek out healthy alternatives are left to contend with the fact that our food is simply not what it used to be. Extra processing, high-heat cooking and pesticides in our soil change the very nature of our food by the time it hits our tables. (49)

Incorporating a multivitamin into your well-balanced diet will help cover many nutritional deficits. (50) Selecting a great multivitamin can be a daunting task, however, considering the plethora of vitamin brands that proliferate in the market. Add to the already confusing mix of general supplements an even wider variety of hair, skin and nail formulas, and most consumers simply get lost in the vitamin shuffle. Consumers in the market for vitamin and mineral supplements should always seek the advice of a licensed medical professional before starting any sort of supplement regimen. Your physician can help you determine which, if any, supplements will work for you given your medical history and current health condition.

Oftentimes, individuals have a hair-focused health approach, consuming vitamins only to boost hair growth. Unfortunately, such a strategy rarely works. Our bodies prioritize areas of nutritional focus. Vital organs receive the bulk of our nutrition to keep critical organs and organ systems functioning. Organs and tissues without vital life-or-death functions (such as hair, nails and skin) receive the remainder of our nutritional allotment. If your diet is lacking, your vital organs quickly take up what is required for basic functioning while hair, nails and skin are left to fend for themselves.

If you plan to include supplements in your healthy hair care regimen, make sure that your brand has been independently tested and verified. Several organizations offer testing services for supplements, and supplement packing often bears seals of approval from the granting organizations. While these seals are not direct endorsements of products or guarantees of their safety and/or effectiveness, they do provide added assurance that the products contain the ingredients on the label in the amounts specified. Seal-granting organizations include the U.S. Pharmacopeia, ConsumerLab.com, NSF International, and the Natural Products Association. (49)

Chapter 14: Working Out on a Healthy Hair-Care Regimen

Many women with textured hair often feel that they have to trade off the health of their hair for the health of their bodies. This point of contention often keeps many choosing their hair and hoping for the best. Keeping your body in tip-top shape is very important for overall health and can prove extremely beneficial to your hair. Exercise increases your body temperature and improves blood circulation to your skin and scalp. Increased blood circulation to the scalp brings important nourishment to the hair follicles and supports healthy hair growth.

The key to working out and keeping the hair healthy is focusing on keeping your regimen as low maintenance as possible. Workout styles should be minimalist. Simple buns, braids, puffs and twists are great styling options. If you work out, products selected for conditioning the hair should be light, inexpensive brands that can serve well for regular high-volume use without creating a hole in the pocketbook.

Workout hair should be cleansed with considerable regularity to remove the sweat and salt that can accumulate on the scalp and abrade the hair's cuticles. Shampooing on a regular basis, however, can cause additional hair problems for textured hair types. The best workout hair regimens for textured hair feature warm water rinsing and conditioner washing as central elements for maintaining the hair. Workouts are a great time to squeeze in moisture and protein conditioning too.

Conditioners contain gentle cleansers that, with a little work and massaging from you, can lift most workout debris and sweat from the scalp.

Because conditioner washing workout regimens tend to be moisture intense, moisturizing conditioners will need to be alternated with protein conditioners on a regular basis. Balancing protein and moisture conditioning in a conditioner washing regimen is paramount. Alternating products will keep your hair from going limp from too much moisture and constant hydrating. As with most conditioner washing regimens, textured hair should be clarified once monthly to lift any lingering conditioner product debris or oils that may have accumulated on the hair fiber over time.

Preworkout   relaxed hair

Before you begin to work out, saturate your dry hair with conditioner or a creamy leave-in conditioner. Use enough conditioner so that the hair is covered but not so much that it begins to drip or run when you move. You can smooth and style your hair in a simple high bun, ponytail or puff so that it is not in your way. For intense conditioning, cover the conditioned hair with a plastic cap and a satin scarf or cap, and begin your workout. If pre-conditioning is not possible, proceed to work out with dry hair, and then rinse and conditioner wash the hair afterward.

Post-workout

Once you have completed your workout, rinse your hair in warm water under the shower. If you have skipped pre-conditioning, you may start your cleansing session now with either a sulfate-free shampooing or conditioner wash. Take note of how the hair feels as you are rinsing. If it feels too soft, limp or weak, follow the rinsing with a protein-based leave-in conditioner or detangler. If your hair feels hard or tough after rinsing, then moisture is required.

After conditioning the hair, give your hair a chance to dry. Post-workout hair may be gently blown dry *on a cool setting* if you will need to wear it straight later on.

Styling Workout Hair   Natural Hair

✳ Unlike relaxed hair, natural hair has an advantage when it comes to workout hair care and styling. Such hair is often quite low maintenance and can simply be misted with water to refresh and restore it to pre-workout condition. Simple hairstyles like buns, puffs, twists and braidouts should be worn to protect all textured hair from breakage during the week. Always moisturize and seal the hair with an oil or butter to protect it from drying out.

For those who press or relax their hair, working out can present a greater styling challenge. Increasing heat use is a common mistake that many people make when they begin to work out, particularly those who are attempting to maintain straightened styles. Those who relax or flat iron their natural hair face a considerable challenge trying to keep frizz and reversion at bay. To preserve hair straightness, pin the hair up high on the head in a large, loose pin curl or ponytail prior to working out. In addition, consider using a light serum or an anti-humectant product on the hair to protect it from premature reversion. Keep in mind that this approach is only ideal for occasions when the hair must be worn straight. Otherwise, if anti-humectant products or serums are applied frequently, they can dry out the hair and contribute to breakage problems.

Daily Workouts

Daily conditioning and keeping the hair wet over long periods of time is not ideal for most types of textured hair. When the hair remains wet constantly from workout to workout with no chance to recover and dry, the hair often begins to falter. The daily manipulation from detangling and arranging hair that is cleansed daily can also prove to be too much for most strands to take. In this case, reducing post-workout hydration to once or twice a week and allowing the hair to dry and recover in between is a better option. Reserve full shampoo and or conditioning sessions for times when the hair has been severely sweated out or soiled.

Textured-Hair Swimmers

After a few laps in the pool, textured hair can begin to feel rough, tangled and hard. While swimming is a great low-impact exercise, it has an extremely high impact on textured strands. The chlorine and other chemicals used in pool water to keep it sanitary are hard on black hair. Relaxed and color-treated hair types are even more adversely affected. Chlorinated water erodes the hair's sebum and disrupts the hair cuticles. With no sebum or protection, the cuticle begins to dry up and split, causing the strands to roughen and tangle terribly. Hair should always be protected before and after exposure to chlorinated water.

Cover and Secure the Hair

The first line of defense against chlorine damage is to secure the hair under a swimming cap. An option is to place a stocking cap under the rubber swimming cap to prevent the rubber or silicone from catching on your hair as you remove it. If you cannot or do not wish to use a swimming cap, plait the hair in a single braid or two. This will keep the hair together, and cut down on tangles significantly.

Wet Hair First

Alternatively, prepare the hair for swimming by soaking it thoroughly in fresh water or a light conditioner product. As you know from the discussion of porosity in previous chapters, our hair is naturally permeable to water but can only take in so much. If you thoroughly saturate your hair with pure water or with an instant conditioner prior to taking your first dive, your hair will be less able to absorb the bad chlorinated water. This pre-soaking method is invaluable to your tresses.

Chelate and Condition

Swimmers must take care to remove all traces of chlorine from the hair. After exiting the pool, always shampoo your hair with a swimmer's shampoo or chelating shampoo formulated to remove chlorine ions from the hair. Look for shampoos that contain the ingredient EDTA, which works well to remove chlorine deposits from the hair. Finish up your thorough cleansing with a moisturizing deep conditioner from the Regimen Builder.

Chapter 15: Final Thoughts

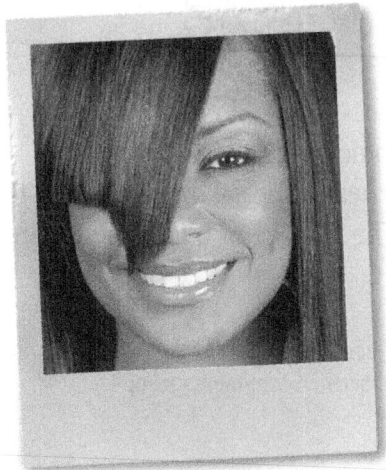

Audrey Sivasothy, author of The Science of Black Hair. Photo Courtesy of Rome Wilkerson, Houston Photography

Years of misinformation have crippled our efforts to grow healthy hair in the black community. Our pro-oil/anti-water rhetoric and high manipulation styling techniques have harmed more than helped our hair growth efforts. Our endless search for quick-grow products and pills has hampered our ability to truly learn our hair and distinguish its true needs. Styling choices that have encouraged temporary looks over long-term substance and condition have also set us back. Finally, chemically altering our hair with regular coloring and relaxing has further disadvantaged our hair -growing efforts. We must begin to take a critical look at these issues in our community. This book is your first step!

Although you do not have to follow every single tip to the letter, understand that close adherence to basic healthy hair care tenets—even in the midst of boredom, will always reap the best hair progress and results over time. Progress monitoring is an invaluable tool for helping you understand which products and techniques work best for your hair and which ones are not good investments. Keeping a hair journal and taking photographs of your progress will help you follow your own hair journey and its achievements. Remember, healthy bodies produce healthy hair. Eat a healthy, well-balanced diet and stay active as much as possible. Keep your body and hair hydrated from within by drinking lots of water throughout the day.

The ability to navigate and control the mysterious interplay of water and protein in black hair fibers is ultimately what determines how our hair responds to hair care product interventions. However, if the perfect hair care product could be packaged and distributed, it would contain one lone ingredient: *time*. Time is the one commodity that has never failed an anxious hair grower, and it is the common denominator in all healthy hair care regimens. Healthy hair, given the proper treatment, will always demonstrate visible length over time.

As you go on to enjoy your textured tresses and build your own successful hair care regimen, remember that flexibility and variety are the keys to healthy hair survival. Our hair care regimens must always be open to change. Try a new product, try a new hair style—enjoy your hair!

Visit the Science of Black Hair on the web at www.blackhairscience.com for more tips, strategies, and information on upcoming hair book titles. Chat with other readers on our hair care forum: www.blackhairscience.com/forum. Be encouraged.

Use your camera phone to scan this barcode to view The Science of Black Hair Website. Scan the code periodically for live updates!

* If you have not installed a bar code reader, visit the Iphone App store, Blackberry Appworld or Android Market to download a free reader.

Use your camera phone to scan this barcode to hear a special message from the author of The Science of Black Hair, Audrey Sivasothy.

Or access her here:
www.blackhairscience.com/message.mp4

References

1. Claude Bouillon and John Wilkinson, *The Science of Hair Care* (Boca Raton, Fla.: Taylor & Francis, 2005).

2. J. A. Swift, "The Histology of Keratin Fibres," in *Chemistry of Natural Protein Fibres*, edited by R. S. Asquith (New York: Plenum Press, 1977).

3. B. Lindelof, B. Forslind, M. A. Hedblad and U. Kaveus, "Human Hair Form: Morphology Revealed by Light and Scanning Electron Microscopy and Computer Aided Three-Dimensional Reconstruction," *Archives of Dermatology* 124 (1988):1358-63.

4. Deborah Dunham, "The Price of Pretty: Women Spend $50,000 on Hair Care Over Lifetime," Stylist, March 29, 2010, accessed November 30, 2010.
www.stylelist.com/2010/03/29/the-price-of-pretty-women-spend-50-000-on-hair-over-lifetime.

5. "Our Mission," Black Owned Beauty Supply Association (BOBSA), accessed December 3, 2010. http://www.bobsaone.org/missionandvalues.php.

6. Christopher Harris, "Scalp Anatomy," *Emedicine,*, July 2009, accessed December 3, 2010. http://emedicine.medscape.com/article/834808-overview.

7. John Halal, *Hair Structure and Chemistry Simplified,* 4th ed. (Milady, 2002).

8. Dale H. Johnson, *Hair and Hair Care* (New York: Marcel Dekker, ,1997).

9. Kathleen V. Roskos and Rich H. Guy, "Assessment of Skin Barrier Function Using Transepidermal Water Loss: Effect of Age," *Pharmaceutical Research* 6 (1989).

10. Bernard Ackerman and Albert M. Klingman, "Some Observations on Dandruff," *Journal of the Society of Cosmetic Chemistry* 20 (1969) 81-101. http://journal.scconline.org/pdf/cc1969/cc020n02/p00081-p00101.pdf,

11. Zoe Draelos, *Hair Care: An Illustrated Dermatologic Handbook* (Boca Raton, Fla.: Taylor & Francis, 2005).

12. Ralf Paus and George Cotsarelis, "The Biology of Hair Follicles," *Mechanisms of Disease* 7 (1999): 341.

13. R. J. Myers and J. B. Hamilton, "*Regeneration and Rate of Growth of Hair in Man,*" *Annals of the New York Academy of Sciences* 53 (1951): 562-68.

14. A. Durward and K. M. Rudall, "The Vascularity and Patterns of Growth of Hair Follicles," in *The Biology of Hair Growth*, eds. W. Montagna and R. A. Edwards (New York: Academic Press, 1958).

15. "Sebaceous Gland," Columbia Encyclopedia, 6th ed. (New York: Columbia University Press, 2008): accessed August 14, 2010. http://www.encyclopedia.com/topic/sebaceous_gland.aspx#1-1E1:sebaceou-full.

16. Byung In Ro and Thomas L. Dawson, "The Role of Sebaceous Gland Activity and Scalp Microfloral Metabolism in the Etiology of Seborrheic Dermatitis and Dandruff," s.l. : *Journal of Investigative Dermatology Symposium Proceedings* 10 (2005: 194)

17. Michael R. Jacobs and Peter C. Appelbaum, "Nadifloxacin: A Quinolone for Topical Treatment of Skin Infections and Potential for Systemic Use of Its Active Isomer, WCK 771," *Expert Opinion on Pharmacotherapy* 6 (2006).

18. "Hormonal Changes and Acne Breakouts," Acne Treatments Guide, accessed December 4, 2010. http://www.acnetreatmentsguide.com/who/hormonal/.

19. S. M. Patil, G. N. Sapkale, U. S. Surwase and B. T. Bhombe, "Herbal Medicines As an Effective Therapy in Hair Loss: A Review," *Research Journal of Pharmaceutical, Biological and Chemical Sciences* (India) 1 (2010): http://rjpbcs.com/pdf/2010_1(3)/90.pdf.

20. Hilda Sustaita, "Chemical Composition of Hair," in *Texas Collaborative: A Close Look at the Properties of Hair and Scalp* (Houston, Tex.: Houston Community College, 2010): accessed August 1, 2010. http://www.texascollaborative.org/hildasustaita/module%20files/topic3.htm.

21. Jutta Maria Quadflieg, "Fundamental Properties of Afro-American Hair as Related to Their Straightening/Relaxing Behaviour," 2003. http://deposit.ddb.de/cgi-bin/dokserv?idn=971528527&dok_var=d1&dok_ext=pdf&filename=971528527.pdf.

22. Lesley Hatton and Phillip Hatton, *Perming and Straightening: A Salon Handbook,* 2nd ed. (Oxford: Blackwell Scientific Publications, 1993).

23. Y. K. Kamath, Sidney B. Hornby, Sidney B. and H. D. Weigmann, "Mechanical and Fractographic Behavior of Negroid Hair," *Journal of the Society of Cosmetic Chemistry* 35 (1984): 24. Tonya McKay Becker, "What's the Scoop on Silicones?", *Naturally Curly,* November 1, 2006, accessed November 30, 2010.
http://www.naturallycurly.com/curlreading/curl-products/whats-the-scoop-on-silicones.

25. Linda Stradley, "Types of Cooking Fats and Oils: Smoking Points of Fats and Oils," What's Cooking America!, accessed August 1, 2010.
http://whatscookingamerica.net/Information/CookingOilTypes.htm.

26. Aarti S. Rele and R. B. Mohile, "Effect of Mineral Oil, Sunflower Oil, and Coconut Oil on Prevention of Hair Damage," *Journal of Cosmetic Science* 54 (2003): 175-192. http://journal.scconline.org/pdf/cc2003/cc054n02/p00175-p00192.pdf.

27. Tonya McKay Becker, "Mineral Oil Versus Coconut Oil: Which Is Better?", *Naturally Curly,,* April 5, 2010, accessed December 5, 2010.
http://www.naturallycurly.com/curlreading/curl-products/mineral-oil-versus-coconut-oil-which-is-better.

28. S. B. Ruetsch, Y. K. Kamath, A. S. Rele and B. Mohile, "Secondary Ion Mass Spectrometric Investigation of Penetration of Coconut and Mineral Oils into Human Hair Fibers: Relevance to Hair Damage," *Journal of Cosmetic Science* 53 (2001): 169-84.
http://journal.scconline.org/pdf/cc2001/cc052n03/p00169-p00184.pdf.

29. Catherine Cartwright-Jones, *Henna for Hair: "How-To" Henna* (Stow, Ohio: Tap Dancing Lizard, 2006).

30. R. Beyak, C. F. Meyer and G. S. Kass, "Elasticity and Tensile Properties of Human Hair: I. Single Fiber Test Method," *Journal of the Society of Cosmetic Chemistry* 20 (1969): 615-26.

31. C. R. Robbins and C. Kelly, "Amino Acid Analysis of Cosmetically Altered Hair," Journal of the Society of Cosmetic Chemistry 20 (1969): 555-64 .

32. Robbins and Kelly, "Amino Acid Composition of Human Hair," *Textile Research Journal* 40 (1970): 891-95.

33. M. L. Tate, et al. "Quantification and Prevention of Hair Damage," *Journal of the Society of Cosmetic Chemistry* 4 (1993): 347-71..
http://journal.scconline.org/pdf/cc1993/cc044n06/p00347-p00371.pdf.

34. Hyung Jin Ahn and Won Soo Lee, "An Ultrastructural Study of Hair Fiber Damage and Restoration Following Treatment with Permanent Hair Dye" *International Journal of Dermatology* 41 (2002): http://onlinelibrary.wiley.com/doi/10.1046/j.1365-4362.2002.01375.x/full.

35. A. N. Syed and A. R. Naqvi, "Comparing the Irritation Potential of Lye and No-Lye Relaxers," *Allured's Cosmetic Toiletries Magazine* 2 (2000): 115.

36. Michael Wong, Gabriela Wissurel and Joseph Epps, *"Mechanism of Hair Straightening,"* Journal of the Society of Cosmetic Chemistry, 45 (1994).

37. "Frequently Asked Questions," American Thyroid Association, accessed October 10, 2010. http://next.thyroid.org/patients/faqs/hyperthyroidism.html.

38. Mary Shomon, "Thyroid Disease 101: The Basics," accessed December 5, 2010.
http://thyroid.about.com.

39. "Position of the American Dietetic Association and Dieticians of Canada: Vegetaran Diets," *Journal of the American Dietetic Association* 103 (2003): 748-65.

40. D. H. Rushton, "Nutritional Factors and Hair Loss,"*Clinical and Experimental Dermatology* 27 (2002): 1282-84. http://www.ncbi.nlm.nih.gov/pubmed/12190640?dopt=Abstract.

41. Leonid Benjamin Trost, Wilma Fowler Bergfeld,and Ellen Calogeras, "The Diagnosis and Treatment of Iron Deficiency and Its Potential Relationship to Hair Loss," *Journal of the American Academy of Dermatology 54(5) May 2006*: 903-6.

42. Vanessa Ngan, "Iron Deficiency," in *Textbook of Dermatology,* 4th ed., eds. A. Rook et al.e, (Location-Oxford: Blackwell Scientific Publications, 2010).

43. D. H. Rushton, R. Dover and M. J. Norris, "Is There Really No Clear Association between Low Serum Ferritin and Chronic Diffuse Telogen Hair Loss?" *British Journal of Dermatology* 148 (2003): 1282-84.

44. Institute of Medicine (IOM), "Source for Acceptable Macronutrient Distribution Range (AMDR) Reference and RDAs," in *Dietary Reference Intakes for Energy, Carbohydrate, Fiber, Fat, Fatty Acids, Cholesterol,*

Protein, and Amino Acids (National Academies Press, 2005. www.nap.edu.

45. U. S. Department of Health and Human Services and U.S. Department of Agriculture, "Dietary Guidelines for Americans," 6th ed. (Washington, D. C.: Government Printing Office, accessed January 2005.
http://www.health.gov/dietaryguidelines/

46. O. M. Metwalli, S. I. Salem and S. L. Abdel-Razik, "Effect of Low-Protein Diet and Its Duration on Hair Composition," accessed December 3, 2010. https://springerlink3.metapress.com/content/h538w36288414k90/resource-secured/?target=fulltext.pdf&sid=k4bq5i551fpfv545ez0exqzy&sh=www.springerlink.com.

47. George Ansstas, Jigma Thakore and N. Gopalswamy, "Vitamin A Deficiency," *Emedicine*, February 12, 2010.
http://emedicine.medscape.com/article/126004-overview.

48. Robert B. Bradfield, "Protein Deprivation: Comparative Response of Hair Roots, Serum Protein, and Urinary Nitrogen," *American Journal of Clinical Nutrition* 24 (1971): 405-10..

49. Robert M. Russell, "The Vitamin A Spectrum: From Deficiency to Toxicity," *American Journal of Clinical Nutrition* 71 (2000).
http://www.ajcn.org/cgi/content/full/71/4/878.

50. Larry E. Johnson. "Vitamin C," in *Merck Manual Online* (Whitehouse Station, N.J.: Merck, Sharp and Dohme, 2007). http:www.merck.com/mmhe/sec12/ch154/ch154i.html.

51. Office of Dietary Supplements, National Institutes of Health, "Dietary Supplements: What you Need to Know," accessed December 3, 2010.
http://ods.od.nih.gov/

52. Janis *Graham,* "Skipping That Little Pill? Big Mistake,"*Fitness Magazine*, accessedDecember 2010. http://www.fitnessmagazine.com/health/body/head-to-toe/multivitamins/.

53. *Roquier D. Se*iler, "Les Defrisage des Cheveux," *Les Actualites Pharmaceutiques* 194 (1982).

54. Centers for Disease Control and Prevention, "Iron Deficiency," *Morbidity and Mortality Weekly Report* 51 (2002): 897-99.

55. Institute of Medicine, Food and Nutrition Board, *Dietary Reference Intakes for Vitamin A, Vitamin K, Arse-nic, Boron, Chromium, Copper, Iodine, Iron, Manganese, Molybdenum, Nickel, Silicon, Vanadium and Zinc (*Washington, D.C.: National Academy Press, 2001).

56. Helena Kloosterman**,** "Essential Amino Acids Search," United States Department of Agriculture National Nutrient Database for Standard Reference (2010), accessed October 10, 2010.
http://www.nal.usda.gov/fnic/foodcomp/search/

57. "Thermal Conductivity," Engineering Toolbox , accessed 2010. http://www.engineeringtoolbox.com/thermal-conductivity-d 429.html.

58. P. Milczarek, M. Zielinski and M. L. Garcia, "The Mechanism and Stability of Thermal Transitions in Hair Keratin," *Colloid and Polymer Sciences. Hair Straightening Temperature*: Clairol Research Laboratories. 270 (1992):1106-1115.

59. R. McMullen and J. Jachowicz, "Thermal Degradation of Hair. I. Effect of Curling Irons," *Journal of the Society of Cosmetic Chemistry*, 49 (1998): 223-44.

Glossary

Afro: A popular hair style worn on natural hair that involves picking and shaping the hair into a large, round halo around the head.

Aloe Vera Gel: A plant-derived gel composed primarily of water. Aloe hydrates, conditions and strengthens the hair and scalp with its healthful mix of amino acids and anti-inflammatory ingredients.

Alopecia: Loss of hair, especially from the scalp.

Alopecia Areata: Hair loss that occurs in patches. Alopecia areata totalis is hair loss that occurs all over the scalp. Alopecia areata universalis is hair loss that occurs over the entire body.

Amino Acids: Small, organic compounds that are the basic building blocks of protein chains.

Anagen: The active growing stage of a hair strand.

Anagen Effluvium: An abrupt shedding of hair in its normal anagen (growing) phase by a traumatic event such as severe illness or cancer treatment (chemotherapy)

Apple Cider Vinegar (ACV): A highly acidic liquid that helps smooth and constrict the hair's cuticles to greatly improve shine and manageability. ACV is often diluted and poured over the hair as a final rinse to seal the hair after conditioning.

Big Chop (BC): Process by which chemically relaxed hair ends are removed from the hair in one step, leaving only natural, unprocessed hair behind.

Biotin: A water-soluble B-complex vitamin. A deficiency of biotin can lead to brittle hair and nails.

Breakage: The physical fracturing of hair fibers due to stress and/or an imbalance of protein and moisture conditioning.

Buildup: Occurs when products, dirt and debris accumulate on the hair fiber over time. Oils and silicone-based products such as serums and conditioners are typical instigators of product buildup.

Butter: A semi-solid fatty oil.

Carrier Oil: A thick oil base used to dilute lighter essential oils before they are applied to the scalp or hair. Jojoba and sweet almond are common carrier oils.

Catagen: Short, transitional stage of the hair cycle that signals the ends of active hair growth.

Ceramides: Fatty acids with lipid components that help the hair and skin retain moisture.

Chelating/Chelator: Ingredients that lift and remove dulling deposits (including metal ions such as copper and iron) from the hair. These ions often build up in water causing hard-water conditions and dry, brittle hair.

Clarifying Shampoo: Clarifying shampoos are formulated to lift product debris from the hair better than traditional shampoos. They often contain EDTA and citric acid and must be followed by a moisturizing conditioner due to their tendency to dry out the hair.

Conditioner: A water-based product formulated to restore the cosmetic appearance of the hair cuticle. Conditioners improve the protein and moisture content of the hair and often confer shine and manageability on the hair fiber.

Conditioner Washing (Co-washing): A hair-washing method that skips the shampoo stage. Hair is simply cleansed with conditioner. Conditioner washing improves comb through and reduces the impact of harsh sulfate-based shampoos.

Cornrows (Canerows): Cornrows are braids that lie flat and tight against the scalp. These braids can be styled in intricate designs, or used simply as a base for a more complex weave hairstyle.

Cortex: The innermost portion of the hair shaft. The cortex houses our hair's color molecules. The cortex also bears the disulfide chains that are responsible for our hair texture.

Cuticle: The shingled, protective outer layer of the hair shaft that is responsible for our hair's cosmetic appearance. The primary role of the cuticle is to protect the cortex from deterioration. The condition of the cuticle determines our hair's ability to take in moisture and affects its ability to reflect light. The thickness of the cuticle layers varies with the coarseness of the hair fiber. Coarser hair fibers have more cuticle layers than fine hair fibers.

Deep Conditioner: A type of conditioner product that contains a combination of light proteins, humectants, oils and ceramides to nourish the hair fiber. These products are left on the fiber for up thirty minutes and often require heat assistance for greater penetration.

Dermal Papilla: The structure at the base of the hair follicle that transports nutrients and oxygen to the early hair and skin cells.

Disulfide Bonds: The important linkages between proteins in the hair cortex that are responsible for our unique curl patterns and textures.

Dreadlocks: See Locs.

Emulsifier: A product ingredient that allows the water and oils in a product to be mixed together without separating. Lecithin is a common emulsifier.

End Bonds: The chemical linkages that join together amino acids into longer protein chains

Erector Pili: Tiny muscles attached to the base of the hair follicle that cause the hair to stand on end.

Essential Oils: Light, water-like oils with natural therapeutic properties for the scalp. These oils are often used as several drops dispersed in a larger volume of oil or water due to their potency and expense.

Fatty Acids: Organic compounds that support the hair's ability to retain moisture.

Follicle: A small sac situated within the scalp from which the hair grows.

Hair: A cylindrical, keratinized fiber that grows from the scalp at the rate of roughly ½ inch per month.

Hair Bulb: Situated at the lowest portion of the hair follicle, the hair bulb contains the rapidly growing cells that ultimately become our hair.

Hard Water: Water with a high mineral content, especially calcium and magnesium.

Humectant: A substance that draws water to the hair or skin from the surrounding air. Sorbitol and glycerin are common humectants.

Hydrogen bond: Hydrogen bonds are linkages that give elasticity and flexibility to the hair. These bonds break temporarily when the hair is wet and reform when the hair is dried.

Hydrolysis/Hydrolyzed: Process by which a compound is made smaller or broken down using water. Proteins are routinely hydrolyzed.

Keratin: Keratin is a fibrous protein found in hair, skin and nails. Hair is almost entirely composed of this high-sulfur protein.

Line of Demarcation: The juncture along the hair fiber where chemically processed hair meets newly-grown-out unprocessed hair. Demarcation lines separate relaxed hair from non-relaxed new growth and colored hair from uncolored hair.

Lipids: Fats, waxes and light oils derived from plants and animals that support the cuticle's ability to retain moisture.

Locs (Dreadlocks): A hairstyle involving the natural, intentional matting of the hair into ropelike strands. Locs may vary in thickness from smaller than a pencil to large, organic, free-form clumps of natural hair.

Lye Relaxer: High pH, sodium hydroxide-based chemical hair straightener.

Melanin: Pigment found in skin and hair.

Neutralizing Shampoo: A low-pH shampoo product that normalizes the hair's high pH just after rinsing a relaxer. These shampoos may change color in the presence of chemical relaxer components.

New Growth: New growth is the untreated hair that grows in after chemical relaxing or coloring has taken place.

No-Lye Relaxer: High pH, hydroxide-based chemical hair straightener.

Peptide: A chain of amino acids.

pH: Scale which measures how alkaline or acidic a given substance is. A pH of 7 is neutral on the scale. A pH of 14 represents the highest level of alkalinity possible, while 0 represents the lowest acidity possible. Acid-balanced products are best for textured hair.

pH Adjuster: Also known as a buffer, pH adjusters regulate the pH of hair products.

Plasticizer: An ingredient that softens the hair or skin and makes it more manageable.

Polar Oils: Oils such as coconut and palm kernel oil that possess polar bonds but are still nonpolar overall. These oils have a slight attraction for other polar molecules including water or proteins, despite their primary non-polarity.

Preservatives: Ingredients that extend the shelf life of hair products.

Pre-shampoo Treatment (Pre-poo): A conditioning treatment done on the hair just prior to shampooing. Conditioners and oils are commonly used as pre-shampoo treatments on the hair to increase its moisture content.

Relaxer: Relaxers are high-pH chemical products that break down the hair's disulfide bonds to straighten the hair. Relaxers are followed by a neutralizer to return the hair fiber to its pretreatment pH.

Saturated Oils: Oils with straight chemical chains that facilitate their passage into the hair fiber.

Sebaceous Glands: The special oil glands in the scalp that produce oily sebum.

Sebum: The hair's natural oil, which is made up of many waxes and triglycerides.

Shedding: Hair that is naturally released from the scalp during the telogen phase of the hair-growth cycle.

Stratum Corneum: Outermost layer of the skin.

Surfactant: "Surface acting agent" used in both shampoos and conditioners. Detergents are the most common surfactants found in shampoo products.

Telogen: Resting phase of the hair cycle during which hair no longer grows but remains within the follicle until it falls naturally. The next new growing hair may push the old hair out of the follicle if it fails to fall free on its own.

Telogen Effluvium: Process of excessive hair shedding that occurs when a large number of hair follicles enter the telogen (resting phase) at one time.

Terminal Hair: A mature scalp hair.

Terminal Length: The longest a hair can grow given the length of its growing phase.

Texlaxing: One of several processes by which hair may be intentionally underprocessed during the relaxing process. Texlaxed hair is generally straighter than texturized hair, but kinkier than fully relaxed hair.

Texturizer: A texturizer is a mild thioglycolate chemical relaxing treatment that processes just long enough to reduce the curl pattern.

Unsaturated Oils: Oils that contain kinks or branching in their chemical structure that inhibit their passage into the hair fiber.

Vellus hair: Shorter, finer, thinner and usually colorless hair fibers. These hairs are commonly found on the face, hairline, and on the backs (non-palm side) of the hands.

Virgin Hair: Hair that has not been treated with chemical processes including colors, perms and chemical relaxers.

Product Ingredients Glossary

If you have ever scanned the back of your favorite shampoo or conditioner bottle, you know that trying to make sense of the ingredients in hair care products can be next to impossible. Very few products today contain easily recognizable ingredients. This ingredients glossary will help you navigate the complex, tongue-twisting chemical compounds, and shed some light on some of the more common chemical product ingredients you may encounter on the quest for a healthier head of hair. To simplify the look-up process, ingredients have been grouped by function. Additionally, since the list of ingredients is ever-changing, this glossary lists key words rather than lengthy chemical names.

Cleansing Ingredients: (Used to lift and remove product build up from the hair)

Look for these key words:
Ingredients ending in –Sulfate, -Sulfonate, -Isethionate, -Xylenesulfonate, -Sulfosuccinate, -Sarcosinate, -Sulfoacetate

Look for these common ingredients:
Ammonium Lauryl or Laureth sulfate
Cocamidopropyl Betaine
Cocoamphoacetate
Cocoamphodipropionate
Decyl glucoside
Sodium Lauryl or Laureth Sulfate
Sodium Tricedeth or Myreth Sulfate
TEA-Dodecylbenzenesulfonate

Moisturizers and Humectants
(Used to increase the moisture content of hair)

Look for these common ingredients:
Acetamide MEA
Alanine
Aloe vera
Carbamide/Urea (also anti-static)
Cocotrimonium chloride
Glycerin/ Glycerol
Honey
Inositol

Panthenol
Propylene Glycol
Potassium PCA
Sodium PCA
Sorbitol

Proteins
(Used to temporarily strengthen and rebuild the hair fiber)

Look for these key words:
Ingredients ending in –amino acid, ingredients starting with "hydrolyzed"

Look for these ingredients and key words
Amino Acids
Collagen
Keratin
Silk Protein
Soy Protein
Vegetable Protein
Wheat Protein

Thickener/Emulsifiers/Stabilizers
(Used to thicken, stabilize, and provide some conditioning benefits)

Look for these key words:
–Chloride, -Stearate, Ceteareth

Look for these common ingredients

Beeswax

Caprylic succinate

Carbomer

Castor Oil

Cellulose

Cetyl alcohol

Cetrimonium chloride

Decyl glucoside

Dicetyldimonium chloride

Dicocodimonium chloride (also anti-static)

Glycol Distearate

Hydroxyethylcellulose

Lecithin (also anti-static)

Polysorbate

Lipids/Oils/Emollients

(Used to improve hair manageability and comb-through)

Look for these key words:

Ingredients ending in -Cone, -Conol, -Col, or -Xane, -butter, Oil

Common Ingredients

Amodimethicone

Aluminum stearate

Behenic acid

Behentrimonium chloride

Cetyl Alcohol

Cyclopentasiloxane (cyclomethicone)

Glyceryl Monostearate

Glycol Distearate

Lanolin

Polyquaternium

Tocopherol

Ph Balancers

(Used to adjust the acid balance of hair products)

Look for these ingredients

Ascorbic acid

Citric acid (also chelating agent)

Lactic acid

Sodium hydroxide

Triethanolamine

Preservatives

(Used to extend the shelf life of hair products)

Look for these key words:

-Paraben

Look for these ingredients and key words

Benzalkonium chloride

Benzoic acid

Carbamide/Urea (also anti-static)

Cocotrimonium chloride

Hydantoin

Paraben

Methylchloroisothiazolinone

Methylisothiazolinone

Sodium benzoate

Stearalkonium chloride (also anti-static)

Index

CPSIA information can be obtained at www.ICGtesting.com
Printed in the USA
LVOW03s1600060314

376324LV00004B/336/P